W9-DBC-947

THE HEAD NURSE

New York

APPLETON-CENTURY-CROFTS

Division of Meredith Corporation

NO LONGER THE PROPERTY
OF THE
UNIVERSITY OF R.I. LIBRARY

RT89
B29
1968

The Head Nurse

HER CHANGING ROLE

JEAN BARRETT, R.N., M.A.

Professor of Nursing, Yale University School of Nursing; Formerly, Professor of Nursing Education, Syracuse University School of Nursing

Copyright, © 1968, by

MEREDITH CORPORATION

All rights reserved. This book, or parts thereof, must not be used or reproduced in any manner without written permission. For information address the publisher, Appleton-Century-Crofts, Division of Meredith Corporation, 440 Park Avenue South, New York, N.Y. 10016.

6127-1

Library of Congress Card Number: 67-27700

PRINTED IN THE UNITED STATES OF AMERICA

M-06476

to my sisters

Mary B. Clyde
and
Harriet B. Finch

Preface

Widespread developments in the health professions during the five years since the first edition of *The Head Nurse* was published have hastened the changes in nursing practice which had already begun. Perhaps the most notable development in nursing has been experimentation in the use of clinical nurse specialists to assist with nursing care and nursing care management in our hospitals. The place of the head nurse in situations where these experiments have been carried on has not always been clear. It seems essential, therefore, in the second edition of this volume to project a role for the head nurse for the years ahead—a role related entirely to nursing and completely free from responsibility for unit management. In so doing, it is realized that role change cannot occur overnight, that many institutions will of necessity move slowly. If this text helps to clarify the need for change, point direction, encourage self-evaluation and experimentation, it will have met its objective.

It is hoped this new edition will stimulate study of the head nurse role in the individual institution for the purpose of increasing the contribution of the key person in the care of patients—the head nurse. Her title may change with her role but there will continue to be need for a competent nurse to assume immediate responsibility for the nursing care of a group of patients and for the coordination of their total care. These have always been the primary responsibility of the person we now know as the head nurse.

Most of the changes in the second edition will be found in Part I. It is here that a concept of a new head nurse role is presented. Since roles cannot be changed without a concomitant modification in the framework in which the role is enacted, this edition has placed increased emphasis on the organization of the hospital and the services it offers. It also suggests the kind of relationships the head nurse must have with other health personnel if she is to achieve maximum effectiveness.

A wealth of reading material related to nursing is available today. Much of the literature deals with mental health, human behavior, and psychological approach. Perhaps this is our greatest need as nurses. In some areas almost no new material has been written in the last several years. In compiling the reference lists it has been impossible to include all relevant writings. The aim has been to select those which will stretch the head nurse's sights without taking her too far afield. Consideration has also been given to the availability of reading material to the head nurse. For this reason most references will be found in nursing periodicals. Because *The Head Nurse* is used outside the United States several Canadian and English magazines were systematically reviewed for pertinent articles. Those selected are felt to have value for head nurses everywhere. References more than five years old have been retained in this edition only if they are considered to have lasting value or if the content has not been dealt with in later writing.

In the spring and fall of 1966, in preparation for revising the text, seven hospitals were visited, and once again most time was spent in observing and consulting with head nurses, conferring with unit managers and nursing service administrators. The purpose of the visits was to learn the philosophy of the hospital and nursing service and to see first hand the way it was implemented in practice.

To the following nursing service administrators and their nursing staffs who so generously gave their time and so freely shared their ideas, I am deeply grateful: Mrs. Lydia Hall and Miss Genrose Alfano, The Loeb Center for Nursing and Rehabilitation, New York City; Miss Barbara Kane, Windham Community Memorial Hospital, Willimantic, Conn.; Miss Sue Kern, The Albert B. Chandler Medical Center, University of Kentucky, Lexington; Mrs. Mary Price, The Johns Hopkins Hospital, Baltimore, Md.; Miss Anne Ryle, Yale-New Haven Hospital, New Haven, Conn.; Miss Ruth Sleeper and Miss Mary Quinlan, The Massachusetts General Hospital, Boston, Mass.; Miss Dorothy Smith and Miss Lucille Mercadante, The J. Hillis Miller Medical Center, Gainesville, Florida.

In addition thanks is given Miss Laura Simms, Department Head, Surgical Nursing, The New York Hospital, for sharing her experiences relative to the clinical nurse specialist; to Miss Eleanor Krohn, formerly Assistant Professor, School of Nursing, Syracuse University, Syracuse, New York, who in a very creative way helped prepare senior students for nursing leadership and who evaluated the first edition of *The Head Nurse* in terms of its usefulness for teaching and for practice; to Miss Grace Eckelberry, Associate Professor, College of Nursing, University of Bridgeport, Bridgeport, Conn., for her valuable assistance in the preparation of the nursing history guide in Chapter 9; and to Miss Margaret Anne Goekler, Administrative Supervisor for Children's Services, Yale-New Haven Hospital, for her help and generous expenditure of time in portraying developments in services for infants and children.

To Mrs. Eleanor Gill, until recently Surgical Supervisor, University Hospital, Boston University Medical Center, Boston, Mass., is extended special thanks for her critical reading of the manuscript and for her valuable suggestions especially in relation to content. Mrs. Gill has had wide experience both in nursing education and nursing service, and because of her involvement in nursing practice at the division level she was particularly qualified for this undertaking. Mrs. Gill will find this same unique experience a valuable asset in her new position as Dean of the University of Connecticut School of Nursing.

Mr. John D. Thompson, Professor of Public Health (Hospital Administration), Yale University School of Medicine, who also has an appointment on the Yale School of Nursing faculty, read parts of the first six chapters and gave very helpful suggestions.

Mrs. Florence Schorske Wald, until the fall of 1967 Dean of the Yale University School of Nursing made time available for the revision of the text and gave encouragement and inspiration every step of the way. It is impossible to estimate the effect of her imaginative ideas on my thinking during the past four years of working with her, but the influence is very real. It was, therefore, particularly appropriate to ask her to read Chapter 6, and her thoughtful comments were deeply appreciated.

I am likewise indebted to my colleagues on the faculty of the Yale School of Nursing, especially those who participated over a three year period in the stimulating discussions on nursing theory. I am grateful also to many members of the Yale-New Haven Hospital nursing staff who gave unstintingly of their time and helped in many ways.

A word of thanks is also given to my sister, Mrs. Mary B. Clyde, who edited the manuscript, provided a layman's critical viewpoint, and helped in innumerable other ways.

Likewise, my sincere appreciation is extended to Mrs. Anna Helfrich who so accurately typed the manuscript, and to my publisher who never failed to give encouragement and understanding when these were most needed.

JEAN BARRETT

Excerpts from Preface to First Edition . . .

The attitudes of the public toward the hospital stem largely from the kind of care patients and their families receive. For this care the head nurse is in great part responsible. Hers is the immediate task of seeing that patient and family needs are met. The magnitude of the head nurse's work has greatly increased in recent years, and the position has become more complex than it was even five years ago. Today many new opportunities for working closely with members of other health professions are opening to the prepared head nurse. It is she, primarily, who makes nursing's contribution to the health team in its search for ways to meet the needs of hospitalized patients.

Many nurse leaders are concerned because head nurses are so involved with unit management activities that patient care administration is being neglected. Much has been written about the need to conserve nursing time for nursing and it is generally recognized that far more emphasis needs to be placed on the head nurse's responsibility for activities related to patient care which the nurse alone has the preparation to perform. Experience in some institutions has shown that a trained lay person is competent to handle the management of the unit or division.

A wealth of reading material is available in professional journals on changes in hospital organization, nurse-patient-doctor relationships, diagnosis of patients' needs, and staff development. Reference lists are included at the end of chapters and should be widely used to supplement the text. Since much of the value to the head nurse will be written in the coming years it is imperative that the reader of this volume study also the current literature. A text can never be more than a foundation which points up areas of study upon which teachers and students build. Hopefully, it stretches the imagination and stimulates the reader to think, experiment, and read further.

This book is designed primarily as a text for nurses who are preparing for positions as hospital head nurses. Nurses who are at present occupying such positions have also been kept in mind as the book has been prepared. It is hoped that some will find help in solving specific problems and that others may gain insight into the many possibilities inherent in their positions.

Administrators within the hospital, at the same time, may be assisted in visualing the scope of the head nurse position and the possibilities for organizing the work entailed. They may be helped to see that the talents of the presumably most capable nurse on the division are being deflected from nursing into activities that do not require nursing skills. It is hoped that this presentation will suggest means by which patient care can be improved and help develop an appreciation of the role the head nurse might play if she were free to do so and were given the help and support needed. Likewise, it is hoped nursing service administrators will find this text a resource in the development of in-service education programs.

The rich and rewarding experience of teaching the principles of ward management to head nurses and prospective head nurses over the past thirty years has provided most of the material on which the content herein is based. In direct preparation for writing this edition eleven hospitals, selected for their recognized excellence in nursing service administration, were visited in the spring of 1961. Most of the time was spent in direct observation of and conference with head nurses. Progressive developments in various types and sizes of hospitals in several parts of the United States were observed. The ideas herein presented are based on the successful experience of many institutions.

Grateful acknowledgement is made to the nursing service administrators and members of their staffs of the hospitals visited for graciously opening their doors to and sharing their experiences with the writer: Miss Thelma Dodds, The Charles T. Miller Hospital, St. Paul, Minn.; Mrs. Harriet B. Klock, St. Luke's Hospital, St. Paul, Minn.; Miss Jacqueline Metcalf, St. Johns Hospital, St. Paul, Minn.; Miss Nina H. Dencklau, Fairview Hospital, Minneapolis, Minn.; Miss Georgia Nobles, Minneapolis General Hospital, Minneapolis, Minn.; Miss Esther T. Roesti, Rochester Methodist Hospital, Rochester, Minn.; Miss Dorothy M. Smith, The J. Hillis Miller Health Center, Gainesville, Florida; Miss Mary Ellen Brown, The Presbyterian Hospital in Philadelphia, Pa.; Miss Ethel A. Brooks and Miss Mary E. Brackett, Hartford Hospital, Hartford, Conn.; Mrs. M. Vera Dormer, The Manchester Memorial Hospital, Manchester, Conn.; Miss Anne E. Ryle, Grace-New Haven Community Hospital, New Haven, Conn.

Special thanks is given to Miss Virginia Earles, Assistant Professor of Nursing Education, Syracuse University School of Nursing, for her critical reading of the entire manuscript and help in the development of the nursing care plan in Chapter 10. Miss Earles' experience includes head nursing, departmental administration, teaching ward management to head nurses on the job as well as to senior students in a university program. The latter involves instruction and supervision of student experience in team leadership and assistant head nursing. In addition Miss Earles has for five years taught the graduate course in Medical-Surgical Nursing in the Syracuse University Department of Nursing Education.

CONTENTS

part 3 THE HEAD NURSE'S RESPONSIBILITY FOR STAFF DEVELOPMENT

THE HEAD NURSE

part 1   **THE HEAD NURSE IN
THE MODERN HOSPITAL**

chapter 1

THE CHANGING ROLE OF THE HEAD NURSE

The head nurse role, probably more than any other in nursing, has been undergoing close scrutiny in recent years. Dissatisfaction of the public, doctors, and nurses with nursing care has been a subject of considerable concern to all who are responsible for care of patients. However, although it is the head nurse who has immediate responsibility for nursing, many believe that the organizational system of the hospital needs changing, that the head nurse cannot be held accountable for the shortcomings of nursing care. Effort is therefore being made in many places to determine what changes in the system are needed. In this endeavor head nurses have much to offer, and much at stake, for out of the study will almost surely come a new head nurse role.

Since young nurses are unaware of many of the developments which have already occurred in the head nurse role these changes will be briefly reviewed.[1] Through looking at the past it is often possible to gain perspective on the present and a vision of the future. It is difficult for the head nurse of today to realize that as late as the 1930's all activities on the patient care division, except medical care, were the head nurse's responsibility. These included housekeeping and dietary service; ordering, cleaning, and sterilizing equipment; maintaining supplies; teaching. The head nurse enjoyed this role because it has brought her many satisfactions:[2] the opportunity 1) for close association with the patient; 2) to work closely with the doctor; 3) to be at the center of activities on the unit; and 4) to participate in the education of nurses.

Little by little these satisfactions were dissipated as certain important responsibilities of the head nurse were transferred to others. Although the head nurse was still the key figure on the unit she no longer had authority over all activities which affected the patient's welfare. So today, for the most part, housekeeping and dietary services are not functions of the head nurse, although in some institutions she may still have responsibility for supervision.

---

[1] A full account of the changes which have occurred in the head nurse's responsibilities since 1920. See: Jean Barrett. The hospital head nurse's changing role, *Nurs. Outlook,* Vol. 11 (November 1963), pp. 800-204.
[2] The first edition of Ward Management and Teaching, the forerunner of this text, published in 1949, discusses satisfactions of the head nurse on pages 13-17.

3

Likewise, it is a rare hospital which does not have a central supply room to package and sterilize equipment, and practically all hospitals provide secretarial help for the head nurse. At first each of these innovations was viewed with skepticism, but doubt was soon dispelled when the head nurse realized that patient care was not jeopardized and efficiency was increased. A second satisfaction keenly felt by earlier head nurses has also greatly diminished during the past twenty years which have seen responsibility for basic nursing education almost completely removed from nursing service. In addition major concern for development of the staff has been assumed by directors of in-service education and department administrators, even though most head nurses feel some responsibility for orientation of the nursing staff, and many make use of opportunities to teach. Few would question the wisdom of these changes nor do they believe that head nurses today have either the time or the preparation to take much responsibility for the clinical aspects of basic nursing education. Nevertheless, divesting the head nurse of any specific part in the educational program of student and staff nurses has meant the loss of one of her four early satisfactions.

Long ago many head nurses gave up accompanying the doctor to see his patients unless he specifically requested that she do so. In medical centers she seldom has time to go on service rounds with residents and interns, and almost never on teaching rounds. Thus the head nurse has had to relinquish another satisfaction, that of working closely with the physician.

Changes in the head nurse role thus far discussed have left her with considerable responsibility for administration of the unit and for coordination of patient care services with both of which she has the help of one or more secretaries; administration of nursing care; coordination of patient care activities; and supervision of personnel. In large, active divisions of today's hospitals these activities comprise an insuperable load, which leaves the head nurse little time for direct contact with the patient. She thus is deprived of still another satisfaction. More serious, however, is the loss to the patient which results from this lack of contact.

Why, when so much has been done to relieve her, is the head nurse still so overburdened? The probable answer to this question lies in the fact that medical care and hospital services have expanded enormously. More and more responsibility has been delegated to nursing service by both physicians and hospital administration. The person at the division level—the head nurse—has been called upon to absorb much of the increased load. For example, the handling of doctors' orders, always a time-consuming activity, has placed a much greater burden on the head nurse than was formerly the case. Added demands result, in part, from the increased number of laboratory and other diagnostic tests, the expanded use of drugs in intravenous solutions, the frequent varying of medications and treatments. All of these require requisitions, transcribing orders, notifying personnel of new or changed prescriptions, preparing and transmitting charge slips for the very large number of items now paid for by the individual patient.

Between all the administrative detail for which the head nurse is responsible and the coordinating function which is hers as administrator of the division, the head nurse has very little time for anything else. She makes rounds to see patients but dares not become involved in talking for fear the administration will get hopelessly behind, and this would result in a disservice to all patients. The head nurse must therefore settle for giving a friendly greeting and asking questions about specific symptoms. Often the patient does not know her name or that she is the head nurse.

We see, then, that the head nurse role has been changing over the years until now she has minimal contact with patients and doctors and almost none with student nurses. The major portion of her time is required to keep the unit functioning, patient care activities administered and coordinated.

Is this the best role for the head nurse—presumably the most able nurse on the division? Is she satisfied with it? A great deal is heard about the desire of the head nurse to "get back to the patient," about her frustration in not being able to have close contact with the patients. If this is true, how does she think this desire can be achieved? Just more nursing staff will not permit closer contact between head nurse and patient unless the staff increase were in professional nurses. A greater number of nonprofessional personnel would require more time of the head nurse for supervision. In today's hectic patient care divisions no one person can manage the unit, coordinate patient care activities, and have time to know patients well enough to administer nursing care as it should be done. If the head nurse is to "get back to patients," it is obvious that her role still needs extensive change.

A few hospitals have made further organizational innovations. In general the three methods they have employed to relieve the head nurse and improve patient care are the centralization of responsibility for providing the unit with linen, drugs, and supplies; the institution of a unit manager system; and the employment of clinical nurse specialists to give consultation and assistance with nursing care. It is hoped these changes, which will be described in later chapters, not only will result in a higher quality of care for patients but will bring back to the head nurse some of the satisfactions which she has lost. No one believes the ideal role for the head nurse has been found. Hospitals and nurses must be willing to examine traditional patterns and cast aside those which no longer meet today's needs. Does the head nurse see herself moving forward with these changes, participating in the development of a new role concept, or will she cling to the present and resist inevitable change?

One of the purposes of this text is to help the head nurse envisage a new and more satisfying role for herself and to discover ways to assist in bringing about necessary change. Certain questions must be answered: Which of the head nurse's responsibilities require professional nurse preparation and which can be carried by someone else? This question has both economic and ethical implications. It is economically unsound for an individual to be employed to perform tasks which could be done just as competently by a person who receives a lower salary. Likewise, it is hardly ethical for professionally educated individuals, especially when they are in short supply, to be given responsibility for activities which do not require the professional preparation which these persons have received. To what extent should the head nurse retain *responsibility* for activities which have been hers through the years even though she may delegate related functions? Should some responsibilities which have been relinquished, either by plan or by default, again be assumed by the head nurse? These questions will be uppermost when attempting to carve out a new role for the head nurse.

Before considering the character of this new role, it is important to review the organization of the hospital—the place where the head nurse works. The next three chapters will, therefore, deal with hospital organization for administration, for patient care, and for efficiency. Chapter 5 will be concerned with organization of the patient care division. It will discuss in detail the problems of coordination which have been touched on in this chapter and ways to alleviate them within the existing organizational structure. Chapter 6 will describe a new role for the head nurse.

SUMMARY

Many, today, are talking about a new role for the head nurse. In looking back over the past twenty years, one realizes that her role has already undergone significant change. Seldom is the head nurse now an assistant to the doctor in performing treatments or in learning about his patients. Nor is she a "mother figure" for the patients or an instructor for students. Infrequently is she the planner for the development of her staff. Instead she is primarily a unit administrator and a coordinator of patient care. The demands in these areas are so great that the head nurse has little time for other activities, including the administration of nursing care or the association with patients which this responsibility demands. As a result of the changes which have occurred in the head nurse role, much of the satisfaction in head nursing has been lost. More important, the nursing talents of the head nurse are not being fully utilized. This violates principles of economics as well as of ethics. Some hospitals are leading the way in changing their organizational structure and developing a new role for the head nurse.

It is imperative that administrators of other hospitals and of nursing service, as well as the head nurse herself, answer several vital questions. These relate to gaps in nursing care, ways in which the gaps can best be filled, and determination of activities which require an education in professional nursing for their fulfilment and which do not. In short it needs to be decided what *should* be the role of the head nurse.

QUESTIONS FOR DISCUSSION

1. What is the difference between patient care and nursing care? What is the head nurse's responsibility in each of these?
2. Which if any of the responsibilities head nurses have relinquished in the past 20 years should be reclaimed when her new role is defined? Give reasons for your answer.
3. At the present time, what blocks stand in the way of instituting a new role for the head nurse?

EXERCISES

1. Before reading further in this text describe the role of the head nurse as you believe it should be. Then put the paper aside to compare with a similar statement to be prepared when you have finished your study of the book and supplementary readings.
2. Head nurses might take note of their own activities for a day or a week while staff nurses and students could observe their head nurse over a specified period of time. List functions performed by the head nurse which could have been done 1) by an aide or practical nurse; 2) by a competent, trained secretary; 3) by a member of the housekeeping or dietary staff. Estimate the time spent on each activity. What was the total time spent in nonhead nurse activities? The daily average?

REFERENCES

Arnstein, Margaret G., Gillan, Ruth I., Tibbetts, Helen G., and Sutherland, Dorothy. The Head Nurse Looks at Her Job, United States Department of Health, Education, and Welfare, Public Health Service, United States Government Printing Office, 1953.
This manual presents a method for studying head nurse activities to determine how her time is being distributed between patient care management—her most important function—and unit management, many aspects of which could be delegated to other personnel. The introduction gives a clear picture of the head nurse's responsibilities.

Barrett, Jean. The head nurse's changing role, Nurs. Outlook, Vol. 11 (November 1963), pp. 800-804.
The history of the head nurse role is traced from the 1920's to the present.

Brown, William King. An administrator's view of the head nurse's work, Nurs. Outlook, Vol. 11 (November 1963), pp. 798-799.
This hospital administrator sees the head nurse as his deputy, as unit manager, role model for her staff, and as a creator of the hospital image in the community.

Bursten, Ben, and Diers, Donna K. Pseudo-patient-centered orientation, Nurs. Forum, Vol. 3 (No. 2, 1964), pp. 38-50.
In attempting to change from task-centered to patient-centered nursing, one must not merely substitute for a physical task the task of "talking with the new patient." Nurses need help with the difficult undertaking of making interactions with patients meaningful.

Canetto, Victorio. T.P.R. q 4h. ad infinitum? Amer. J. Nurs. Vol. 64 (November 1964), p. 132.
A nurse with an inquiring mind made a month's study of T.P.R.'s on ambulatory patients and learned that 97 percent of the temperatures were within normal range. Of the 56 elevated temperatures, 36 were in four patients. Her conclusion was that "temperature measurements, made as they are now in a traditional and casual manner, constitute a substantial waste of time. . . ."

Christman, Luther. The influence of specialization on the nursing profession, Nurs. Science, Vol. 3 (December 1965), pp. 446-453.
Nursing must make up its mind whether it wishes to move in a clinical (ie, practice) direction or in a managerial direction (giving care through others). Hospital nursing is organized vertically—not horizontally as in medicine. With the development of well-prepared clinical nurse specialists will it be possible or advisable for hospital nursing to change its organizational pattern?

Corrigan, Shirley M., and Julian, Florence. Head nurse, maternal or executive? Nurs. Res., Vol. 15 (Summer 1966), pp. 214-217.
A study of characteristics of head nurses showed them to be of the "executive" type. "However, if her responsibility shifts and requires expertness in nursing diagnosis, the planning of individualized care, and the implementation of direct care, we might expect a concomitant alteration in the perception of desirable personal characteristics."

Hall, Lydia E. A center for nursing, Nurs. Outlook, Vol. 11 (November 1963), pp. 805-806.
A description of Loeb Center for Nursing where nurses only nurse.

Mauksch, Hans O. Nursing dilemmas in the organization of patient care, Nurs. Outlook, Vol. 5 (January 1957), pp. 31-33.
There is probably no more complex and frustrating job in existence than that of head nurse. She is responsible to doctors who are present much of the time in

large numbers and to the hospital administration through the nursing service administrator or supervisor who are seldom present. She thus represents to patients and other groups both medicine and administration. She needs to be prepared for and accorded the power to be the coordinator and administrator.

Pellegrino, Edmund D. The changing role of the professional nurse, Hospitals, Vol. 35 (December 16, 1961), pp. 56-62.
Written by a doctor, this thought-provoking article describes the professional nurse of the future. He sees her returning to the bedside, not as a "19th century lady with a lamp" but as a clinical specialist who will determine the patient's needs, observe him, and supervise less well-prepared individuals in carrying out the functions of nursing. Excellent reading.

——— The nurse must know; the nurse must speak, Amer. J. Nurs., Vol. 60 (March 1960), pp. 360-363.
An excellent article by a doctor who sees the nurse in a new and highly different role from that of a few years ago. If the nurse is to take her place on the health team, she must know comprehensive nursing and be able to share in the planning of patient care. Administrative activities will need to be handled by someone else to free the professional nurse to meet the rightful demands which will be made of her in the future.

Scheffler, Gustave L. The nurse's role in hospital safety, Nurs. Outlook, Vol. 10 (October 1962), pp. 680-682.
Many dangers which exist in the hospital are described and the need for the nurse, who is the one person present for 24 hours, to know their causes and implications.

Simmons, Leo W. Past and potential images of the nurse, Nurs. Forum, Vol. 1 (Summer 1962), pp. 16-33.
Images of nurses as held by themselves and others.

——— What is the potential role of the nurse in patient care?, Nurs. Outlook, Vol. 10 (February 1962), pp. 103-105.
A sociologist, who has for many years been associated with hospitals, nurses, physicians, and patients, describes the changes which have occurred in our way of life which are affecting nursing. The potential role of the nurse is still a question. The thoughtful head nurse will find this stimulating reading.

Skipper, James K. Jr. A further note on research communication, Nurs. Forum, Vol. 1 (Summer 1962), pp. 7-10.
"Role" has two meanings in social science: 1) actual behavior and 2) expected behavior. To differentiate, Skipper calls the first "role behavior," the second "role."

——— and Leonard, Robert C. Social Interaction and Patient Care, Philadelphia, J. B. Lippincott Company, 1965.
A compilation of papers by nurses and behavioral scientists, this paper back volume contains a wealth of thought-provoking, highly interesting information for nurses in all types and levels of practice. Reference to several individual papers is made in this text when especially applicable to a subject under consideration.

Talking about patient care, Amer. J. Nurs., Vol. 61 (May 1961), pp. 56-59.
"At four A.N.A. conferences across the country, nurses raised questions and sought ways to improve their practice."
Frances Reiter suggests that "professional nurse power" should be conserved for direct care of and communication with patients. She promotes the idea of a nurse clinician in place of a head nurse or supervisor (p. 56).

chapter 2

THE HOSPITAL IN WHICH
THE HEAD NURSE WORKS

The hospital exists primarily to diagnose the ills of people, to care for individuals when they are sick, to restore them to health if possible, to teach them self care, and to help them learn how to keep well or to live with a disability. In addition the hospital serves as a learning field for many groups of health workers—doctors, nurses, dietitians, medical social workers, and technicians of all kinds. The hospital also is a rich field for research in many areas—primarily medicine, nursing, sociology, psychology, and administration. The extent to which each hospital functions in these various fields depends upon the type of hospital, its size, facilities, and the like.

TYPES OF HOSPITALS

Hospitals are classified according to service and ownership. In the former there are three types: 1) psychiatric, 2) tuberculosis, 3) general and other special. In the United States in 1965, 90 percent of the hospitals fell into the third category. This group is subdivided into short and long term care institutions.

In the classification by ownership, hospitals are either governmental or nongovernmental. The former, which includes federal, state, and local hospitals, comprise approximately 35 percent of the total number. Nongovernmental hospitals are designated either voluntary or proprietary. The latter are privately owned profit-making institutions (see Table 1).

Voluntary or community hospitals, as they are sometimes called, are owned and operated by a nonprofit corporation. Church hospitals and those belonging to a fraternal organization fall into this category. Table 1 shows that voluntary hospitals make up 51.5 percent of all hospitals. Approximately 95 percent of these are for short term care (Table 2). Voluntary hospitals are financed by patients' fees, earnings of the departments, endowments, donations, and community chest contributions. The government may subsidize the care of the medically indigent in a community hospital. By so doing, however, it has no control over the functioning of the institution.

10

table 1.   CLASSIFICATION OF HOSPITALS*

CLASSIFICATION	TYPE	% HOSPITALS	% BEDS	% ADMISSIONS
SERVICE	Psychiatric	7.4	42.9	2.0
	Tuberculosis	2.6	2.4	0.2
	General and other specialties	90.0	54.7	97.8
	TOTAL	100.0	100.0	100.0
TYPE OF OWNERSHIP	Nongovernmental			
	Voluntary	51.5	32.4	66.3
	Proprietary	13.6	3.2	6.6
	Total	65.1	35.6	72.9
	Governmental			
	State and local	28.7	54.2	21.4
	Federal	6.2	10.2	5.7
	Total	34.9	64.4	27.1
	TOTAL	100.0	100.0	100.0

* Figures taken from Guide Issue, *Hospitals* (August 1), 1966.

Although many hospitals have educational programs for health personnel a so-called teaching hospital is one whose facilities are used by a university for the education of medical students, interns, and residents. More often than not, a teaching hospital will also have one or more schools of nursing associated with it. The teaching hospital may be government controlled if it is part of a state university medical center. On the other hand, a teaching hospital may be an institution operated by a private university for its medical school, or a voluntary hospital whose facilities a school of medicine contracts to use.

table 2.   CLASSIFICATION OF NONFEDERAL, VOLUNTARY, GENERAL HOSPITALS* BY LENGTH OF STAY†

CLASSIFICATION	NO. HOSP.	%	NO. BEDS	NO. BEDS IN VOL. HOSP.	%
Short Term	5,736	95.2	741,292	515,374	96.2
Long Term	283	4.8	65,897	20,272	3.8
TOTAL	6,019	100.0	807,189	535,646	100.0

* This includes most all the voluntary hospitals.
† Figures taken from Guide Issue, *Hospitals* (August 1), 1966.

The principles of nursing care administration with which this volume will be concerned are applicable in all hospitals. The head nurse's responsibilities and problems may vary, however, depending upon the type of service and ownership of the institution in which she is working. Since general hospitals comprise 90 percent of the total number in the United States, since 55.9

percent of general hospitals are voluntary (Table 3), and since 96.2 percent of voluntary hospital beds in this country are for short term care (Table 2), this text will be concerned primarily with the organization and responsibilities of head nurses in voluntary, short term, general hospitals.

table 3. SUBCLASSIFICATION OF GENERAL AND OTHER SPECIAL HOSPITALS*

	% HOSPITALS
Voluntary	55.9
Proprietary	13.6
Government	30.5
TOTAL	100.0

* Figures taken from Guide Issue, *Hospitals* (August 1), 1966.

ADMINISTRATIVE ORGANIZATION OF THE HOSPITAL

Every hospital, large or small, has a basic system for the coordination of its vast number of activities. The head nurse needs to know how she fits into the system. Therefore, let us look at the formal organizational structure of the hospital, that is at the people who carry out its functions and their formal relationship to one another.

At the head of the hospital is the administrator, appointed by and responsible to a board of directors or governing board which represents the owners. The administrator is responsible for maintaining standards of service and patient care established by the board. He should be given free reign to carry out the functions of the institution in accord with the philosophy and established policies set by the governing board. To help with the administration of various departments the administrator usually has one or more assistants. One of these may have responsibility for professional services, one for business and operational services, and a third for special services (Fig. 1). Each of these departments has a specialist at its head to manage its affairs. The directors of large departments have assistants with whom to share their loads.

Line Organization

Line organization is commonly found in hospitals, schools, and military services. In this type of organization each individual takes orders from and is responsible to the person on the next higher administrative level. Thus the head nurse who is in charge of a division is responsible to the depart-

HOSPITAL ADMINISTRATION - CHART OF ORGANIZATION

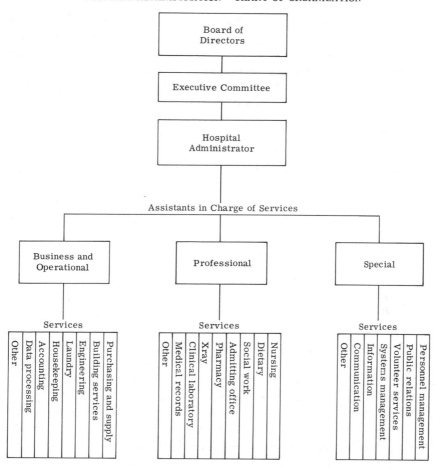

Fig. 1. A typical plan of organziation for administrative services. Many services have a department head. Others are the direct responsibility of the assistant administrator.

ment administrator,[1] the latter to the nursing service administrator or one of her assistants. Members of the division staff take directions from the head nurse and report to her. We thus see that in line organization responsibility is delegated down the line to the person or persons who are under an administrator's immediate jurisdiction.

Line organization may be operated in an autocratic or in a democratic way. Administration will be autocratic if an administrator at any level considers it his sole prerogative to designate the rules or enforce policy. This is true also if a small committee or group sets up regulations by which others are expected to operate. An organization will be democratically managed if responsibility for leadership is shared by administrators at all levels, if all persons have a part in setting goals, in establishing the method for achieving them, and in differentiating the authority necessary. In democratic administration, there is provision "for broad assumption of responsibility, for leadership, ample freedom for exercising initiative, and means of cooperative self-evaluation."[2]

Line organization can be pyramidal or flat in structure. The former has many levels of responsibility with a short span of control for each individual, which means each administrator has few persons reporting directly to him. For example, the head nurse may have eight or ten staff members responsible to her; the department administrator, four or five head nurses under her jurisdiction; an assistant nursing administrator, four to six department administrators reporting to her, and the nursing service administrator, only her assistants communicating directly with her. In this pyramidal pattern with its many levels, there is little contact between top and bottom. Problems in communication result. Usually the lower a person is on the hierarchical ladder, the more rules and regulations there are to control his behavior, the closer his supervision, and the less he has to say about how his work is to be done. Policies and procedures are established to furnish standards and direction for his behavior on the assumption that individuals will "assume their accountability" if they are given specific direction and are checked periodically. Research has shown that often these assumptions are false, that individuals perform better when they are able to increase their self-esteem and sense of personal worth. Opportunities for these satisfactions do not necessarily occur when persons are told exactly what to do. Chris Argyris,[3]

[1] This individual is usually called a "supervisor." Since many persons including the head nurse have supervisory functions, the term is confusing and will not be used in this text to denote a position.

[2] John A. Rorer. *Principles of Democratic Supervision,* New York, Teachers College, Bureau of Publications, Columbia University, 1942, p. 150.

[3] Chris Argyris. *Interpersonal Competence and Organizational Effectiveness,* Homewood, Illinois, The Dorsey Press, Inc., Richard D. Irvin, Inc., 1962, pp. 27-34.

who has studied and written widely on the effects of organization on personality, finds that the pyramidal type organization (which is essentially autocratic) increases dependence and, for those at the bottom of the line, leads to frustration and conflict because the workers wish to be creative and independent and cannot, due to the system.[4]

Another criticism made of pyramidal organization is that although responsibility is delegated, accountability is retained by the delegator.[5] Thus the head nurse may delegate the administration of medications to a staff nurse who will be responsible for accuracy and promptness. Should an error be made, however, the head nurse bears a share of the responsibility and is accountable for the mistake because she made the assignment to a nurse who, in this instance, was not entirely competent. Also the head nurse presumably had control over circumstances making for safety—correctness of medicine card, correct labeling of patients and their beds, prevention of confusion at the medicine closet. Actually, however, the head nurse has no control over the selection of her staff (though she may have some choice of whom she assigns to administer medications) and very little control over the environment. Therefore the department administrator and nursing service administrator who do have control over staffing are also accountable for medication errors. In the final analysis, accountability goes straight to the top, that is, to the board of directors who partially control staffing through standards, salary scales, and personnel practices. The fact is that each person in the line is accountable to the extent that he has authority or power to carry delegated responsibility. Likewise, responsibility cannot be given unless it is accepted. Both giver and recipient need to be clear about the limits of responsibility accepted.

In contrast to pyramidal organization, the so-called flat pattern has fewer levels of responsibility and broader span of control.[6] This means that many persons report to one individual, which results in his giving them greater responsibility and less detailed supervision. Instead of checking performance, which he does not have time to do, he judges by results. Because there is less supervision *persons with unusual competence are needed in management positions*. They function under broad guidelines and objectives but are given freedom to determine how the objectives are to be met. They are held accountable for their actions. It is quite obvious that the flat organization is more likely to result in democratic administration. Fig-

[4] Chris Argyris. *Personality and Organization*, New York, Harper and Brothers, 1957, p. 95.
[5] Argyris, *op. cit.*, 1962. pp. 3, 34.
[6] George Strauss and Leonard R. Sayles, *Personnel—the Human Problems of Management*, Englewood Cliffs, New Jersey, Prentice-Hall, Inc., 1960, pp. 378-394.

ures 2 and 3 illustrate the pyramidal and flat organizational types in a hospital setting.

Pyramidal organizations in which important decisions must go up through many levels are said to be *centralized,* whereas, in the flat type, authority is *decentralized.*[7] In the pattern shown in Figure 3, the head nurse would have much more authority or power to make decisions than would the head nurse pictured in Figure 2. For this reason, of course, she would need to be a highly capable individual who had the education, maturity, and judgment to carry the responsibility delegated to her. Because many more persons would be reporting directly to the assistant nursing service administrator—for example, 15 head nurses (Fig. 3) instead of three department administrators (Fig, 2)—the assistant would have considerably less time for close supervision. In some hospitals the nursing department is moving in the direction of decentralization. This trend will be discussed in Chapter 6.

Line and Staff Organization

Usually an institution which has line organization also has persons who are in a staff relationship to an administrator. Staff officers are employed to perform special service functions rather than those of an administrative nature. These individuals have little, if any, line authority except over their own staffs. The system is called line and staff organization. Thus a nursing service assistant in charge of inservice education is a staff, not a line officer. Her responsibilities are educational. She does not have responsibility for nursing service although she works with nursing service personnel. She does, however, have line responsibility for her assistants.

The Informal Organization

The formal organization of the hospital which we have been discussing is necessary for the record and for handling problems. However, in healthy situations a large percentage of the work gets done through informal relationships and direct contact, not through the administrative line.[8] For exam-

---

[7] *Ibid.,* p. 388.
[8] Lyndall F. Urwick. The nature of line and staff, In *Readings in Management,* Koontz, H., and O'Donnell, C. New York, McGraw-Hill Book Co., Inc., 1959, p. 117.

PYRAMIDAL TYPE ORGANIZATION OF NURSING SERVICE

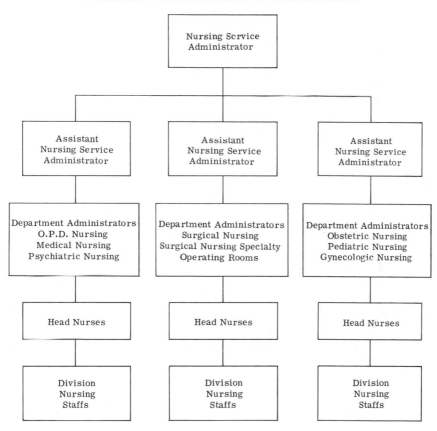

Fig. 2. Pyramidal type organization with five levels of personnel. (Evening and night assistant nursing service administrators are not shown.) This is the most common pattern except in very small hospitals. In very large institutions assistant department administrators could create a sixth administrative level.

"FLAT" TYPE ORGANIZATION OF NURSING SERVICE

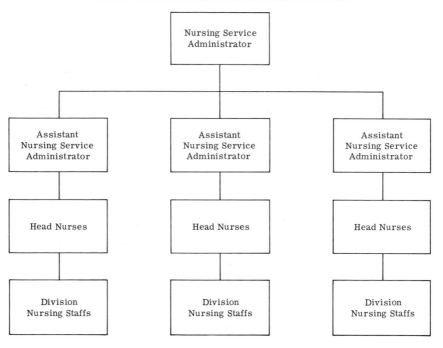

Fig. 3. In this flat type organization the position of department administrator has been eliminated. Head nurses are directly responsible to an assistant administrator. In smaller hospitals, the assistant administrator may also be omitted from the line.

ple, head nurses on adjacent floors may plan their staff time together in relation to needs of both divisions, so that one could help the other in an emergency. So too, a minor matter may be settled between the head nurse and ward dietitian. If more than one division is concerned or a policy change is involved, the head dietitian and nurse administrator need to be brought into the discussion. Together they may decide that one of the hospital administrators should be involved. Whether to do so is a mutual decision. Informal working and problem solving across, rather than up and down, administrative lines are called horizontal (as opposed to vertical) relationships.

Informal relationships also operate through small groups which form an informal organization and can bind together many individuals with varying backgrounds and interests. Man is a social being and needs to "belong." He is usually a member of many groups—at work, at home, at play. A staff nurse, for example, may be a member of a group of young women with whom she shares an apartment, a member of a bridge club, and of a church. At work she may belong to more than one group—the staff of the division on which she works, the staff nurses of the hospital, or those of the pediatric service. If a staff nurse (or other employee) is not accepted as a member of a group in the hospital, she will feel herself isolated, will fail to have job satisfaction, and as a result will not be able to function at her best.[9]

Informal groups exist at every level. They are supportive of their members, and loyalty to the group may be stronger than to the larger organization. In the hospital, aides may compose an informal group. If they feel they are appreciated and respected, they will help one another retain that status. If they are considered to be lazy and to have no interest in their work, as a group, they will find ways to avoid their responsibilities through absenteeism or excessive time in the rest room and will encourage one another in these practices.[10] Administration, therefore, cannot deal only with the individual but must take into account the group or groups to which the person belongs. There is strength in groups which can be used for constructive purposes, and hospital administration would do well to encourage their development. The existence of small groups has potential for increasing output and maintaining morale. The head nurse who is able to develop her staff into a group finds they will work as a team and that in stressful times the group will consolidate its efforts to see that the work is done. Likewise, if the department administrator gives the head nurses on her service an

[9] For this reason some nurses are very unhappy as P.R.N.'s. Floating between a few divisions rather than anywhere in the hospital, however, may make it possible for a P.R.N. nurse to "belong."
[10] Strauss and Leonard, *op. cit.*, p. 45.

opportunity to work together on common problems, they will in all likelihood form a group willing to help one another with loan of staff when unexpected demands, illness, or absence places a heavy load on one division. The attitude of the head nurse toward the group of her fellow head nurses and toward her own staff group will determine the willingness of one of her nurses or aides to help out on another floor. Needless to say the small group theory has implications for the way in which staffing is planned for the entire nursing service. These will be considered in Chapter 8.

THE DEPARTMENT OF NURSING

Nursing is the largest department in the hospital. At its head is the nursing service administrator who is variously called director of nursing, head of the department of nursing, chief of nursing practice. It is customary for her to have at least one assistant for each period of the day, since the nursing department is staffed for 24 hours. The department of nursing also has clinical specialists to administer at least some of its services, such as pediatrics, maternity, and operating room. Every service has two or more divisions each of which has a head nurse in charge. The head nurse, in turn, has helpers who have varying types and degrees of preparation. All these individuals are part of the line organization. We have seen that the nurse administrator may also have assistants in staff positions such as the director of inservice education. Although this organizational pattern is the most common today, other designs are being used in some hospitals which are not satisfied with traditional arrangements. Some of these patterns will be discussed in Chapter 6.

Responsibilities of Nursing Administration

To the administrator of nursing service has been delegated the responsibility for setting standards and providing good nursing care to the patients in the entire hospital. She employs and places the personnel who help in this undertaking. Orientation and development programs are instituted for staff at all levels. Through nursing service, safe, effective nursing techniques are devised; new equipment is tested and evaluated. The nursing service administrator holds each department head responsible for the quality of nursing in her area. The department administrator's responsibilities thus involve defining standards for nursing practice on the service and appraisal of its quality; counselling head nurses in regard to nursing care; development of the staff and evaluation of personnel performance; staffing the divisions; and serving as liaison between the nursing units and the nursing service administrator. The department administrator should be expected to instigate studies for the solution of nursing problems and make use of experimentation to find better ways of nursing the patients on her service.

The head nurse is immediately responsible for providing good nursing for the patients on her unit 24 hours a day, for carrying out the medical care delegated by the doctor, for coordinating patient care activities. She also has responsibility for the orientation, instruction, supervision, and evaluation of members of her staff. In most hospitals, the head nurse is still responsible for managing the unit. She keeps the department administrator informed of the needs of patients for unusual amounts of care, of inadequate staffing and of accidents, injuries, and complaints. The head nurse is often relatively inexperienced and needs the guidance and help which the department administrator can provide. There should be a very close working relationship between the two.

Relationship of the Head Nurse to the Nursing Service Administrator

Between the administrator of nursing and the head nurse there is an employer-employee relationship. As her employer the administrator customarily expects the head nurse to comply with hospital and nursing policy. Usually this policy is made at the top and transmitted down the line. Sometimes, however, the head nurse has the opportunity to help make regulations which affect the activities of the patient care division. When this is true and when the head nurse is free to function in her own way, she must expect to be held responsible for results. Usually this responsibility proves to be a challenge to the head nurse and frequently leads to a deeper commitment. The nursing service administrator considers it important that the head nurse not only carry out the day by day activities of the service but that she make a more lasting contribution to the institution by improving the quality of patient care, making suggestions for the good of the entire nursing service, improving herself professionally, and contributing to the growth and development of the personnel on her division. The head nurse is expected to give her loyal support to the institution and to the individuals by whom she is employed. Because the head nurse sets the tone and establishes the values for the unit, she greatly influences the attitudes of the public toward the hospital.

Relationship of the Head Nurse to Her Staff

The head nurse needs to recognize that she is part of hospital administration and, through the line from the administrator, carries both responsibility and authority. Remembering this fact will help her understand her relationship to her nursing staff. In the same way that the head nurse has obligations to top administration through the various levels of nursing administration, so the staff nurse and the aide have definite responsibility through her to those in the higher echelons of administration.

The head nurse's relationship to her staff should be that of a leader who by her knowledge, ability, ideals, and the force of her personality makes people want to live up to her expectations. A leader recognizes the value of group participation in settling problems and in making plans and policies. She does not, however, shrink from decision making, taking a stand, or being directive when the occasion demands. (See Chapter 6 for further discussion of her leadership role.)

The best relationship between the head nurse and her staff is usually attained when she is one *with* the members of the division personnel but not one *of* them. She is friendly and warm, dignified but approachable; she is neither chummy nor authoritative. If her relationship were too close, it would be difficult to maintain impartiality and to evaluate the personnel objectively.

Fairness and consideration for each staff member are essential to good working relationships. Important also are recognition and appreciation of effort and achievement. The head nurse who has a personal interest in the members of her staff finds it much easier to be understanding. She cannot, however, assume the personal worries and burdens of each person. She must expect that the staff nurse or aide, if she is able to be on duty, will put her mind on her work and not complain or discuss her problems with others while on the division. There are many ways in which the head nurse can show her understanding and interest without letting the atmosphere become demoralized by making a great many adjustments or exceptions for one or two people.

The line between friendliness and too much sociability is difficult to draw. It is important, however, that the staff not use the division as a place for more than occasional exchanges of conversation about personal matters. Few would wish to return to the stiff, rigid "professionalism" of yesterday, but when the pendulum swings too far in the opposite direction minds are apt to be distracted from the important business to be done. Impressions of laxness may be conveyed to families who are concerned about their loved ones and to members of the medical staff who may have much on their minds and would appreciate a little more assistance. Dignity and courtesy rather than formality and deference, and freedom from tension instead of laxity in manner are the objectives to be achieved. It is this atmosphere which is conducive to good patient care and good public relations.

THE PLACE OF THE DOCTOR
IN THE HOSPITAL ORGANIZATION

The reader may have noted that the doctor has not been mentioned in the discussion of hospital organization. The reason for this omission is that the doctor has an entirely different relationship to the hospital than do members of any other professional group. He is not a part of the line organization unless he is an employee of the institution as are some specialists such as roentgenologists, physiatrists, and pathologists. The physician is an independent practitioner who utilizes the facilities of the hospital. He functions as an individual and not as part of the institution, as does the nurse. However, because of his high status the doctor wields an enormous amount of influence.

To be a member of the medical staff and have the privilege of using hospital facilities, a physician must be approved and appointed by the board of directors of the hospital. The board, however, is not qualified to judge the competence of a doctor and must be advised by the medical staff. Likewise, the medical staff must advise regarding the standards of care to be given by legally qualified physicians. Guided by the staff's judgment the board sets standards and establishes hospital policy. While "it is a universally accepted principle that no layman should tell a physician how to treat his patient—the board, as a group of laymen, is legally responsible for the quality of medical service performed by a group of physicians." [11] To exert this control the board makes certain that the medical staff has a sound system of self-government, that it sets up rules and regulations which make the standards of patient care specific. Each staff member is pledged to comply with these regulations. The board expects the staff to establish disci-

[11] John R. McGibony. *Principles of Hospital Administration*, New York, G. P. Putnam's Sons, 1952, p. 154.

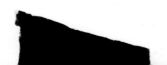

plinary procedures and to prevent derelictions.[12] The medical staff is thus self-governing and self-appraising.

Most of the work of the medical staff is done by committees which are elected or appointed by the chief of staff. Three of these committees will be mentioned here. 1) An elected executive committee coordinates activities and acts for the staff under specified circumstances. 2) The joint conference committee is composed of three members of the hospital board of directors, three from the active medical staff, and the hospital administrator. This is a highly important committee which serves as the liaison between the three groups represented. It advises on problems, interprets reports, and discusses recommendations of the medical staff to the board. 3) A medical audit committee evaluates medical care through a study or audit of medical records to learn, for example, the accuracy of preoperative diagnosis as judged by postoperative diagnosis, x-ray and pathological findings, or to judge the thoroughness of physical examination from the procedures used.

A hospital may have two types of members—a courtesy staff made up of private practitioners who are permitted to use the hospital's facilities to care for their patients, and the attending or active staff which is concerned with maintaining standards and with internal staff government. In addition to their private patients the attending staff cares for patients who do not have physicians of their own. In teaching hospitals the attending staff is made up of university professors. The teaching hospital and other large institutions have a resident staff composed of resident physicians who are eligible for licensure, assistant residents, and interns. Internships and residencies are part of the medical education program.

RELATIONSHIPS AMONG THE HOSPITAL ADMINISTRATOR, THE DIRECTOR OF THE NURSING DEPARTMENT, AND THE MEDICAL STAFF[13]

To the hospital administrator, the board of directors delegates responsibility for carrying out its policies and for upholding standards in the care of patients. The administrator, in turn, delegates responsibility for nursing care to the director of the department of nursing whom he has employed and who is directly responsible to him. On the other hand, the medical staff, as we have seen, selects and evaluates its own members and is

[12] *Ibid.*, p. 154.
[13] Malcolm T. MacEachern, *Hospital Organization and Management,* Chicago, Physicians Record Company, 1957, pp. 96-103.

responsible directly to the board of directors, not to the hospital administrator, for the quality of medical care. The administrator, nevertheless, as the appointed executive of the hospital, must see that the policies of the board are followed and that physicians do not violate staff rules and regulations.[14] One important staff rule pertains to standing medical orders. These orders are formulated in a conference between the medical staff or its representatives and the hospital administrator.[15] Although the latter is expected to see that these orders are carried out, he is in no position to do so directly. He therefore holds the director of nursing service, his representative in the line organization, responsible for seeing that doctors comply with regulations. The implementation, however, is usually the responsibility of the head nurse and it frequently places her in an ambivalent position. For instance, a common standing order in most hospitals is that medical orders shall be written, and given orally only in an emergency. Upon the head nurse falls the onerous duty of enforcing this directive. But she also has another responsibility—that of carrying out certain aspects of medical care which the doctor delegates. For this, she is professionally responsible to the physician. It is not uncommon that hospital policy which the head nurse is expected to enforce conflicts with an order or directive for patient care given by the doctor. This and other problems resulting from the differences in relationship of the two major health professions to hospital administration will be discussed further in Chapter 5.

A word needs to be said here concerning the employed medical staff which heads such departments as x-ray and physical therapy. For proper functioning of these departments the physicians in charge are responsible to the hospital administrator in the same way the head of the nursing department is responsible to him for providing safe, effective nursing care. The doctors in such positions, however, are responsible to the medical staff for sound professional practice. The residency staff also has a dual responsibility—to the hospital administrator who employs them and to their medical chief.

SUMMARY

Care of the sick and injured, promotion of health, education of health personnel, and research are the functions assumed by hospitals. The amount of emphasis on the last three varies according to the type of institution.

[14] Recent legislation (Medicare Act) requires that each hospital have a utilization committee to determine that beds are being utilized for the proper patients at any given time. The administrator must implement committee decisions.
[15] *Model Medical Staff By-Laws, Rules and Regulations,* Chicago, Joint Commission on Accreditation of Hospitals, revised 1957, p. 13.

Hospitals are classified in two ways, by type of care given and according to control. The general voluntary hospital is by far the most common in the United States. A hospital which is used for education of medical students, interns, and residents is often called a teaching hospital.

In many ways a hospital is organized like a business. A governing board representing the owners is legally and financially responsible for the institution. The board appoints an administrator to operate the hospital, holding him responsible for its services and for the care given patients. Size of hospital, in part, determines the number of assistants the administrator needs. Experts are placed in charge of departments, and they in turn employ their own personnel. Most hospitals function under line and staff organization, which can operate autocratically or democratically. In the former, authority is centralized; policies are made by a few at the top, with those in the lower echelons expected to comply. Supervision is close, opportunity for initiative and creativity limited. In a democratically operated institution, authority is usually decentralized; individuals help make the policies under which they work; they have greater independence and usually gain greater job satisfaction. In line organization, persons in charge at each administrative level may operate in a democratic manner in the areas where they are not bound by autocratic policy. Likewise, in line organization each administrator has responsibility for the development of the staff under his immediate supervision. The head nurse is an administrator even though she is near the bottom of the hierarchical ladder.

The head nurse is responsible for nursing care, for certain prescribed medical functions, for coordination of activities on the division, and usually for unit management. The division staff takes orders from and is directly responsible to the head nurse while she in turn is responsible to the department administrator and through her to the director of nursing. The latter, head of a hospital department, functions immediately under the hospital administrator or one of his assistants. The head nurse is thus one of the administrative arms of the hospital.

The relationship of the head nurse to the hospital organization is entirely different from that of the doctor. Except for the resident staff and a few physicians employed by the hospital as department heads, doctors are independent practitioners who use hospital facilities but are not a part of the institution. Nevertheless, they exert enormous influence. Appointed by the governing board of the hospital and responsible to it for meeting standards established by the medical staff, the doctor is not under the jurisdiction of the hospital administrator. Nonetheless the board expects the administrator to see that physicians adhere to its policies regarding medical practice. Since the head nurse is the extension of hospital administration and is on the scene where the doctor practises medicine, it is often she who is expected to keep him from breaking the rules. The difficulty in her doing so is compounded by the fact that the head nurse is responsible to the physician for performance of medical procedures which he delegates to her.

In addition to the formal line or line and staff organization, every institution has an informal organization through which much of the work is accomplished. Individuals of all levels working with one another across lines, i.e. horizontally, solve problems and get matters cared for that would require much more time if they had to go through channels up one line—say, to the director of nursing—across to another department head and down his line to an individual low in the hierarchy.

The informal organization works also through small unorganized groups of persons who have common interests. Membership in a group can help the individual gain satisfaction in his work and give him status. Small groups by supporting their members are powerful forces for good or ill, and the wise administrator promotes and takes them into account.

QUESTIONS FOR DISCUSSION

1. What individuals or groups in your hospital wield considerable influence? How does this informal organization function?
2. Is a head nurse ever justified in breaking a rule or failing to obey a hospital policy? If your answer is affirmative, describe such a situation and tell how the head nurse should handle it.
3. Describe the behavior of the most democratic head nurse you have known; the most autocratic. Was each aware of her behavior? What was the effect on the staff working in each situation?
4. Is it possible for a head nurse to be too democratic? Explain.
5. In line organization to whom is the division night nurse responsible—the head nurse or the associate nurse administrator for nights? What is the rationale for this relationship?
6. Is your hospital more centralized or decentralized? Would changes in organization be helpful to the head nurse? If so, explain.

EXERCISES

1. Diagram the formal organization of your hospital.
2. Using the same diagram show how the organization really functions.

3. During a week's time observe yourself, if you are a head nurse, or, if not, the head nurse of your division, for conflicts between loyalty to the doctor and to the department administrator or nursing service. For each situation consider the cause of the conflict, the way it was handled, the results. How could such conflicts in loyalty be prevented?

REFERENCES

Argyris, Chris. Interpersonal Competence and Organizational Effectiveness, Homewood, Illinois, The Dorsey Press Inc., Richard D. Irwin Inc., 1962, pp. 1-37.
The effects of an organization on human behavior and the social responsibility of institutions are presented. Assumptions underlying presently accepted principles of organization are considered questionable.

——— Personality and Organization, New York, Harper and Brothers, 1957, pp. 53, 61-63, 177-224.
The author's description of the effects of total organization of an institution on the individuals in it and the behavior of those persons under different types of organizational structure will help the head nurse to understand the behavior of her staff member.

——— Diagnosing Human Relations in Organizations, New Haven, Yale Labor and Management Center, 1956.
Human personality, or the individuals which make up an institution, is not separate from the "organization," ie, the institution, and they cannot be considered apart from one another in analyzing the problems of management.
This is the report of a study of the management of a world-famous hospital in relation to its nursing department. All hospital nurses as well as hospital administrators should find it very revealing particularly in its discussion of the reasons for existing attitudes and behaviors on the part of nurses. Supervisors, head nurses, and staff nurses are compared.

Bloom, Samuel W. The Doctor and His Patient, New York, Russell Sage Foundation 1963.
This volume has many values for nurses not the least of which is a better understanding of the attitudes and behaviors of doctors and of patients. The "sick role," its obligations and privileges, circumstances which affect one's playing the "sick role," the doctor's privileged role in the hospital, and the reasons for it —all have implications for nursing.

Brown, Esther Lucile. Nursing and patient care. In The Nursing Profession: five sociological essays, Davis, F., ed. New York, John Wiley and Sons, Inc. 1966, pp. 176-203.
Dr. Brown shows deep insight into the problems of nursing. Patients' needs and expectations are portrayed. Responsibility for failure to meet them is laid at the doors of both nursing education and nursing service.

——— The social sciences and improvement of patient care, Amer. J. Nurs., Vol. 56 (September 1956), pp. 1148-1150.
"The inflexibility of the hospital's formal social structure has frequently been

the cause of its failure to improve the morale of hospital personnel and the quality of the care which they give to their patients." Contains much that is of immediate concern to the head nurse.

Clingman, Arthurline, and Kriegel, Julia. A nursing service without a director, Nurs. Outlook, Vol. 14 (November 1966), pp. 34-35.
A very interesting account of the way in which a hospital which tripled in size has maintained the character and advantages of the small hospital. Five directors of nursing have autonomy in a section of the hospital. An administrator serves as coordinator.

Corona, Dorothy F. Sedatives and stimulants to creativity, Nurs. Outlook, Vol. 12 (July 1964), pp. 24-26.
"Nursing service organizations should not only *permit* creativity, but should exercise every effort to *encourage* it." This article expresses a philosophy of organization and is filled with positive ideas of value to the head nurse as well as to nursing service administrators.

Covington, Robert N. Moral and legal responsibilities of surgical nurses, Nurs. Forum, Vol. 4 (No. 3, 1965), pp. 19-26.
To whom is the nurse legally responsible? A lawyer answers this question and illustrates some of the nurses' legal responsibilities. Of special interest to head nurses will be the matter of the permit to operate.

Guide Issue, Hospitals, August 1, 1966.
Gives statistical data on all types of hospitals.

Hill, S. G. Rules that bend aren't often broken, Mod. Hosp., Vol. 92 (June 1959), pp. 69-71, 168-169.
Although rules are probably more essential in a hospital than in other types of organization where life is not at stake, it is preferable to permit some initiative and flexibility in order to achieve good relationships. To some degree, efficiency is less important than contentment, and efficiency does not always result in effectiveness.

——— The Salmon report: a group secretary's views, Nurs. Times, Vol. 62 (July 15, 1966), pp. 931-932.
An interestingly written account of the report of a several-year study of nursing in England. Recommended are sweeping changes in nursing administration and a plea that nurse administrators not get too far removed from nursing.

Howland, Daniel. Approach to nurse-monitor research, Amer. J. Nurs., Vol. 66 (March 1966), pp. 556-558.
Research being conducted at Ohio State University aims "to provide hospital system designers and managers with information on the probable consequences of their resource allocation decisions, that is, their decisions on types and distribution of machines and manpower." It is expected that "the functions of nurse, physician, and patient will be made explicit in a patient care model which describes their interaction."

MacEachern, Malcolm T. Hospital Organization and Management, Chicago, Physicians' Record Company, 1957.
Although outdated in some respects, the third edition of this voluminous text contains much information useful to the head nurse in understanding the administrative organization of the hospital and the organization and functioning of the medical staff.

Masur, Jack. Goals for American hospitals, Hospitals, Vol. 35 (November 16, 1961), pp. 56-58.
Dr. Masur states 14 objectives or goals toward which hospitals should be working.

Mauksch, Hans O. It defies all logic—but a hospital does function. Reprinted from Mod. Hosp., October 1960. In Skipper, James K. Jr. and Leonard, Robert C. Social Interaction and Patient Care, Philadelphia, J. B. Lippincott Company, 1965, pp. 245-251.
A sociologist compares the organization of a garage with that of a hospital making the point that the increasing complexity of the hospital demands that the hospital administrator "must emerge as the mainspring of coordination and the center of responsibility. . . ."

McGibony, John R. Principles of Hospital Administration, New York, G. P. Putnam's Sons, 1952.
An easily read description of hospital administration and organization.

Miller, Doris I. Administration for the patient, Amer. J. Nurs., Vol. 65 (July 1965), pp. 114-116.
A nurse administrator suggests three steps "crucial in administering a nursing service based on a decision-making theory of administration."

Model Medical Staff By-Laws, Rules, and Regulations, Chicago, Joint Commission on Accreditation of Hospitals, revised 1957. (Pamphlet.)
Guidelines to be adapted to the individual hospital are described.

Roethlisberger, F. J., and Dickson, William J. Management and the Worker, Cambridge, Mass., Harvard University Press, 1939.
Described are the so-called Hawthorne studies which were concerned with the relation between conditions of work, fatigue, and monotony. The last chapter deals with the formal versus informal organization and its effect on work output.

Rorer, John A. Principles of Democratic Supervision, New York, Bureau of Publications, Teachers College, Columbia University, 1942.
Principles in this book are clearly and succinctly expressed.

Rourke, Anthony J. J. Joint conference committee should be vital, not perfunctory, exercise. Mod. Hosp., Vol. 107 (July 1966), p. 119.
The head nurse should gain a better understanding of the functions of the medical staff by reading this article.

Standards for Organized Nursing Services, Amer. J. Nurs., Vol. 65 (March 1965), pp. 76-79.
Although they are primarily the concern of nursing service administrators, the 16 standards which have been established should be of interest to head nurses.

Strauss, George, and Sayles, Leonard R. The Human Problems of Management, Englewood Cliffs, New Jersey, Prentice Hall, 1960.
Chapter 15, "The supervisor: man in the middle," pp. 338-352.
The supervisor has loyalties to top management and to his staff. His own supervision by management should be general in nature, he should have freedom to act, and should work for the good of his men.
Chapter 17, "Minimizing the human problems of large organizations," pp. 376-394.
Productivity depends on organizational structure as well as on patterns of supervision and the qualifications of personnel. Line and staff organization is discussed as is decentralization of authority. Although this chapter is especially valuable for nursing service administrators, the head nurse also will find it interesting.

The professional care and treatment of nurses, Nurs. Forum, Vol. 1 (Summer 1962), pp. 77-86.
In spite of new demands on nurses the doctors' attitudes toward them have changed little. The nurse—the head nurse, especially—is caught at the crossroads of medical expectations and administrative policy.

Uris, Auren. The three basic methods of leadership, In Readings in Management, Koontz, H., and O'Donnell, C., eds. New York, McGraw Hill Book Company, Inc., 1959, pp. 223-227.
An interesting description of democratic, autocratic, and free-reign leadership. The author suggests that a leader uses all three types and that leadership skill lies in knowing when to use which method.

Urwick, Lyndall F. The nature of line and staff. In Readings in Management, Koontz, H., and O'Donnell, C., eds. New York, McGraw Hill Book Company, Inc., 1959, pp. 114-118.
The number of formal organization relationships are three rather than the two usually considered. These are 1) line relationships, 2) specialist relationships, and 3) general staff relationships. Each is explained

——— The manager's span of control. In Readings in Management, Koontz, H., and O'Donnell, C., eds. New York, McGraw Hill Book Company, 1959, pp. 40-53.
The writer is responding to criticism of the theory of "span of control" (ie, the number of persons directly responsible to an executive) on the basis that the plan is undemocratic.

Venger, Mary Jane, and Yourman, Julius. Modern management theory applied to nursing service, Nurs. Outlook, Vol. 14 (November 1966), pp. 30-33.
A description of the way in which one nursing service has reorganized its manner of functioning to comply with modern management principles wherein administration is concerned about workers' motivations, satisfactions, and morale as they affect production.

Wilson, Robert N. The social structure of a general hospital. In Social Interaction and Patient Care, Skipper, J. K. Jr., and Leonard, R. C., eds. Philadelphia, J. B. Lippincott Company, 1965, pp. 233-234.
The doctor and the patient, the "two chief figures are in the (hospital) organization but not of it." The doctor's role in the hospital, its formal and informal structure, and the nurse's role are presented in an interesting way.

chapter 3

ORGANIZATION OF THE HOSPITAL
FOR PATIENT SERVICES

The preamble to the Constitution of the World Health Organization states that health is the right of every human being. Providing health involves many things, including sanitation, nutrition, inoculation, physical examination, medical and nursing care, health supervision and education, and institutional care. Some countries through insurance or taxes provide medical and hospital care for all their citizens regardless of economic status. In the United States the year 1966 saw the institution of medicare with its provision, under the Social Security system, of partial hospital and medical care for persons aged sixty-five and over. Long before medicare, however, city, county, and state institutions had provided outpatient and inpatient services for those unable to pay for any, or only a small part of their care. Notwithstanding this, many recipients of free service are ashamed to accept such help which they consider "charity." One great advantage of medicare is that it has removed any feeling of stigma for those in the upper age bracket who receive financial help. Welfare provisions of the Medicare Act, Title 19, vary from state to state for persons under sixty-five who are unable to pay. Some states are beginning to provide financial assistance for families of moderate means. This is fortunate since a serious illness usually depletes family savings and often puts its members deeply in debt. Not infrequently in this situation a family is eventually forced to accept help from a community social welfare agency.

Regardless of an individual's ability to pay, however, not all hospitals are equable in the services they offer. Nor is it necessary that highly technical services be provided in all institutions as long as a hospital with these facilities is located within a reasonable distance. Such a hospital, perhaps part of a medical center, may be a base to which other hospitals in the area send their patients who require complicated diagnosis or therapy. The outlying hospitals concentrate on giving the more usual, less involved medical and nursing care.

This chapter will consider patient services, most of which are available today in larger institutions although many are also found in smaller community hospitals as well. The head nurse regardless of the institution in which she is employed will want to be informed about different ways in which hospitals may be organized to care for their patients, the philosophy behind the different systems, the demands they place on nursing service.

EMERGENCY SERVICE

The service which is common to all hospitals is the care of the sick and injured. Some institutions have a very active emergency service where persons who have been injured or taken suddenly ill may be brought for diagnosis or care. An emergency room is prepared at all times for immediate action. Emergency equipment in working order is ready for instant use. Competent nurses and doctors staff the emergency room around the clock. It is imperative that the emergency room nurse be able to remain composed, to set intelligent priorities, and to delegate responsibility clearly. She must be highly skilled in every emergency procedure which the law and the hospital's policy permit nurses to perform. In endeavoring to meet the needs of the patient and of the doctor who may be under severe stress, the nurse should under no circumsances forget members of the family or friends who have accompanied the patient. They desperately need information and frequent confirmation that everything possible is being done. If at all possible, a relative should not be left alone when the patient's condition is serious. It might be suggested that he call another member of the family, a friend, or his clergyman to be with him. It is especially important that he be seen frequently and kept informed of the situation.

The emergency room makes heavy emotional demands upon both doctor and nurse. Ability to cope with these demands and be concerned with the needs of both patient and family is an important criterion in the selection of an emergency room nurse. In addition, it needs to be remembered by administrators that nurses in anxiety-producing situations themselves need understanding and psychological support.

Not all persons who come to a hospital emergency room are seriously ill or hurt. An individual may be given care and discharged. He may be referred to a private physician or asked to return to the hospital outpatient department for a follow-up visit. Many patients cared for in the emergency room are admitted to the hospital as inpatients.

OUTPATIENT SERVICES

Clinics

Many hospitals offer outpatient as well as inpatient services. Persons who cannot afford a private doctor may be followed by a hospital clinic which is staffed with doctors and nurses who specialize in a given service—ophthalmology, gynecology, urology, medicine, metabolism, surgery, dermatology, obstetrics, and other specialties. Clinic patients admitted to the hospital return to the clinic for after care. Complete histories and records provide continuity in medical care between clinic and hospital or clinic and clinic. Fees for clinic visits are charged according to a sliding scale. Medications prescribed are sold at reduced rates or are given free if the patient is unable to pay. Many clinic patients who were formerly medically indigent now have medical coverage through medicare and various types of insurance.

Usual services rendered by outpatient clinics are concerned with diagnosis, prescription of therapy, dispensation of drugs and appliances, and with administration of therapy which can be handled on an outpatient basis. Services such as these, many of which require regular clinic visits and self care at home, make it imperative that the patient understand the purposes of tests and treatments, their importance to his health and well-being, and the procedure to be used. Likewise, the patient needs help in learning the causes of ill health, its prevention, and ways to keep himself and his family in optimum health. Teaching, then, is one of the most important functions of both doctors and nurses in the clinics. Many communities have a public health nursing department or a visiting nurse service which will help the patient to carry out instructions at home. In some places, the public health nurse is based in the hospital where she is in touch with clinic patients and clinic nurses. In other instances, the clinic nurses go into the home to follow the patients who need their assistance.

Because home conditions, family relationships, and economic problems may prevent a patient from carrying out the instruction he has received, a medical social worker is available in the clinic to investigate, advise, and assist the family with the solution of social problems. Social workers, doctors, and nurses form a close working team. In many instances, there is no clear cut line where the function of one ends and that of another begins. This is especially true in dealing with psychosocial problems and in teaching.

Many special types of service are offered to patients and families on an outpatient basis. A few will be described.

Consultation Services

Medical centers and teaching hospitals usually provide diagnostic and consultant service for a broad geographic area—a whole state, a section of the country, or even the entire country. In this way excellent medical counsel for obscure clinical conditions can be provided by a specialist in the field or by a team of experts. For example, patients travel far to obtain diagnosis and consultation for cancer, neurological disorders, cardiac and kidney disease. Individuals are usually referred by a private physician. The patient may return home for therapy, or if special skills are needed, he is treated at the medical center.

Family Health Care Clinic

One of the newer services provided by at least one hospital in the United States is the family health care clinic. Established in a medical center[1, 2] primarily to help the junior or senior medical student gain a concept of family health and the social, economic, and interpersonal forces which impinge upon it, this clinic was also designed to meet a community need. Its purpose is to provide health maintenance and family-centered care through a team of health workers.

The family health care clinic provides for the total health needs of a limited number of selected families who have expressed a desire to participate in the program. When a family has been selected for the service, a study is made of the environmental and social factors affecting its health and welfare. Each member undergoes a complete medical evaluation and, if necessary, a social work evaluation is made. A detailed family health plan is then developed. Through complete records and frequent meetings, members of the health team are kept informed. The clinic is a general one with a medical student "family physician," supported by an internist and a pediatrician who serve as preceptors, composing the medical staff for a group of families. Consultative service by other specialists or a medical social worker is used when necessary. A neighborhood health aide, who

[1] Jerome S. Beloff and E. Richard Weinerman, Yale Studies in Family Health Care, I. Planning and Pilot Test of a New Program, *J.A.M.A.* Vol. 199 (February 6, 1967) pp. 383-389.
[2] Yale-New Haven Medical Center. For a discussion of forerunners of this service in other institutions See: Parnie S. Snoke and E. Richard Weinerman. Comprehensive Care Programs in University Medical Centers, *J. M. Educ.,* Vol. 40 (July 1965), pp. 625-657.

introduces the program concept to the family, and a public health nurse complete the team. Thus every family has its own doctor, its own nurse, and a member of its own community, each of whom knows each family member personally. A member of the medical staff, student-physician or preceptor, is always available for emergency calls.

The clinic nurse (a public health nurse) is a participant in the over-all planning, management, and evaluation of the project. Initial discussion of the service with a family, arranging for health evaluations, surveying the home with the student-physician, clearing calls from family members, and contacting the physician when necessary are the clinic nurse's specific administrative responsibilities. In addition, she is a team member together with the student-physician and neighborhood health aide for a group of families. Visits are made to the home on occasion, and family members who are admitted to the hospital are visited by members of the team who do not, however, give care in the hospital. The intimate knowledge of the patient held by the clinic nurse is of inestimable value in providing individualized care when this information is conveyed to the hospital head nurse.

Parents' Classes

A fairly common service of hospitals to the community are mothers' classes and parents' classes which may be part of a preparation for parenthood program. Prospective mothers and fathers learn from obstetricians about the development of the fetus, the importance of antepartal care, and the birth process. Mothers' classes are taught by a nurse and include personal hygiene, antepartal breast care, relaxation and exercise, expectations during labor and the puerperium, a tour of the labor and delivery area of the hospital, and care of the baby. Mothers also learn about follow-up care for themselves so they will remain in good health and rear a healthy baby. A well-versed and dedicated maternity nurse, with ability to teach and to relate to people, is essential if classes with mothers are to be successful.

Counselling for Parents of Children for Whom Open Heart Surgery Is Recommended

A service provided by some hospitals, usually through a special clinic, is destined to increase as it becomes more widely recognized that parents can help or hinder the recovery of a child who is to have open heart or other major corrective surgery. The child is usually followed in the cardiac clinic over a period of time before the surgeon concludes that surgery is the best course to follow. The very difficult decision—to have surgery or not to have it—must be made by the parents. If the clinic nurse who knows the family visits in the home, giving the mother and the father an opportunity to express their doubts and fears and to have their questions answered, she can often, if skilled in interpersonal relationships, help them become clear on the best course to follow. If the parents can resolve their own anxieties, they will be better able to support the child through hospitalization.[3] In supporting a child, no nurse is equal to the mother who has gained control of her own emotions.

INPATIENT SERVICES

The usual practice in hospitals has been to assign the patient to a patient care division in accord with the field of medical specialization in which his physician is practicing—obstetrics, pediatrics, medicine, surgery, or psychiatry. In large hospitals each of these services may be subdivided; for example, the neurosurgical patients will be on one surgical floor, eye patients on another. In small hospitals and those in which many of the medical staff are general practitioners, the obstetric service may be the only one segregated. With patients assigned to beds according to medical services a doctor's patients are consolidated in a relatively small area of the hospital. In recent years another way of assigning patients has been promoted; it is called "progressive patient care."

Progressive Patient Care

Since about 1958 some hospitals have felt they could make better use of facilities and personnel by organizing services around nursing and medical needs of patients instead of segregating patients according to medical specialties.

The type of care and equipment required by a critically ill person differs

[3] Roberta Fitzgerald. *The Role of the Public Health Nurse in Helping Parents of Children Having Open Heart Surgery.* (Master's Report) New Haven, Conn., Yale University School of Nursing, 1966.

from that needed by an ambulatory patient capable of self care or from that of the chronically ill individual who may need rehabilitation or custodial care. Lifesaving measures vary less with the disease than with the patient's physical condition.

In this type of organization, as the patient's needs change, he is transferred to another unit which has the personnel and facilities necessary to care for him in the best possible way. Progressive patient care, as this method of serving patients is termed, has five elements, although to date only a few institutions have more than one or two. Hospitals have named these elements or stages of progress according to their concepts of the services needed by their clientele. The five elements are 1) self care, ambulatory, minimal care, or special service, 2) intensive, maximum, or special care, 3) intermediate care, 4) long-term care or rehabilitation, 5) home care or extension service. All, with the probable exception of obstetric patients, can be cared for during at least part of their hospital stay in progressive patient care units in which there is no segregation by diagnosis or service. The child, during a period of critical illness, may be better cared for in an intensive care unit, but for the remainder of his hospital stay he will be sent to the pediatric division. Those who strongly support the progressive patient care philosophy believe that lives are saved, patients are happier, and nurses better satisfied under this system of organization. A great deal has been written on the subject. A brief overview will be given here.

Self care unit. A large proportion of people who are admitted to the self care unit are in the hospital for diagnosis. They may be undergoing a series of tests and, for one reason or another, it is preferable that they be hospitalized rather than be at home during this period.

Another group found in the self care unit is made up of patients who come from other parts of the hospital when they are almost, but not quite, ready to go home. The patient may have recovered from a myocardial infarction and his doctor thinks he will adjust better to home life if he has a few days of supervised activity in the self care unit. Here the atmosphere more nearly resembles that with which he will have to cope when he goes home. The patient with diabetes or a colostomy who needs a bit more concentrated instruction may also find several days in this unit a good transition between hospital and home. Here he can become adjusted to selecting his own food, wearing street clothes, and taking full care of himself in a restricted atmosphere.

Patients in the self care unit usually go to the hospital cafeteria where a dietitian helps them as necessary with food selection. Sometimes they are served in a dining room on the unit. If the patient is to have tests, the nurse explains the procedure and the preparation that is necessary. Usually he is also given an attractive booklet explaining the test in simple terms (Fig. 4). When it is time for his test or treatment he walks to the department unaccompanied, except perhaps by another patient.

Your doctor has requested an examination of the stomach. This is an examination, by use of X-ray, of the esophagus, stomach, and part of the small bowel.

The following preparation is necessary to insure a satisfactory examination:

1. You are not to have anything to eat or drink after 10:00 P.M. the evening before, nor the day of the examination until the X-ray is completed.

2. Refrain from smoking in the morning until after the X-ray is completed.

3. You will be required to wear a hospital gown and will be taken to X-ray as soon as that department notifies us.

4. In X-ray you will be given a flavored barium mixture to drink. The doctor will then examine you under a fluoroscope in a darkened room.

5. Following this, several X-ray films will be taken. The length of time for this examination varies.

6. A technician will be there at all times to help you.

7. You will be returned to your room after the X-ray examination is completed. Please leave the card given to you in the X-ray department with the secretary at the station desk. The nurse will notify you when it is permissible for you to eat or drink.

We thank you for your cooperation in this examination.

Form 300K 6-61

Fig. 4. Informtaion for patient who is to have stomach x-ray. Folds in half to make booklet and has an attractive cover. Different colored leaflets with information for all types of tests are available. (Courtesy the Charles T. Miller Hospital.)

Rooms in the self care division are like those in a hotel or motel with low daybeds, lounging chairs, private showers, and toilets. Maids instead of aides care for the rooms. Some hospitals provide accommodations for the patient and his family to be together during the few days the patient needs to be hospitalized. This is especially helpful when the hospital is part of a medical center which services a wide geographic area.

A sitting room where patients can gather to socialize, watch television, or play cards is essential. A hospital library serves this division as well as others. A snack room for patients, with an electric plate and a refrigerator stocked with milk, fruit juice, and soft drinks, helps give the unit a homelike atmosphere.

Although a large number of nurses may not be needed for the self care unit, those assigned should have special skill in teaching and in detecting real concern underneath a gay, carefree front. Probably most patients admitted for diagnosis have some deep underlying fear concerning the findings which tests will reveal. The nurse needs skill in purposeful listening and in creating an atmosphere in which the patient feels free to express his concerns. She needs to recognize the importance of making and taking time to converse with each patient alone. He may have misconceptions which can be cleared up by the nurse. Just the opportunity to talk may release tension. A gifted nurse or perhaps two or three is therefore necessary to staff the self care unit during the day and evening hours. Very often a practical nurse can meet any needs the patient may have at night.

Intensive care unit. A great variation exists among hospitals in the degree of illness of patients assigned to the intensive care unit. Some accept only the critically ill such as the patient with acute coronary thrombosis, a severely bleeding peptic ulcer, or meningitis, neurosurgery, cardiac surgery or pulmonary surgery. Other hospitals, which have few patients in such acute condition, admit to the intensive care unit less ill persons who require considerable care for a few days, such as those who have had cholecystectomies or gastrectomies. Men, women, and children, too sick to notice or care, are placed in the same room.

The purpose of the intensive care unit is life saving. Patients are sent here only if it is anticipated that concentrated medical and nursing care will restore them to health. All kinds of emergency equipment are close at hand. Each patient's unit has piped-in oxygen, wall suction, and a sphygmomanometer. Monitoring equipment for continuous recording of heart beat, blood pressure, pulse, and respiration is available. A defibrillating machine, emergency drug cart, and positive pressure machine are near at hand. The bed is equipped with side rails, irrigating poles, and gatches. Folding wall shelves provide places for treatment trays and are out of the way when not in use. No call signal is necessary for the patient as a rule, but one is available in every unit for the nurse should she need assistance in a hurry. Sufficient skillful help is available day and night (sometimes averaging 12 hours per patient in 24 hours) to make close observations, give the necessary care, and keep the patient comfortable. Especially competent practical nurses are sometimes used to assist with bathing, turning, and feeding patients in this unit.

The patient is under constant observation of professional nurses highly skilled in detecting change in condition, making quick, sound decisions; nurses who do not become overly depressed by being continuously surrounded by very ill people. The nurses' station is central and from it, ideally, all patients can be seen and heard. Patients find comfort and security in having a nurse in view at all times. At least one hospital [4] has made this

[4] Manchester Memorial, Manchester, Conn. See: Report on progressive care—it works, *Mod. Hosp.,* Vol. 90 (May 1958), pp. 73-79.

possible by placing a stool at a high chart desk in sight of four patients in each of two rooms. Another hospital [5] has built a circular unit with the nurses' station in the center and the patients' rooms on the periphery. All rooms in this unit are single with double doors made of glass. Other valuable features of this architectural arrangement are described in the literature.

The families of critically ill patients need a comfortable place adjacent to the unit where they can rest day or night. In some hospitals members of the immediate family are permitted to go to the bedside once an hour for a few minutes, but they may look at him through the window or door as often as they wish. Recognizing the intensity of the care and observation the patient is receiving usually gives the family such confidence that they may not feel the need to visit even this frequently. Families of patients in the intensive care unit need every consideration that can be shown them. Often a wife or father or son or sister may not leave the hospital for a week or more when a loved one lies near death. If the hospital has not made regular provision of couches or lounging chairs with pillows and blankets for persons unable or unwilling to leave the hospital at night, nurses on the division must assume responsibility for making them comfortable in the visitors' room. The head nurse should make sure this same room is not used during the night hours by medical and nursing personnel for smoking, drinking coffee, and socializing. The staff needs a place for a comfortable break but can they not use the office or the kitchen in preference to depriving fatigued, worried families of much needed rest? Older hospitals which have converted space for intensive care units are not always able to provide for both families and staff to the degree they would desire. A considerate staff will recognize this and sacrifice a degree of their own comfort for that of anxious families.

The intensive care unit has been the most commonly adopted of the five elements of progressive patient care. So important has this unit become that some hospitals which have not accepted the philosophy of progressive patient care are organizing intensive care units in conjunction with the different services—one for intensive cardiac care connected with medical divisions; one for surgical patients, and one or more in the pediatric department. (See Services for Children, p. 50.)

Intermediate care unit. The intermediate care units are more like the hospital divisions as generally known except that the acutely ill, the individuals able to care for themselves, and those who require long-term care are not present. This greater homogeneity makes possible more con-

[5] Methodist Hospital, Rochester, Minn. See: Madelyne Sturdavant. Intensive nursing service in circular and rectangular units compared, *Hospitals,* Vol. 34 (July 16, 1960), pp. 46-48, 71-78.

sistent care. Many patients are admitted to and discharged from this division although some may come from the self care or intensive care units. Likewise some are transferred out. Individuals in the intermediate care units may be quite ill for a time; most are ambulatory for short periods and are beginning to participate in their own care.

Professional nurses, practical nurses, and aides staff these divisions preferably working in nursing teams in order to utilize to the full the capabilities of each person. With fewer fluctuations in patient requirements than exist under the typical pattern of organization, the nursing load is more predictable and staffing therefore more regular. A problem, however, in attracting staff for this type of unit is apparent. Nurses miss the drama of acute illness and the challenge of "major, major surgery." Too frequently they are ill-prepared to identify and deal with the psychosocial, rehabilitative, and teaching needs of patients. The head nurse on the intermediate care unit, therefore, faces a real challenge in keeping her staff stimulated to develop their ability in these truly professional aspects of nursing.

Long-term care unit. The long-term care unit is designed to serve two groups—those who can be rehabilitated for return to a productive life, or at least to partial self-sufficiency, and those who are terminally ill. Individuals who have had cerebral vascular accidents, fractures, poliomyelitis, or other crippling diseases spend many weeks on this division in intensive rehabilitative procedures. The terminally ill include aged persons who are physically worn out and need a great deal of loving care, as well as the individual in the last stages of carcinoma or other chronic illness.

Assigned to the long-term care unit are nurses and aides who are challenged even when progress is slow, and those who enjoy making patients physically comfortable, giving "tender, loving care," and bringing a little cheer and comfort to persons who are tired and discouraged and have little for which to live.

Home care. The least developed stage of progressive patient care is home care. Its purpose is to extend medical and nursing services to the home, making it possible, in some instances, to reduce the length of hospital stay. The patient becomes a candidate for this service when the physician believes he can receive adequate medical and nursing service at home. While the patient is still in the hospital, he and his family are helped to think through the adjustments which will have to be made in the home preparatory to the patient's return. These sometimes entail a visit by a hospital-employed home care nurse. She discusses with the patient's nurse his needs for instruction and may at times assist with the teaching that is required. She makes contacts with the state or local vocational rehabilitation service and with insurance companies concerning provision of supplies when such services are needed.

In some communities a public health agency may give the nursing service after the patient has returned home, in which case a referral is made by the hospital home care nurse with the help of the patient's nurse. In other situations it may be preferable to have the home care nursing service handled entirely by the outside agency working in close cooperation with the hospital. In this plan, instead of the hospital employing a home care nurse, a public health nurse from the local agency visits the patient prior to discharge and makes suggestions for his instruction. In each case nursing service is coordinated with medical and allied home care services. The patient is saved considerable expense when he can be cared for in his home. He is usually happier there, and through this type of service, hospital beds are freed for other patients.

The home care nurse should have had experience in public health nursing. She needs to have initiative in seeking out patients who would benefit from home care, enthusiasm for the service, and the ability to work cooperatively with many different groups.

Questions Raised Relative to Progressive Patient Care

Head nurses may well ask:
1. How do patients feel about transferring from one division to another, perhaps two or three times? Are they troubled about leaving the staff and surroundings with which they have become familiar?
2. How can continuity of care be maintained when patients are transferred?
3. How do nurses feel when they are unable to see the patient through the various stages of illness?
4. How can the student be taught "total" nursing care when her experience with the patient is interrupted by his transfer?
5. Does not the extensive transfer of patients and their belongings make for confusion and a greatly increased work load?

Let us see how those who have worked within the system answer these questions.

1) *How do patients feel about transferring from one division to another? First,* nurses will wish to know whether patients and their families are

frightened when the doctor suggests transfer to the intensive care service. When it is explained that the care is of such quality that private duty nurses are neither needed nor permitted, people tend to be convinced that exacting care will be provided, that everything possible will be done to heal and comfort. It is important that patients are not sent to this unit to die, although it is inevitable that some acutely ill patients may die here despite the best medical and nursing care. If the unit has the reputation of saving lives the public will have faith in the care given there. Even when the occasional person must be sent back to intensive care after being moved out, he *knows* he is sicker and is confident in going back to the division where once more he will be restored and where he will have enough nursing care to keep him comfortable and secure.

Second, how do patients feel about being transferred out of the intensive care unit? It is the experience of some nurses that patients on leaving the intensive care area are encouraged in knowing they no longer need the close attention. They feel they have been "promoted." Families comment, "The doctor feels he is better. He is being moved out of intensive care." To which the quick response comes, "Good!" Spirits are lifted. Some of the weight of worry and concern is removed when this transfer occurs.

On the other hand, many patients react with fear to the prospect of moving—of leaving the nurses who literally saved their lives and with whom they closely identify. The importance of preparing patients in advance for the transfer and moving them in a nonemergency fashion cannot be overemphasized. They should feel they are being transferred because their condition is improved, not because the bed is needed for someone else. Transfer under the latter circumstance becomes "preferential treatment" and patients have been known to regress when the move has been made under these conditions. It is very important, too, that the patient have the difference in care and facilities thoroughly explained by the doctor as well as the nurse so that he will not be disturbed by the change. Many nurses are greatly concerned lest the patient suffer from lack of continuity in his care when he is moved from one unit to another.

Third, it has been observed that some patients who are transferred from the intermediate to the self care unit are at first uncertain whether or not they like the situation. It does not harmonize with their concept of a hospital. They have formed friendships with roommates whom they do not wish to leave, and sometimes they are lonely. Those consulted seemed to have no particular feeling about leaving the nursing staff—a possible reflection on the great amount of functionalism in nursing today. Any loneliness or unhappiness, however, is usually rather quickly dispelled as the newcomer socializes with other patients and finds he has many of the freedoms of home life. Nurses who are aware of the tendency for the transfer patient to feel lost and uncomfortable can help by taking time to talk with him, orient him to the facilities, and introduce him to other patients who have common interests. Preparation of the patient for the changes he will find and explanation of the advantages for him in the new unit are important to his adjustment.

2) *How can continuity of care be preserved when the patient is moved from one division to another?* Continuity of care may be defined as the smooth carry-over from hour to hour and day to day of a well-thought-out nursing care plan based on knowledge of the patient, understanding of his behavior and his needs, and a feeling of empathy toward him as a person. To provide continuity of care the same nurse needs to be in close contact with the patient long enough to know him. The knowledge she gains and the resulting plan for his care are transmitted in full to the persons who will be responsible for him in her absence. When the patient is to be transferred to the care of a nurse in another unit of the hospital or to one who will assist him at home, full communication is essential if the patient is to be understood, his needs well met, his care efficient. This transfer of information can be rather time consuming when patients are continuously moving from one unit to another in a program of progressive patient care. The values in this organization of services will be lessened, however, unless arrangements for communication between head nurses of the divisions are provided within the system.

A written nursing care plan describing the patient's behavior and the nurses' approach to him, the objectives for his care, the plan for meeting them, and the problems involved, as well as specific instructions for carrying out nursing measures, should be sent with the patient to the new division. In addition, the head nurse or the nurse who knows the patient best should accompany him, introduce him to the nurse in charge, go through the care plan and medical orders with her. In this way continuity of care is provided.

3) *How do nurses feel when they are unable to see the patient through the various stages of illness?* The advantages for the patient resulting from continuity are obvious but many satisfactions for the nurse also are inherent in providing, for patients, care which is coordinated and continuous. She comes to know her patients and to develop a real interest in them and their families. Unfortunately many nurses have never experienced giving this kind of care. Due to the functional method of assignment so frequently used, they have had no opportunity to give complete care to patients or to help plan it. Many, therefore, do not object to the lack of opportunity to see the patient through his illness. With the hope of eventually ending the system of the functional method of assignment and of helping nurses

appreciate the values in continuity of care, some schools of nursing are providing their students with experience in long association with individual patients.

4) *How can the student be taught "total" nursing care when her experience with the patient is interrupted by his transfer?* If hospitals organize their entire service on the progressive patient care basis, schools of nursing will find it necessary to change the method of providing clinical experience for students. To care for an individual patient through varying stages of his illness will necessitate the student travelling from unit to unit with her patients rather than being assigned to a specific floor or division for a block of time. The student might have a combination of experiences spending some time in the various units of progressive patient care in which she will have opportunity to transmit to others the nursing care plans which she has made. She will also learn by receiving care plans made by other nurses for other patients. During other parts of her program the student could follow the patient about the hospital giving the care herself. There will be many educational experiments in the next few years with which head nurses will be asked to assist and in which all will be greatly interested.

5) *How can the extensive transfer of patients and their belongings be accomplished without confusion and a greatly increased work load?* For many hospitals the problem of transferring the patient's clothing and other belongings when he is moved to another unit is already serious. Some have simplified the procedure considerably by asking the patient to sign a release from liability for the loss of any article kept in his possession. Although the hospital has a moral obligation to prevent loss or theft, this policy simplifies the procedure enormously because the clothes slip does not have to be checked and signed at every move. The patient coming in for surgery with the possibility of being transferred to the intensive care unit can be encouraged to leave or send home all but a minimum of personal effects until such time as he is ready to use them. The need to have some personal items should be recognized. Special bags or cases in which clothes can be stored and transported have been simply designed. Baskets to hang on the bed are useful for transferring toilet articles and other small items. The ideal solution is yet to be found for transporting personal possessions of patients who spend time in several different units during a single hospitalization. The time and effort involved in the transfer process is only one facet of the problem, however. Another is the double amount of linen which is used when the patient occupies a bed on two divisions in the same day. It is not possible to move the patient in his bed since a different type is used in almost every division. The many transfers resulting from progressive patient care greatly increase the amount of laundry to be handled in a day.

Life Saving Services

Lives are of course saved in all patient care divisions, but four services are geared especially to achieve this purpose. Of the four, the emergency room and the intensive care unit have already been considered. A third service of this nature is the postoperative recovery room which many general hospitals have established. Adjacent to the operating theater, the recovery room is usually open from 8 AM to about 4:30 PM. Recovery room nurses may be part of the operating room personnel or may be a separate staff. Surgical patients remain here under the supervision of the anesthetist until they have recovered from anesthesia and their vital signs have become stabilized. Judgment is of extreme importance in the recovery room just as it is in the other situations in which change in condition can be instantaneous, and prompt measures may save lives.

The fourth life saving service, the cardiac arrest team, is relatively new. Respiratory and cardiac arrest can often be dealt with effectively and a life saved if symptoms are recognized immediately and resuscitative measures started within two to three minutes. Nurses in intensive care units and other areas where arrests would be most likely to occur are taught mouth-to-mouth breathing and external cardiac massage. Drugs and equipment are ready and at hand for instant use. When a patient anywhere in the hospital has respiratory or cardiac arrest a coded emergency call is placed and goes out over the page system. The cardiac arrest team arrives within three to five minutes during which a doctor who was present or the nurse who detected the arrest starts resuscitation procedures. The composition of the team varies somewhat from institution to institution, but basically it includes an attending physician or resident, one or two interns, and an inhalation therapist. Sometimes an anesthesiologist and one or more pharmacists also respond to the emergency call. The nurse may assist the team by loading syringes (if a pharmacist is not present), keeping a record of drugs administered, and providing any supplies or equipment not present. The patient will need her when he has revived. During the resuscitation procedure, it is very important that the head nurse or the patient's nurse talk with members of the family, especially those who may have been present when the patient arrested and were sent from the room. She needs to explain what is happening and give support as necessary. No member of the family should be left alone for more than a few minutes without a report from the nurse. Waiting at such a time can seem an eternity.

Clinical Nurse Specialist

There is a new trend in hospitals toward the employment of a clinical nurse specialist—variously called liaison nurse, nurse therapist, nurse coordinator, or nurse clinician—to assume responsibility for portions of the nursing care of selected patients.[6] A clinical nurse specialist in some hospitals is concerned with patients who have a common diagnosis or type of surgery; for example, specialty areas for clinical nurse specialists are open-heart surgery, colostomies, coronary thrombosis. The nurse is not confined to a specific unit or assigned specific hours to work but makes and maintains contact with the patient wherever he is in the institution at whatever time she is needed. Her functions include orienting the patient to the hospital, explaining the plan for his care, teaching, providing support for the patient and his family throughout hospitalization.

The clinical nurse specialist has freedom to practice and to try out new methods of nursing. She enjoys a collaborative relationship with the doctor. Responsible to the department administrator or director of inservice education, the clinical nurse specialist is not part of the unit staff. However, she counsels the division nurses regarding the patient's care and interprets to them his needs which, in her role, she has had time and opportunity to discover.

The patient, without doubt, receives considerable benefit from care given by a clinical nurse specialist. In most instances, this service has been instituted for patients who are suffering from conditions or facing situations which are especially anxiety-producing. In the qualified clinical nurse specialist,[7] the patient finds an individual to whom he has opportunity to relate and from whom he can gain a sense of security. She provides continuity throughout the patient's hospital stay. Having depth of knowledge and full awareness of the doctor's plans, the clinical nurse specialist is in a position to help the patient understand his pathology, the therapy prescribed, and his part in it. Her skill in communication frees the patient to raise questions, express fears and doubts, and helps the patient deal effectively with them.

---

[6] For details of the way the service functions in various institutions see references at end of chapter to articles by Laura Simms, Nancy Scully, Hildegarde Peplau, Louise Anderson, Doris O'Connor and Faye Hagan, Bernard Bressler, and an editorial in *Nurs. Forum,* Vol. III, 1964.

[7] Qualifications of the clinical nurse specialist will be discussed in detail in Chapter 6.

Social and Diversional Opportunities for Patients

In providing for recreation, hospitals for the patient with long-term illness are minimally expected to have sitting rooms where patients may visit with one another and with families and friends. Some institutions, of course, furnish much more than the minimum. In self care units numerous facilities are available for the patient's use. (See p. 38.) In the acute divisions of general hospitals, however, much less attempt has been made to provide for the personal and social needs of patients. Dr. Esther Lucile Brown[8] advocates a hospital which is as much like the home setting as possible. Patients should have a comfortable, attractive lounge large enough for ambulating patients to get necessary exercise and for small groups to visit or play games. Lamps for reading, television, and growing plants all help to create an atmosphere conducive to relaxation. A beautiful view from the windows of the lounge and patient rooms adds pleasure and bolsters the spirits of the convalescent as well as contributing to hope during the more acute phase of illness. If it is far enough away to limit noise, a view of traffic, while not as interesting to most persons as is a garden or a stretch of landscape, is nevertheless preferable to looking at a blank wall. Could anything be more uninspiring than that? A "symbol of normal living," lounges on the patient care division alleviate boredom, loneliness, and depression. Concomitantly, having a place for patient recreation relieves the staff of "harassment by bored patients seeking attention." [9]

Almost as important as a lounge in Dr. Brown's opinion is a small dining room on the division where patients who are able to be up can socialize during mealtime. It is remarkable what eating with a group can do to improve the appetite. Table service would add to the pleasure for many.

In place of or in addition to socializing, some patients may wish quiet. This too should be available to all. It should not be necessary for anyone to listen to a radio or television or to the chatter of others when he does not wish to do so.

Although the head nurse may not be able to change architectural design of existing hospitals she can promote investigation of the possibility for desirable change and insist that her ideas be considered when new construction is being undertaken. If she is to be influential she must give serious thought to the physical and social environment which would be beneficial

[8] Esther Lucile Brown. *Newer Dimensions of Patient Care,* Part I: The Use of the Physical and Social Environment of the General Hospital for Therapeutic Purposes, New York, Russell Sage Foundation, 1961, pp. 30-54.
[9] *Ibid.,* p. 42.

to her patients. In the meantime, with very little effort but a good deal of insight and caring, it should be possible for nurses to individualize much of the care of patients and improve their environment. Most patients except the critically ill are more comfortable and at ease if they have around them a few personal possessions to make a "home" in the hospital. This is true although the patient may be in only for a few days. Even though space is limited, and it often is, a patient should be encouraged to keep a few personal items with him: a photograph, a clock, toiletries, a negligee or robe— something he really wants. Separation from family and friends is easier when the patient has some personal possession as a tangible tie to normal living.

Services for Children and Their Families

Until recently it has been customary to organize pediatric services according to medical specialties. In institutions large enough to have two pediatric divisions, sick infants and children up to sixteen years were cared for by pediatricians on a medical pediatric division.[10] Children admitted for surgery were assigned to a surgical pediatric unit where they were treated by surgeons, not pediatricians. The present trend is for children's services to be organized according to the age of the child and to his medical and nursing needs. Pediatric floors as a whole are likely to be under the direction of the department of pediatrics, while patient care is the responsibility of the doctor on the service to which the child was admitted, such as urology or surgery.

Organization of Services by Age and Condition of the Child. In this new plan of organization one may find units for infants to age five, for five to ten year olds, and for children aged eleven to sixteen. Advantages of placing children according to age rather than medical service are many. The environment can be suited to his care. The nursing staff becomes more aware of the needs of the child at a particular age level. The toddler, for instance, requires a greater amount of supervision than the older child. Recreational needs vary with age. The young child wants opportunity for creative play while the older child is more interested in crafts.[11] Older children

[10] In earlier years a separate unit was provided for children with communicable diseases.

[11] It is not infrequent to find hospitals employing a trained person at each of these levels to be responsible for directing play activities. Nurses participate in the program. Student nurses often spend a few days with the play director learning to apply principles.

are more responsible. Disciplinary problems are less frequent when children over ten are grouped together, separated from toddlers who come along and upset a partially completed jigsaw puzzle which has been temporarily set aside. However, development of a psychosocial spiritual program is essential to make sure that the needs of the older child are met.

When children are assigned to patient care divisions by age there may be an intensive care section in connection with each unit; or a single division for care of the acutely ill may be established for children of all ages. Except in very large pediatric departments, medical and surgical patients are cared for in the same unit. Sometimes special divisions are provided for patients who have open heart surgery. Here children and adults may be assigned to the same division.

The special care unit for infants from birth to one month is one of the newest pediatric services to be developed.[12] A revolutionary new wash technique for infants and personnel, developed through intensive research, has made it possible to assign to the same room all infants, including prematures who need special care.[13, 14] Cross contamination poses no problem. Parents, using the same precautions as the staff, come into the unit to learn to care for their babies. Since many infants with birth defects are sent to the newborn special care unit, a social worker is attached to the division to work with the families on the solution of social and economic problems. Here the care is truly family centered. In addition to being taught to care for their child before taking him home, parents are helped to accept his condition. They learn about corrective measures which may be taken when the baby is older. The entire staff recognizes that the child's life adjustment will be determined in large part by the attitude of his parents.

It is obvious that a newborn special care unit such as that described needs to be staffed with professional nurses who can make sensitive observations, an ability which results from knowledge broadened by experience. Due to the closeness of observation which is necessary, the immense amount of parent instruction required, the scrubbing and gowning called for in the special precaution technique, the nursing staff should be proportionately large and highly stable in addition to being competent. This need is intensified if interns, for whom the service on the newborn special care unit is but a small part of their educational experience, spend only about one month in the division. When this occurs, the stabilizing effect of a ma-

[12] The service described is that developed in the Yale-New Haven Medical Center.
[13] Infants with weeping skin lesions are the only exception.
[14] Louis Gluck and Harrison F. Wood. Staphylococcal colonization in newborn infants with and without aseptic skin care, *New Eng. J. Med.*, Vol. 268 (June 6, 1963), pp. 1265-1268.

ture well-informed head nurse is often necessary to present an unwitting change in an infant's carefully balanced regimen.

A much less common grouping of children who are not assigned according to age occurs in medical centers where research in childhood disorders is carried on. Since the child must be in his best health before he can be admitted, physical care is minimal. Most children are up and about. They often wear their own clothes and may leave the hospital on passes. Nursing is focused on helping the child accept his disorder, his prognosis, and the hospital. Not infrequently research units are financed by federal funds.[15] Nurses who choose to work in a research division tend to be perfectionists. They are meticulous in detail and concerned about having time to function in this manner.

Rooming in by Parents. Another service for children and their families is rooming in by a parent. In modern hospitals restrictions on visiting have been lifted and for some time parents have been encouraged to participate in their child's care. Opportunity for rooming in by a parent of the young child is being provided in some hospitals where it is recognized that a child, especially the eighteen month to five year old, may feel abandoned and suffer serious deprivation if his parents leave him alone among strangers. With the five to ten year old a mother or father often needs to room in, more for the parents' peace of mind than for the child's. Understandably, parents of children who have undergone surgery or been injured tend to use the rooming in facility more than others. Rooming in and unlimited visiting hours provide a rich opportunity for teaching the family. To help with parent education at least one hospital [16] employs a social worker, skilled in group work, as part of the staff on the division for five to ten year olds. She meets the families on admission and holds group sessions two evenings a week to which parents of all children on the division are invited. Since the social worker knows the children, she can anticipate problems that will be of common interest. She invites questions and discusses subjects helpful to parents, including growth and development and the effects of illness on the child's behavior. This service is of real benefit to parents and places emphasis where it belongs—on the child as part of a family upon which he is dependent for emotional, social, and spiritual support. When a social worker is employed to help in parent education, it is easy for nurses to let her do all the teaching and handle all the problems because she has the necessary time. However, the farsighted head nurse will recognize that the pediatric nurse has an essential role in teaching and supporting parents

[15] The National Institutes of Health presently make grants to institutions in the United States for construction of pediatric research units. It also pays a large percentage of the operating costs. There is no charge to the family for hospital or medical care of the child.
[16] Yale-New Haven Hospital, New Haven, Conn.

which must not be relinquished to anyone. Nurse and social worker in the situation observed complement one another in serving families.

The Care-by-Parent Unit. A very new service for families is known as "care-by-parent." In the institution[17] which is known to have developed such a program, a child from the pediatric clinic who needs a series of tests, teaching for home care, or special tests is assigned with his mother or father to a special division where they are given a private room with private toilet and shower. Here the two live for as long as is required for the tests to be completed. The parent—usually the mother, but not always—is instructed and supervised by the pediatric clinic nurse and takes full care of her child. She takes his temperature, gives him medications, supervises his eating, plays with him, sleeps on a bed beside him. A play room with toys is provided for the children, while a kitchen with washing machine, dryer, iron, and ironing board are available on the unit for the mother who takes care of her own and her child's personal laundry. A unit manager is in charge of the division. She gets acquainted with parents and children but does not participate in the physical care. Child care assistants who are specially trained, competent aides are available on the unit during the day and evening hours. Parents are encouraged to consult them and ask for help whenever they have problems or questions. The child care assistant teaches temperature taking and other procedures if the parent needs instruction. She keeps records of medications and temperatures. The responsibility for the care of the child, however, lies with the parent. The purposes served by this unit are many. Tests are carried out accurately under controlled conditions, children are not separated from their parents, expense of care is relatively low. Perhaps most significantly, parents learn the importance to the child's health of accurately carrying out instructions, of fostering good eating habits, of protecting the child from unsafe toys and other objects. They see the stress laid on placing medicine in a high cupboard under lock and key.[18] Keeping herself and her child clean and well groomed, made easy in the hospital, encourages hygienic habits and pride in appearance.

SUMMARY

Increasing awareness of the needs of patients has resulted in improvement of existing services and the development of new ones. Common to all is emphasis on bringing the family into planning and care. The patient can-

[17] The Albert B. Chandler Medical Center, Department of Pediatrics, University of Kentucky, Lexington.
[18] The parent has a key to a medicine closet in their room and gives all medications except injections which the clinic nurse administers.

not be considered apart from his family. In this chapter, an attempt has been made to give the head nurse an idea of the types of services available to patients and their families. No attempt has been made to be exhaustive. From the picture given, however, the head nurse can see that many hospitals are experimenting with new and better ways to serve people.

Emergency room service is expanding as a result of the modern way of life. Here the most demanding responsibility of the staff is life saving. However, the psychological needs of both patient and family are at a high level in the emergency room. Unfortunately this aspect of the service is all too frequently neglected. There are times when all hands are necessary to care for the sick or injured. This is not always the case, however, and when needs of families are accepted as an integral part of the emergency room nurse's responsibility, it will be a rare occasion when at least a few minutes cannot be spared periodically to provide information and support for the family.

Outpatient departments are not new, but the number and type of services offered to families are increasing. Classes for expectant parents, family health care clinics, and nurse conferences with parents of children for whom open-heart surgery has been recommended are a few of the ways in which outpatient services assist parents in the healthful rearing of their children as well as with their own physical and psychological well-being.

Conspicuous developments are occurring in the hospital proper. While progressive patient care continues in some places, the two elements which have been most widely adopted are the self care division and the intensive care unit. The latter, especially, is accepted almost as a necessity, and many hospitals now have several divisions for the care of the acutely ill. Coronary care units, special care divisions for newborn infants, intensive care units for patients undergoing open-heart surgery are among the newer intensive care services. Monitoring devices are an accepted part of the equipment for these divisions. Cardiac arrest teams are considered indispensable, at least in large hospitals. Again nurses must not forget that at these times and places of crisis, families, too, need intensive care. Failure to provide this care cannot be attributed entirely to lack of time. On the other hand, it is imperative that nurses who work in these anxiety-ridden services receive the understanding and support of those who supervise and direct them.

Services to patients which have been given too little attention are those which attempt to provide a homelike atmosphere in the general hospital. Comfortable lounges and dining areas on the divisions in addition to a place where quiet is preserved could do much to relieve boredom and depression. Valuable also is provision of individual space for each patient to have with him a few personal possessions.

Services for children and their families have received prominent consideration in recent years. One of the most significant developments has been the reorganization of services to provide placement of children on the basis of age. Other noteworthy innovations are rooming-in for parents, care-by-parent units, and special divisions for care of children who have common needs. All these services provide excellent opportunities for the teaching of parents. Time to give this service must be considered in arranging staffing. Implications for staff development are inherent in these new programs and will be considered in later chapters.

Certain hospital experiences such as open-heart surgery are more threatening than others to patients. To assist them in accepting such experiences with a minimum of psychological trauma and thus to contribute to their recovery, a new service for patients is being introduced. Clinical nurse specialists as used by some institutions serve the patient wherever he is in the hospital and interpret his needs to the unit staff.

QUESTIONS FOR DISCUSSION

1. Suppose you were entering the hospital for about a week's stay, what personal possessions would you wish to keep with you? Do you think you should be permitted to have these things?
2. A patient is brought into the emergency room with a gunshot wound in his head. He is unconscious. What could the head nurse in the emergency room do for the patient's wife who was with him when the shooting occurred?

EXERCISES

1. Survey the division on which you are working to see what reasonable changes could be made in organization of facilities or in structure to improve services to patients and to families. Consult patients and members of the staff. Draw up a list of suggestions or a plan for change.
2. Select any one of the services depicted in this chapter, or another service with which you are familiar. Pretending you are a patient or a parent in the situation, describe the nursing (in addition to that related in the text) which you would wish to receive.
3. In your hospital observe what happens to members of a family under one of the following (or similar) circumstances:

a. The patient is being treated for cardiac arrest.
b. The patient is in intensive care. His nearest relative has not left the hospital since his arrival. It is between midnight and 5 AM.
c. A mother is rooming in with her child.
d. The patient is in the emergency room with a probable cerebral accident, myocardial infarction, or other medical emergency condition.

What was the head nurse (or charge nurse) doing at the time of your observation? Evaluate the part that the *head nurse* played in the situation which existed.

REFERENCES

A community hospital rehabilitation unit, Nurs. Outlook, Vol. 13 (February 1965), pp. 40-41.
   A rehabilitation unit connected with a general hospital provides an organized program in which patients quickly learn to become self-dependent. Families participate actively in the program.

A pictorial report on the expanded role of one professional nurse, Nurs. Forum, Vol. 3 (No. 4, 1964), pp. 21-28.
   With pictures and captions the role of nurse therapist as practiced in a Veterans Administration hospital is depicted. She is responsible for the care of patients—regardless of their location in the hospital—who are admitted for colostomies.

Abdellah, Faye G., and Strachan, E. Josephine. Progressive patient care, Amer. J. Nurs., Vol. 59 (May 1959), pp. 649-655.
   A report on the Manchester, Conn., studies of progressive patient care. The five elements of progressive patient care are described including the patients cared for in each unit and the kind of staffing required. Implications for both nursing service and nursing education are presented.

Adam, Antoinette. Revise and consent, Amer. J. Nurs., Vol. 64 (January 1964), pp. 85-87.
   Nursing procedures "are man-made and not sacrosanct." Continuous questioning and review in light of principles is the responsibility of professional nurses. "As guardians of the public health we must recommend, advise and continuously inform until conditions which require change are changed to meet acceptable standards." A real challenge to head nurses.

Anderson, Louise C. The clinical nursing expert, Nurs. Outlook, Vol. 14 (July 1966), pp. 62-64.
   In an experiment at the National Institutes of Health, some of the nurse supervisors have been relieved of administrative responsibilities and serve as clinical nursing experts. Their functions are described as is the philosophy behind the change.

Angrist, Shirley. Nursing care: the dream and the reality, Amer. J. Nurs., Vol. 65 (April 1965), pp. 66-69.
   A sociologist believes that nursing care on an individual basis is outmoded and

unrealistic and that in actuality the professional nurse is becoming more a technician and manager.

The thoughtful nurse will raise some serious questions relative to this point-of-view.

Beghtel, Genevieve, and Akins, Charlotte. Hospital nursing service coordinates home nursing program, Amer. J. Nurs. Vol. 64 (May 1964), pp. 97-99.
A reorganization of nursing services in a county general hospital has resulted in the hospital director of nursing being responsible for the home care phase of nursing.

Beloff, Jerome S., and Weinerman, E. Richard. Yale studies in family health care, I. Planning and pilot test of a new program, J.A.M.A., Vol. 199 (Feb ruary 6, 1967), pp. 383-389.
Objectives, concepts, planning, and design of a project which provides complete health service to a group of families in a neighborhood near the hospital.

Blumberg, Mark S. Cardiac monitors work—but they should report more than they do, Mod. Hosp., Vol. 106 (January 1966), p. 58.
Minor irregularities in heartbeat may be precursors to more serious ones. Nurses will be expected to take increasing responsibility for the detection of such irregularities.

Bressler, Bernard. The psychotherapeutic nurse, Amer. J. Nurs., Vol. 62 (May 1962), pp. 87-90.
A psychiatrist trained a nurse to work with medical-surgical patients in a hospital division. The way in which she was prepared, the manner in which she functioned, and the values to the patient are described. The nurse, Mrs. Mary Ella Vause, has written her evaluation of the experience on pp. 88-89.

Brown, Esther Lucile. Newer Dimensions of Patient Care, Part 1: The use of the physical and social environment of the general hospital for therapeutic purposes, New York, Russell Sage Foundation, 1961.
This small paper back volume is filled with suggested ways for helping the patient at a very trying time in his life—hospitalization. Although many of Dr. Brown's ideas must be instituted by administration, a point of view is expressed which can make head nurses question present practices. A great many suggestions can be initiated and put to use by head nurses.

Cowan, Linda. Emergency! Amer. J. Nurs., Vol. 64 (April 1964), pp. 123-125.
Many years of experience in emergency room nursing are reflected in this description of the responsibilities of the nurse at this trying time for patients and families. Every emergency room experience is a crisis for the patient.

Davidson, Ramona. A medical intensive care unit, Amer. J. Nurs., Vol. 64 (December 1964), pp. 79-80.
Five beds within the medical unit have been set aside for intensive care. Its functioning is described.

Durbin, Richard L., and Brewer, Myrdas. 24 hour pharmacy is best prescription, Mod. Hosp., Vol. 104 (June 1965), p. 126.
When service is provided by the pharmacy throughout the 24 hour period, the pharmacist becomes a member of the health team. The article lists activities assumed by the night pharmacist in one hospital. Much of the relief provided is to nurses.

Erickson, Florence. When 6- to 12-year-olds are ill, Nurs. Outlook, Vol. 13 (July 1965), pp. 48-50.
The school-age child is a "middle child" who appears to have fewer needs than infants, toddlers, and adolescents. However, he has many fears, and his behavior needs to be understood so that he may be helped to help himself.

Errera, Paul, and Dye, Mary C. Emotional steam clouds emergency care, Mod. Hosp., Vol. 104 (February 1965), pp. 87-92.
A psychiatric study of the treatment of the emergency room patient as a human being has a message for all nurses as well as doctors. "Injury—not fear—gets attention."

Fagin, Claire M. Why not involve parents when children are hospitalized? Amer. J. Nurs., Vol. 62 (June 1962), pp. 78-79.
A nurse-mother suggests that parents can be of immense help both to their hospitalized child and to the staff and should be encouraged to remain with him.

Falls, Caroline E. Nursing in the ambulatory services, Nurs. Outlook, Vol. 13 (February 1965), pp. 42-46.
The nurse has a unique opportunity in the ambulatory services (emergency room and clinics) to detect fears and needs, and help the patient and his family cope with them.

Farrisey, Ruth M. Clinic nursing in transition, Amer. J. Nurs, Vol. 67 (February 1967), pp. 305-309.
A change has been made in the role of the head nurse in a large medical center clinic from that of clinic manager to a role in which she is responsible for nursing service and for medical administrative tasks.

Fields, Sister Mary Lucida. The C.P.R. team in a medium-sized hospital, Amer. J. Nurs., Vol. 66 (January 1966), pp. 87-90.
A cardiopulmonary resuscitation team reaches the patient with cardiac arrest within minutes. Resuscitation measures started by the unit staff are continued until the team arrives.

George, Joyce Holmes. Electronic monitoring of vital signs, Amer. J. Nurs., Vol. 65 (February 1965), pp. 68-71.
Much accurate information about vital signs is available through monitoring devices, but their ultimate value depends on the nurse's capability, her acceptance and use of the tool.

Gilbert, B. M. Mothers in hospital, Nurs. Outlook, Vol. 7 (December 1959), pp. 690-692.
Importance of maintaining the mother-child link through permitting the child to visit his hospitalized mother is convincingly expressed in this interesting article.

Gluck, Louis, and Wood, Harrison F. Staphylococcal colonization in newborn infants with and without antiseptic skin care, New Eng. J. Med., Vol. 268 (June 6, 1963), pp. 1265-1268.
Extensive research relative to the transmission of staphylococci in newborn infants has revolutionized nursery care in one hospital.

Imboden, Clarence A., Jr., and Wynn, Jane E. The coronary care area, Amer. J. Nurs., Vol. 65 (February 1965), pp. 72-76.
Coronary care areas, which combine monitoring equipment with expert nursing care, are responsible for saving the lives of many patients who have had myocardial infarctions.

Kilpatrick, Helen M. The frightened patient in the emergency room, Amer. J. Nurs., Vol. 66 (May 1966), pp. 1031-1032.
Patients in the emergency room, because they have had no time to adjust to their mishap, are especially in need of an understanding nurse who is confident enough in her technical functioning to have time to think of the patient.

Lambertsen, Eleanor C. Nurses have been trained to nurse people, not machines, Mod. Hosp., Vol. 105 (October 1965), p. 144.
Why should the nurse be the one to take on the responsibility for the new

machines? "The problem is to keep the benefits of automation in appropriate balance with the skills of professional workers."

Mahaffy, Perry R., Jr. Nurse-parent relationships in living-in situations, Nurs. Forum, Vol. 3 (No. 2, 1964), pp. 52-68.
Important guidelines for the nurse in helping living-in parents to function effectively. Pediatric nurses will find this a stimulating article.

Nightingale, Charles H. Distribution of drugs on the nursing unit, Nurs. Forum, Vol. 4 (No. 2, 1965), pp. 93-97.
Two points are stressed as important in a drug distribution system:
1) The doctor's order should go direct to the pharmacist and not through the nurse. 2) Drugs should be prepared by the pharmacist for distribution to the patient.

O'Connor, Doris, and Hagan, Faye. Liaison nurse, Amer. J. Nurs., Vol. 64 (June 1964), pp. 101-103.
A liaison nurse in the University of Kentucky Hospital is in a "staff" rather than a "line" position in the nursing service and is a member of the medical care team.
The reader is impressed with the program described but even more with the amount of interdisciplinary planning and consultation which appears to take place in this medical center.

Peplau, Hildegard E. Nurse-doctor relationships. Nurs. Forum, Vol. 5 (No. 1, 1966), pp. 60-75.
Miss Peplau, ably and in an interesting way, portrays the historical development (1900-1966) of relationships between doctors and nurses. She discusses "trends in the general disintegration of previous relationships and believes that "Interdisciplinary colleagueship based upon shared power and focused on health needs of people is evolving."

Pinneo, Rose. Nursing in a coronary care unit, Amer. J. Nurs., Vol. 65 (February 1965), pp. 76-79.
Nurses who man the coronary care units must be skilled nurse practitioners who have, in addition, the knowledge needed to read the monitor and the judgment to decide on appropriate action.

Rousseau, Olivia. Mothers do help in pediatrics, Amer. J. Nurs., Vol. 67 (April 1967), pp. 798-800.
Mothers who remain with and help in the care of their children make the situation much less traumatizing for the patients and in turn make nursing much easier.

Ruhlman, Rose G., and Ishiyama, Toaru. Remedy for the forgotten back ward, Amer. J. Nurs., Vol. 64 (July 1964), pp. 109-111.
A story of the amazing changes that took place in a custodial ward when hospital staff, patients, and community joined in a dynamic interrelationship. A thought-provoking article for head nurses as well as nurse administrators.

Scully, Nancy Rae. The clinical nursing specialist: practicing nurse, Nurs. Outlook, Vol. 13 (August 1965), pp. 28-30.
A complementary article to that of Laura Simms of same date. Presents the problems, especially of staff resistance, as well as the satisfactions in the role.

Short-term hospital serves hearty bedtime snack, Hospitals, Vol. 39 (April 16, 1965), p. 96.
Patients' suggestions led to the provision of substantial snacks—sandwiches, cupcakes, milk, fruit, etc.—at bedtime and solved the problem of patients going to bed hungry because of the early supper hour.

Simms, Laura L. The clinical nursing specialist: an experiment, Nurs. Outlook, Vol. 13 (August 1965), pp. 26-28.
Description of a very interesting innovation in nursing service—the use of a clinical nurse specialist. Describes her responsibilities and her place in the organization.

Snoke, Parnie S., and Weinerman, E. Richard. Comprehensive care programs in university medical centers, J. Med. Educ., Vol. 40 (July 1965), pp. 625-657.
Report of a study which attempted to discover whether a specially organized family health care unit is required for truly comprehensive medicine to be demonstrated and at the same time an effective educational environment achieved.

Spencer, G. T. Diagnosis of cardiac arrest: a non-nursing duty?, Nurs. Times, Vol. 61 (December 3, 1965), p. 1663.
This letter-to-the-editor is in response to a preceding article on cardiac arrest. The writer (anesthetist) contends that ventilation of the lungs is more often the correct procedure when sudden collapse occurs and should always be the first emergency measure. The question remains: Is cardiac arrest a nursing duty?

Wolford, Helen G. Complemental nursing care and practice, Nurs. Forum, Vol. 3 (No. 1, 1964), pp. 8-20.
In complemental nursing care a very able nurse practitioner contracts with a patient to assume responsibility for his care during and following hospitalization until he and his family are ready to take over.
An editorial (pp. 21-26) which follows the article, "Toward real continuity in patient care," recommends that nurses read the article carefully and think about the feasibility of experimenting with its application.

chapter 4

ORGANIZATION OF THE HOSPITAL FOR EFFICIENT MANAGEMENT

Since the end of World War II, widespread change has taken place in hospital service. This change can be attributed primarily to five developments: 1) progress in medical science resulting from research in drugs, surgery, radiation, and other modes of therapy and diagnosis; 2) increase in the use of ancillary workers such as aides, technicians, and clerks; 3) scientific developments which have resulted in the production of disposable materials of many kinds; 4) use of computers for data processing; and 5) changes in hospital design to provide greater safety in patient care and increased efficiency in service. The entire institution has been affected by these developments. Hospitals have become "big business," huge operating concerns, which has necessitated extensive reorganization of services. In attempting to utilize material and personnel resources to the full, care has been needed to protect the patient from possible harmful effects, such as the psychological trauma of feeling himself a mere cog in a machine, which could result from reallocation of functions. New hospitals are fortunate in being able to design their pattern of organization, utilizing results of research and experience, experimenting boldly with new ideas and philosophical concepts. In established institutions, however, change has had to be superimposed on existing organizational and architectural structure. Since in these hospitals changes have not occurred all at once but have extended over a period of years, the various innovations have not always been coordinated. Likewise a hospital which has made many technical improvements may still be using archaic methods in part of its services. Recognizing this, some large institutions are establishing systems management services and employing industrial engineers or methods analysts to study and recommend ways to increase efficiency.

This chapter will describe some of the more universal changes which have been made in hospital organization, mostly during the past ten years, as well as innovations which have not yet come into general use. Changes will be considered from the point of view of their purposes—safer care for patients, efficient use of personnel and equipment—and the effect of reorganization on the operation of the patient care division. Developments in the areas of communication, transportation, handling supplies and equipment, dealing with needs for small repairs, and sharing patient care with technicians and other professional groups will be considered.

CHANGES RELATED TO COMMUNICATION AND TRANSPORTATION

Messages, requisitions, materials, and patients flow in a ceaseless stream from one part of the hospital to another. The promptness with which communication and transportation are accomplished has potential for preventing frustration, saving large amounts of time, and even for saving lives.

Communication Devices

One means of transmitting messages between patients' rooms and the central desk is the voice intercommunication system, commonly known as the "intercom." This device makes it possible for the secretary or head nurse to respond to a patient's call immediately and to inform his nurse that he needs her.[1] Likewise an intercom between the treatment room or office and other departments permits requests to be honored without delay for a treatment tray from the central supply room or a glass of milk from the diet kitchen.

Another device for sending messages is the radio page, a pocket radio receiver which transmits a "beep beep" or, in more expensive models, a voice message. The radios are carried by persons who may be needed promptly but are not always within hearing of the switchboard page system. This might include doctors, engineers, transportation personnel, or hospital administrators on call at night. Messages are sent by dispatchers located in the departments whose personnel carry the radios. When the signal is heard the receiver calls his dispatcher from the nearest telephone. The head nurse may never be directly concerned with a radio page system except if it is used in such emergency settings as the intensive care unit to call the cardiac arrest team (see p. 47).

[1] An interesting study indicates that although the intercom is intended for patient-nurse communication, it of necessity becomes a staff paging system because the person designated to answer patient calls cannot leave the desk to perform the requested service. See: John D. Thompson, John F. O'Connor, and Hugh J. Maher. This study shows who really uses the nurse-patient communication system, *Hospitals*, Vol. 33 (February 1, 1959), pp. 40-44, 92.

Transportation and Messenger Service

Newly constructed hospitals, as well as some built with foresight several years ago, provide pneumatic tubes for sending requisitions and reports, dumbwaiters and conveyer belts for delivery of sterile supplies, drugs, and store items. Most hospitals, but especially those which do not have mechanical conveyers, need a messenger service to pick up and deliver requisitions, reports, and small items of all kinds. In addition to a general messenger service which sends couriers to all units and services, as often as once an hour during the day, some departments have persons on their own staffs who make rounds at periodic intervals. The record room, for example, may collect clinical records of discharged patients while the laboratory collects specimens.

Transportation of Patients

Patients are usually transported by wheel chair, stretcher, or in their beds. It is customary for the operating room and the x-ray service to handle their own transportation while other departments may depend on a centralized transport service. It is becoming more common for ambulatory patients to walk to x-ray or other departments; directions are usually indicated by colored guide lines. Likewise patients who are able to walk are discharged directly from the division in custody of family or friends.

Values of Transport Services

Organized messenger and transportation services have great value in preventing disruption of activities in the patient care division, although constant study and vigilance are necessary to keep the services functioning efficiently. Sometimes head nurses find it easier to bypass them and send a clerk or aide from the division on an errand. However, transport services will not, indeed *cannot* be improved unless the persons responsible for their administration are kept aware of the problems and given opportunity to solve them.

CHANGES RELATED TO SUPPLIES AND EQUIPMENT

Hospital administration has taken many steps to relieve the division nursing staff of responsibility for ordering and handling supplies and equipment. Various departments which supply the division—the laundry and central supply room and, in some instances the pharmacy and laboratory —send representatives to the floors to take inventory and then, according to a standard,[1] to make up and deliver the order. Bundles with the day's linen supply for each patient, packaged in the linen room and distributed to each patient's stand, provide the nursing staff with necessary materials in the place where they will be used. Complete sets of linen to make up cleaned units may also be packaged and distributed to the division or, preferably, to the housekeeping department for the maids who make the beds. Some institutions have gone much farther than others in thus supplying the nurse with the materials she needs, when and where she needs them.

Medical Supplies and Equipment

Probably in a majority of hospitals today, equipment is ready for use when it reaches the nurse, and it can be predicted that in a few more years this situation will exist in all hospitals. The widespread use of disposable materials has revolutionized the handling of medical supplies and equipment and enormously reduced the time spent by nurses and other personnel in handling these items. Articles such as catheters and gloves are packaged individually, used once and discarded. Treatment and dressing sets are prepared in compact bundles by the central supply service; extra sponges and pads are done up in separate small packages to be added to sets if necessary. Available in a warming cupboard are sterile solutions for irrigations. Since modern rapid transportation delivers sterile sets within minutes after they are requested, when this service is available it is unnecessary to store much sterile equipment on the unit. When rapid transportation is not available, however, considerable storage space is needed. This has often become a problem due to the enormous increase in the amount of material that must be available in the divisions. Not only is there the regular standard for treatment sets and dressings which needs to be maintained, but, due to the tremendously expanded use of injectable drugs and parenteral fluids, it is imperative that syringes and needles of all sizes and an ample supply of sterile tubing and intravenous solutions be

[1] A standard is an established quantity which is required to meet the needs of a particular division. Standards are based on many factors and are frequently set by nursing service or hospital administration. If not, the head nurse should calculate needs on her unit and establish standards for the items which she orders.

immediately accessible. In addition, space is needed for containers to hold discarded equipment, soiled dressings, disposable medicine cups, and other waste, as well as for a receptacle in which to place equipment to be returned to the central supply room.

The heavy volume of material needed for modern medical practice, the lack of mechanical conveyers, and the inadequate space for storage which is commonplace in older hospitals combine to produce a steady flow of people and delivery trucks down the corridors of the division, in and out of service and storage rooms. In addition, accumulation of large quantities of waste and its removal have posed a problem. Trash chutes are a great help, but many hospitals were not built with this facility, and a porter must collect the waste several times a day. This in turn increases traffic on the unit.

Some hospitals have been able to eliminate this traffic and resulting confusion in the patient care area by developing a central station near a service elevator adjacent to the unit. Easy wheeling trucks with linen, sterile supplies, and store items can be promptly moved from the central station to the storage area on the division by an aide or a unit helper if one is assigned to the floor. This entails the division staff unloading the trucks and shelving the supplies unless the truck, instead of shelves, is used for storage. This latter system has proved very effective. Two compartmentalized trucks are available for each unit for each type of supply, that is, linen, sterile goods, store items. Supplies are handled only once by the maid, aide, or clerk in the issuing department who stocks the truck according to the standard for the floor. One truck is kept on the division, the other in the supplying department. Once or twice a day or once a week according to schedule the truck on the division is replaced by a fully stocked one. Under this system provision must be made for obtaining needed items promptly should the supply on the unit be depleted unexpectedly. Likewise, it is important that standards be increased or decreased as needs change. The truck should be stocked for maximum usage. When a plan of this kind is instituted it is imperative that head nurses cooperate to the full and not decide to remove from the truck, prior to its exchange, several pieces of linen or certain much-used materials in the fear that the supply might run out. When this practice is engaged in, it is possible for large quantities of material to lie dormant in hiding places all over the hospital. Since head nurses are inveterate hoarders (often with good reason under old systems), those who have completely transferred to a secretary or other helper the responsibility for keeping the division adequately stocked admit that they have no need to hide "extras" against a "rainy day."

Other successful systems for providing supplies and equipment to the nurse at the time and place needed are also in use; for example, treatment room cupboards and linen closet shelves open into a central station or hall corridor. The department delivering the supplies places them directly on the shelves. The unused items which remain in the cupboard are pushed forward toward the door opening into the treatment room. A similar system is used in newer hospitals in which cupboards in patients' rooms have two-way openings. The daily supply of linen and the equipment to be used for treatments can be placed in the cupboard from the corridor, without having to disturb the patient. The equipment is at hand for the nurse when she is ready to use it.

Large Items of Equipment

It is customary today to keep on a division only the general equipment which is in use daily, such as wheel chairs. However, an oxygen tent and suction machine should be housed on divisions where these are used consistently. Less frequently used items—inhalators, foot boards, cradles, special beds and mattresses—are kept in a central store room and called for when needed. In this way clutter is prevented on the unit, and large amounts of storage space are unnecessary. The central service which delivers and collects this equipment is responsible for cleaning and keeping it in repair.

CHANGES RELATED TO PLANT MAINTENANCE

To varying degrees, head nurses are responsible for requisitioning or reporting needed small repairs such as a dripping faucet, squeaking door, broken light bulb, hard-to-open window, loose tile. Calling the building services department may be done by the secretary, but days or longer often elapse before nonemergency requests are handled. Although nurses should not have to be concerned with plant maintenance, it is usually they who discover the needs, and an easy way to report them is necessary.

Some plant service or maintenance departments have solved this problem, to the great satisfaction of head nurses. In one such instance, repair needs are listed on a special sheet which hangs on a clipboard in the division office. The list includes small repairs required for wheel chairs, beds and the like as well as for fixed equipment. A "handy-man" makes rounds staying on a division until he has completed the work noted.

SHARING RESPONSIBILITY FOR PATIENT CARE

The doctor has, over the years, transferred to the nurse many functions which he originally performed. However, hospital nursing service has varied from institution to institution in the activities it has been willing to accept as the responsibility of its regular nursing staff. In order for nursing personnel to have more time for nursing responsibilities and patient care, some institutions have employed teams of specialists who carry out many of the functions previously performed by the nurse.

Special Therapists

In some institutions where the state law permits, professional nurses routinely give infusions and transfusions. In others these responsibilities have been delegated to a team of specially trained nurses who go all over the hospital to start intravenous therapy. The nurses on the division are responsible for observation, changing flasks, adding medications, removing needles, recording amounts. Nursing service administrators are now doubting whether an education in nursing is a necessary requisite for administration of intravenous therapy. Why could not technicians be trained by medical personnel and perform this medical function under the supervision of a doctor as do laboratory technicians? Manual, observational, and interpersonal skills are needed but these can be learned in a much shorter time than that required for the education of a nurse. Regardless of the composition of the team, the patient's nurse should prepare the patient for the treatment, support and comfort him as necessary during and after the venipuncture.

Many larger hospitals have established departments of inhalation therapy with a physician in charge who is responsible for all inhalation therapy in the institution. Technicians under his direction and supervision are responsible for the administration of positive pressure and oxygen. They keep equipment in good working order and administer the therapy. If the treatment is to be continuous, the therapist starts it and checks functioning of the system once or twice a day. The nurse makes sure the patient understands the purpose of the treatment and his part in its success. She positions him, maintains his comfort, observes his condition, and interrupts or discontinues the inhalation in accord with the doctor's prescription and the patient's needs. The therapist is called if mechanical difficulties arise or supplies need to be replenished.

"Prep" Team

An operating room "prep" team composed of orderlies and aides may be trained to do skin preparation on all patients who are to have surgery. Division nurses are thus relieved of responsibility for this rather time-consuming procedure. However, the head nurse must realize that though shaving may be a simple, routine task, for many patients abdominal-perineal shaving is a psychologically traumatic experience. Explanation of the procedure cannot, therefore, be left to the nonprofessional member of the "prep" team. This is a nursing responsibility which needs to be performed by a nurse skillful in detecting patient concern and, if necessary, in helping him accept the need for shaving to be done. For a patient who has had objections to the procedure his nurse or the head nurse must instruct the aide or orderly in an acceptable approach and be present when the procedure is begun. At times it may be imperative that the nurse herself do the shave. When a "prep" team is used a competent individual is needed to supervise the members and schedule their work. The head nurse will wish to make sure that shaving has been done before the patient leaves for the operating room.

Pharmacist

At the present time, in all but a few hospitals, the customary procedure for dispensing drugs, preparing them for administration, and recording them is somewhat as follows: A supply of medications sufficient for multiple doses is distributed by the pharmacy either as stock drugs or as prescriptions for individual patients. The nurse pours the prescribed number of tablets or capsules and measures the prescribed amount of fluid due at a given hour. A medicine card transcribed from the doctor's order sheet is used as the prescription when pouring, as the indentification for each patient's medicine during administration, and as the record of drugs given when charting. Literally hours of nursing time are required in the pouring of medications, checking and double checking to be sure the drug and dose are correct. The actual administration of the medication requires a relatively short period of time. Charting in the usual present day procedure is time-consuming as is keeping track of orders for drug changes and transmitting these to the pharmacy.

In recent years some hospitals have experimented with methods to increase efficiency and safety in the handling of drugs.[2] As a result the pharmacist in these institutions has assumed more responsibility for preparation of drugs for administration thus relieving the nurse of time-consuming detail.

The purposes of new systems which have been instituted are to place responsibility on the pharmacist for preparation of individual doses to be administered at a given hour; to eliminate error of which there is a great deal under the present system;[3] to save nurses' time for nursing; and to give the pharmacist a direct part in patient care. The following steps in new procedures aim to achieve these purposes:

1) A carbon copy of the doctor's order is sent to the pharmacist who transcribes it on a medication record of the individual patient, which is kept in the pharmacy.

2) The head nurse or clerk on the division transcribes the orders on medicine cards or on an individual medicine sheet for the patient.

3) The pharmacy sends, to the unit at the proper time, single doses of medications in form for administration.

Most common drugs are prepackaged in unit doses industrially or by the pharmacy—tablets in cellophane strips, capsules in envelopes, and liquids in medicine glasses or small capped bottles from which the patient drinks, subcutaneous and intramuscular drugs in syringes.

4) The nurse checks the labeled doses against the medicine cards or list and upon finding them in agreement administers the medication. Otherwise, she checks the doctor's order sheet.

The medications to be given at a specified hour may come to the division by dumbwaiter, on a tray together with the medicine cards which the nurse had sent to the pharmacy, or the drugs may arrive in a medicine chest which has an individual drawer for each patient. In the latter case, a medicine list for each patient is used. Lists are filed in a loose leaf notebook which accompanies the medicine chest as it is wheeled to the patient's room.

5) As soon as the patient has taken the medicine it is charted on his medicine sheet which becomes part of the permanent record when the patient is discharged. When medicine tickets are used the nurse returns with them to the office, records the drug on the patient's cardex or chart or both, and files the cards.

[2] Two hospitals known to have done extensive study in this area and to have instituted radically different medication procedures are the University of Kentucky Medical Center, Lexington and the J. Hillis Miller Health Center, University of Florida, Gainesville.

[3] Kenneth N. Barker and Warren E. McConnell, How to detect medication errors, *Mod. Hosp.*, Vol. 99 (July 1962), pp. 95-106.

This procedure saves time in at least four ways: 1) preparation time is eliminated, 2) there is no combining of medicines or calculating fractional dosages, 3) ordering drugs is eliminated since medications are not kept on the division, 4) drug charges and credits are handled by the pharmacist, 5) narcotic records are no longer a nursing responsibility.

The pharmacist gains greater satisfaction from this system. His talents and training are more fully utilized, for he knows all the drugs a patient is receiving and has opportunity to detect and advise the physician on any incompatibility between drugs which have been ordered. Although this system for handling medications has proved highly successful in some institutions, certain problems inhibit others from making similar changes. The chief blocks are a shortage of registered pharmacists in some areas, and a lack of equipment for packaging, for data processing of medication cards in the pharmacy, and for vertical transportation. Each hospital must work out its own method for handling drugs. Some are waiting for methods analysts to study the entire hospital organization and make their recommendations before instituting a new procedure. For whatever changes are made the purposes stated (page 69) should be used as a guide. Every precaution possible must be taken to protect patients because medication errors can be tragic. It should be emphasized, however, that in addition to procedural safeguards there is still the need for an intelligent, scientifically prepared, conscientious nurse who knows the action and normal dose for each drug she administers, why it is prescribed for the particular patient, and how it is expected to affect him. There is no substitute for the brain and conscience of the nurse in administering drugs. It is for this reason some hospitals will not permit medicines to be given by practical nurses even though they have been trained in this function. It needs to be remembered that the licensed practical nurse, conscientious and reliable though she may be, has not the scientific knowledge for understanding the physiological effects and chemical changes which drugs induce. Some pharmacists believe it to be a very dangerous practice to permit practical nurses to administer drugs. When a practical nurse does give medications the professional nurse who delegates the function to her (as well as those on up the hierarchical ladder) retains responsibility and accountability. Are professional nurses aware of this fact? Are they willing to be responsible for the acts of one who lacks scientific preparation particularly when many of the new drugs are still experimental and their side effects not wholly known?

Nurses have questioned the safety of giving drugs poured by another and their liability under the law should an incorrect medication be given. However, there is no more danger in a nurse administering a glass or syringeful of medication *prepared and labeled by a pharmacist* than there is in her pouring from a stock bottle which a pharmicist has filled and labeled. In both instances the pharmacist takes the responsibility for the correct drug and dosage; the nurse for knowing the drug the patient is receiving and its purpose, for checking the label on the individual dose with the medicine ticket, for administering the drug to the right patient, and for recording it on the patient's chart.

SUMMARY

Scientific developments over the past two decades have necessitated many organizational changes in hospitals. New hospitals are constructed to accommodate such change while established institutions have often had to be more conservative. Perhaps the newest addition to the hospital administration staff is the methods analyst, an industrial engineer, employed to study the organization as a whole and recommend ways to increase efficiency.

This chapter has considered four areas of change which result in centralization of activities thereby relieving the head nurse of certain non-nursing functions. First, transportation and messenger services alleviate the need to send division personnel off the floor. A second area of change deals with supplies and equipment. Great strides are being made in the development of disposable materials and in relieving the unit staff of the responsibility for ordering and stocking supplies. However, the resulting increase in traffic and large amounts of waste create problems on the divisions in older buildings. Hospitals presently being constructed are providing for direct automatic transportation for supplies and central delivery stations for large items of equipment. Third, minor repairs to plant and unit equipment are promptly cared for by a roving "handy man" from the department of building services. By the fourth change, nurses are relieved of some of the technical functions which can be better handled by specially trained groups of therapists or technicians. The more extensive participation of the pharmacist in patient care relieves the nurse of responsibility for preparation of medications for administration.

QUESTIONS FOR DISCUSSION

1. Where are the loopholes in the medication procedure used in your institution? What would the head nurse need to do to eliminate them? Is it

practical or possible to follow the procedure? Explain. What changes would make the procedure more practical while still being safe?

2. A method for building maintenance has been suggested. Is your hospital using a different perhaps more effective one?

3. What satisfactions do you believe nurses gain from being members of an I.V. therapy team?

4. Would you feel safe giving a hypodermic of drug prepared by the pharmacist? Identify the source of your feelings about this matter.

EXERCISES

1. What problems in relation to supplies and equipment exist in the hospital with which you are associated? Define the problem. What are the factors contributing to the problem? What are the effects on patient care? What suggestions to alleviate the situation could be instituted without a major reorganization of services? Could or should a head nurse make such suggestions? To whom?

2. Confer with relatives or personal friends whom you know well who have had abdominal or perineal surgery. Determine their reactions to the surgical shave. If any were disturbed, do you believe a perceptive nurse could have eased the situation?

3. Study the nurse practice act of your State. What are the legal limits of practice for the R.N.? the L.P.N.? What is the responsibility of the R.N. for the acts of nonprofessional members of the nursing staff?

REFERENCES

Barker, Kenneth N., and McConnell, Warren E. How to detect medication errors, Mod. Hosp., Vol. 99 (July 1962), p. 95-106.
    Various means were used, in the research reported here, to determine medication errors, known and unknown to the nurse administering the drugs. The findings are interesting and disturbing.

DeMarco, James P. Automating nursing's paper work, Amer. J. Nurs., Vol. 65 (September 1965), pp. 74-77.
    Describes the use of a computer for transcribing orders, requisitioning supplies and services, preparing medicine tickets, recording action, writing reports. Further uses are projected for the future such as nursing care plans, nurses' notes, inventory of supplies, etc.

Drew, Jacqueline A., and Blumberg, Mark S. What happens to medication orders?, Amer. J. Nurs., Vol. 62 (July 1962), pp. 59-61.
A survey of the procedure for handling medication orders showed a wide variation between hospitals and within the same hospital. Standardization is recommended as is a form which calls for specific and complete information for the written order.

Friesen, Gordon A. A mechanized supply system provides supplies where needed, Hospitals, Vol 40 (May 1, 1966), pp. 109-112.
A hospital consultant describes plans for mechanizing delivery of supplies and equipment so the nurse will have them when and where she needs them. Automating communications is also discussed.

Kleinmann, Kurt. How the pharmacist can lighten the nurse's workload, Hospitals, Vol. 39 (January 16, 1965), pp. 94-102.
More and more hospitals are safeguarding patients and relieving nurses by having the pharmacist perform many functions traditionally handled by the nurse. Practices actually in use are described and should be considered by other hospitals.

Kron, Thora. Stepping beyond the 5 rights of administering drugs, Amer. J. Nurs., Vol. 62 (July 1962), pp. 62-63.
To individualize the administration of medications the nurse must know not only their action and expected effects but what she can do to enhance their effect, both physiologically and psychologically.

Lapniewska, Janina B., and Martinetti, Mary O. Working smarter (not harder), Nurs. Outlook, Vol. 10 (December 1962), pp. 812-813.
Values and techniques of work simplification.

Noroian, Edward H. Efficiency and Effectiveness, Nurs. Outlook, Vol. 12 (May 1964), pp. 46-48.
The meaning of these two words is compared. Important for head nurses is the fact that idle equipment can be equated in terms of time and of dollars.

Parnell, Marie A. Medicines at the bedside, Amer. J. Nurs., Vol. 59 (October 1959), pp. 1417-1418.
To help make mothers, who are generally healthy young women, self-dependent, one hospital provides the newly delivered mother with her medications to be taken as needed. All concerned like the system.

Payne, L. C. Medical automation: a professional necessity, Nurs. Mirror, Vol. 120 (May 14, 1965), pp. V-VII.
The potential for medical automation is great and many innovations could be made with present knowledge if funds were available. Valuable man-hours can be saved for patient care by the use of such devices as computers for calculating diets; sub-pharmacies for dispensing prepackaged drugs; monitors for taking vital signs. A unique nurse's station—a center for electronic devices, observation, coordination—is described.

Schwartau, Neal, and Sturdavant, Madelyne. A system of packaging and dispensing drugs in single doses, Amer. J. Hosp. Pharm., Vol. 18 (September 1961), pp. 542-559.
A very interesting report of a study in which medications were prepared for administration in the pharmacy thus relieving the nurse of this time-consuming procedure.

Smalley, Harold E. Professional methods improvement is ultimate path to more efficient hospitals, Mod. Hosp., Vol. 105 (September 1965), pp. 107-110.
More hospitals need to employ industrial engineers to improve the efficiency of the organization. Work simplification with which many hospital nurses have been involved is a beginning step in the direction of methods improvement. Head nurses

need to be informed of these trends and ready to cooperate in a program of methods improvement when it is undertaken.

Stryker, Ruth Perin. Precepts for a method study, Nurs. Outlook, Vol. 13 (May 1965), pp. 65-67.
Method studies are sufficiently important and needed in hospitals to justify the employment of a nurse for this specific function. The hospital and nursing administrators must believe in studies and expect broad participation by staff if studies are to be effective.

Thompson, John D., O'Connor, John F., and Maher, Hugh J. This study shows who really uses the nurse-patient communication system, Hospitals (February 1, 1959), pp. 40-45.
Findings in this study showed the intercommunication system is used primarily by the staff. Suggestions are made for reducing the need to page staff members.

Trites, David K., and Schwartau, Neal W. Nursing or clerking?, Nurs. Outlook, Vol. 15 (January 1965), pp. 55-56.
A researcher and pharmacist have made an extensive study of the clerical aspects of the medication procedure. In all but a few instances, the largest amount of this work is handled by the nurse. An interesting, factual report.

Vere, D. W. Some errors in drug administration, Nurs. Times, Vol. 61 (May 14, 1965), pp. 673-675.
Mistakes increase as work load increases. A study revealed the circumstances under which drug administration errors occurred. The need for determining the "saturation limit" of the nurse's capacity and for cooperative planning between nurses, administrators, and doctors, to lessen the burden of medication administration, is presented.

Webb, John W. Mosaics, Amer. J. Nurs., Vol. 65 (January 1965), pp. 105-108.
The title stands for Medication Order Supply and Individual Charge System. The article describes the way in which one hospital has decreased the administrative load of the patient care division by transferring certain responsibilities to the pharmacist.

chapter 5

ORGANIZATION OF THE PATIENT CARE DIVISION

Previous chapters have considered the organization of the hospital as a whole. It is now time to look at the patient care division, the people who work there, their relationships to one another and to those who, though they have responsibility for patients on the unit, carry out their functions elsewhere.

In the patient care division are centered the most important activities of the hospital. Here the purposes of the hospital are expected to be achieved for it is on the division that patients are cared for, clinical research conducted, health personnel educated. It is in the patient care division, primarily, that the hospital and the public meet. Here a very large part of the hospital dollar is spent. Here most members of the largest department in the hospital —nursing—spend their time.

Activities Carried Out on the Division and Persons Responsible

It will be well to review briefly the activities which are executed on the patient care division and the persons or groups which perform them. The first is medical care. This service is carried out only in part by doctors. Technicians and medical students perform many of the functions, while much of the prescribed medical care is given by the nursing staff. In fact nurses have come to think of this as *nursing*. However, while administering medical procedures has become a function of nurses, this care is to be differentiated from nursing. Nursing is ministering, that is, caring for a patient's personal needs, providing services necessary for life, health, and comfort, both physical and mental, which, were he able, the patient would perform for himself. It is helping the patient to function at the highest level of which he is capable, to obtain the greatest possible value from the resources open to him. Nursing then is the second of many activities carried out in the patient care division. Although responsibility for it rests with the head nurse, most of the actual nursing care is given by others—professional staff nurses, practical nurses,

75

student nurses, and aides. The administration or management of nursing care is a third activity of the division. It involves determining needs for care, planning, delegating, teaching, supervising, and evaluating. These responsibilities will be discussed in Part 2.

In addition to medical care, nursing, and the administration of nursing care, activities which take place on the division include dietary service, maintenance of the physical environment, clerical work, sending and receiving telephone messages, reception of visitors, and traffic control. For these the head nurse has varying degrees of responsibility depending upon the institution in which she is employed. Some head nurses are still responsible for making sure the diet served is correct, for carrying and collecting food trays, but more and more the dietary department is assuming this responsibility. The head nurse, as part of nursing, sees that patients are prepared for meals and receive assistance as needed. Housekeeping is most often the responsibility of a separate department, but the head nurse must be concerned that the environment is conducive to health and comfort. If a clerk or secretary[1] is employed she is an assistant to the head nurse and, therefore, responsible to her. Care of the telephone and direction of visitors, among other things, are the clerk's responsibility in all but a few hospitals. Of the seven activities listed, for only three—medical, diet service, and housekeeping—is someone other than the head nurse held accountable, and in all three of these, she has some degree of responsibility.

Other activities performed on the division are of a different nature. They are more general and cut across all the specific activities mentioned. These general functions include coordination of patient care and unit coordination—both head nurse responsibilities in most hospitals—supervision, and teaching. For the last functions, others besides the head nurse also have responsibility, each in his own area. The head nurse supervises and informally teaches her nursing staff. She sometimes participates in a class or conference for medical students new to the division.

Relationships of Personnel Who Work on the Division

In Chapter 2 the relationships of the head nurse within the nursing service and the comparative relationships of the nurse and the doctor to

---

[1] The terms clerk and secretary tend to be used interchangeably. Actually a secretary should be able to carry more responsibility than a clerk. A secretary is competent to do a clerk's work, but a clerk is not always prepared to do the work expected of a secretary. Some hospitals employ both in which case the clerk may take directions from the secretary.

TRADITIONAL RELATIONSHIPS OF THE HEAD NURSE

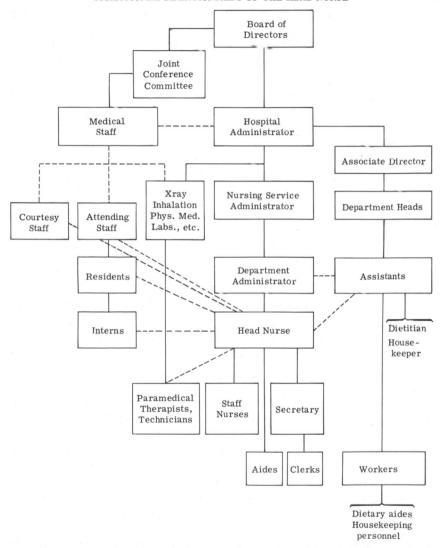

Fig. 5. Traditional relationships of the head nurse. Solid lines indicate administrative lines of responsibility. Dotted lines show professional relationships. Note that the nursing staff is in the administrative line organization; the medical staff is outside the line.

the hospital administrator were discussed. Figure 5 diagrams the organization of the unit showing the head nurse's administrative and professional relationships. Looking at the chart the head nurse can see that very few persons in the top three echelons function on the unit, or even appear on the division except under unusual circumstances. These are the individuals who carry the over-all responsibility for patient care. Of the persons in the lower three levels, only the head nurse and her staff are continuously present on the unit. Others have additional responsibilities elsewhere. They come and go on the division at their own convenience, some merely in a supervisory capacity. The unit nursing staff, bound by time and space, and by the organizational structure, maintains continuity in patient care.[2] As a result of the nursing staff being present 24 hours a day their designated leader, the head nurse, has of necessity become coordinator of patient care and of unit activities. In the patient care coordinator role she must see that the medical care activities prescribed by many different doctors mesh with one another and with nursing, that each is carried out at the proper time or, in case of conflict or insufficient time, decide which shall receive priority. This is an integrating function which requires judgment and decision-making.[3] In her unit administrator role, the head nurse coordinates activities of many individuals who come to perform tasks on the patient care division. She also sees that reports are made, records kept, supplies and equipment provided—that all these are carried out properly and on time so the machinery of both the division and the hospital will function smoothly. In addition, the head nurse is expected to coordinate unit and hospital administration with patient care activities. At times these two types of responsibility are in conflict and it falls to the head nurse to make a choice or in some way resolve the problem. For example, hospital policy may dictate that one division shall not borrow equipment from another. The doctor needs an ophthalmascope, but the instrument belonging to the division has a burned-out bulb and no extras are at hand. The head nurse must decide what to do. To solve the problem she may let the doctor, if he is an intern or resident, go to the next floor to borrow the item, for the medical staff does not feel bound by the rules. Otherwise the head nurse either has to disregard the policy or fail to meet the physician's needs.

As another illustration of conflict between responsibility for coordination of patient care and hospital or nursing administration, the department

[2] Hans O. Mauksch. The organizational context of nursing practice, In *The Nursing Profession,* Davis, F., ed. New York, John Wiley and Sons, Inc. 1966, p. 122.
[3] *Ibid.,* pp. 127-128.

administrator may be waiting to receive the afternoon report, the staff time sheet for the next day needs to be prepared, and narcotics have to be counted. A doctor wishes to do a sigmoidoscopic examination and requires the assistance of a nurse. At the same time patients are returning from the postoperative recovery room; they must be seen and their condition checked. The head nurse has to decide which demands upon her time shall take precedence—patient care or administrative responsibilities.

That problems arise from the present organizational pattern of patient care divisions is understandable. Problems center around three situations, two of which (1 and 3) are obvious if the chart in Figure 4 is studied. *One* of these problems results from centralization of services which necessitates supervision of workers by many different departments. A *second* problem has resulted from the increased volume of administrative functions performed on the division and the delegation of more and more technical medical procedures to nursing. The *third* problem relates to the head nurse's dual role as representative of hospital administration and as deputy of the physician. Although not new, this third problem as a result of the other two is taking on larger proportions.

These problems will be discussed in turn after which possible ways to solve them will be considered.

PROBLEMS ARISING FROM THE ORGANIZATION OF THE PATIENT CARE DIVISION

Problems Resulting from Centralization

The centralization of services and development of numerous therapy teams, described in Chapter 4, have increased traffic on the division and greatly extended the problem of coordination. The coming and going throughout the day of large numbers of workers from other departments, and their supervisors, has increased the activity on the unit to such a degree that it is confusing and wearing for patients and personnel alike. To direct this array of individuals to proper places and to keep them from getting in one another's way is a time-consuming and often frustrating coordination activity. It is one with which a clerk often assists but in most present-day hospitals, the problems which arise must be settled by the head nurse.

Problems Resulting from Increased Administrative Load

Although hospital administration in certain instances, as described in Chapter 4, has done a great deal to ease the burden of the head nurse, in other ways her load has been increased due to many hospital-wide innovations. New administrative demands are being made on the head nurse's time 1) by the increasing number of reports and charges resulting from medicare and other forms of insurance, as well as from the need for the patient to pay for items too expensive to be included in a flat rate, and 2) by the many different forms to be completed because of computerized data processing. In situations where the head nurse is still responsible for ordering, storing, and keeping track of drugs and equipment, the ever-expanding amounts used have also increased her burden.

The head nurse's responsibility has been extended in other ways as well. The doctor's prescriptions have become more complex as new tests and treatments of many kinds have come into common usage. Handling these prescriptions is the responsibility of the head nurse. It is she who must prepare and send the requisition to the proper department, see that the patient is prepared for the test, follow through to be sure it is performed at the specified time, see that the report is received and filed and that, when the test has been completed, prior therapy (diet, medications, and the like) is reestablished. A competent clerk can help with some of these administrative activities, but it is a rare occasion when the head nurse is not deeply involved. The head nurse is also responsible for coordinating the timing of diagnostic and therapeutic procedures performed by other departments with medical and nursing measures carried out on the patient care division.

In addition to the increase in unit administrative and coordinating activities, nursing service has accepted for performance by its staff many medical procedures formally administered by interns, medical students, or the patient's private physician. Although the division nursing staff carries out the procedures, the head nurse must delegate them, make sure they are being properly done, and must observe the over-all results. This is patient care coordination but only a small part of the total responsibility in that area.

What is the result of the head nurse's time being largely taken up with unit administration and with coordination and management of patient care services? Even with a capable clerk or secretary to assist her the head nurse has little choice but to keep the unit functioning, the medical care administered. To do otherwise would mean chaos. Many head nurses enjoy this managerial-coordinating role but those who are deeply concerned about nursing are not satisfied unless they also have time to plan and supervise nursing care, which cannot be accomplished adequately without considerable direct patient contact. The result of the head nurse not knowing patients well enough to plan their care intelligently, of not supervising and teaching personnel is less than satisfactory patient care and a frustrated head nurse. The result may also be a dissatisfied nursing staff, or worse, a complacent one, resigned to the situation. Only when there is a will to solve a problem can an answer be found.

Problems Resulting from the Dual Role of the Head Nurse

As the extension of hospital and nursing service administration the head nurse is expected to see that administrative policy is carried out, that patients are well nursed, that doctor's prescriptions—even those assigned to other departments such as x-ray or cardiology—are carried through. Yet the head nurse shares very little if at all in making policy which is supposed to govern her actions. Likewise, she has little heart for enforcing directions which she does not understand and with which she is not in sympathy. The problem is more difficult when a doctor's prescription is involved, for the head nurse, in addition to being the representative of hospital administration, is also the deputy of the physician. He, as well as the administrator, expects the head nurse to carry out medical orders. However, never is the head nurse responsible to but one doctor, and each physician is concerned only with his own patients. The result often is more orders written than can be carried out and one doctor's prescriptions precluding the following of another's orders. In addition some medical orders are in opposition to institutional policy and hence not legitimate. The procedure prescribed by the doctor may not have been accepted as a nursing function in the particular hospital (for example, starting intravenous fluids), or there may be risk of legal suit should the patient by any chance be injured. (Use of an electric heating pad might fall in this category.) When a physician prescribes or requests something which is prohibited by the hospital policy, the head nurse is expected by administration to adhere to the policy. However, if she believes the prescription will help the patient, or if she wants to please the doctor, the head nurse because she is divided in her loyalties will be torn as to the course to pursue. The doctor on the other hand has no such compunctions. Since he is not responsible to the hospital administrator from which directives emanate, he does not have to go through channels as does the head nurse. He feels free to break the rules if he believes his patient will be benefited.

When a doctor's order conflicts with policy the head nurse because she plays a dual role must make a decision. She has several choices. She can tell the physician she is unable to carry out his order[4], in which case he may go to the hospital administrator to request that an exception be made, or, since he does not like to be told by a nurse what he can and cannot do, he may report to the nursing service administrator that one of her staff is insubordinate. The nurse administrator may support the head nurse, thus accepting part of the blame, or perhaps she will feel free, the physician having told her the circumstances, to take responsibility for making an exception. This, of course, would put the head nurse in a poor light with the doctor and perhaps induce her to make such decisions herself in the future.

A second way in which the head nurse might handle the conflict between policy and prescription would be to disregard policy and comply with the doctor's order. Were she to do so she might keep still about it, trusting the matter would not be discovered, or she could report that she had broken the policy. In the latter case, the head nurse stands the chance of being punished. Another alternative would be for the head nurse to refer the matter to the department administrator and let her handle it. This is probably the most frequent course of action, but the head nurse in so doing is relinquishing responsibility for her patient's welfare. Furthermore, she is admitting her lack of authority, and this she might not wish to do, for it weakens her relationship with the doctor.

None of these courses of action is satisfactory. Perhaps, under present organizational structure, the head nurse would be wisest to suggest to the doctor an alternative, indicating that a different prescription would be safer or more convenient for the nursing staff. In so doing, it may not even be necessary for her to quote the rule. However, this method of handling the problem is not satisfactory either, if the head nurse believes the doctor's original order would be best for the patient. In so doing she would be abdicating her professional responsibility. As long as the present hospital organization is as it is, the head nurse's dilemma will continue to exist. Each head nurse will solve the problem of nonlegitimate doctor's orders in her own manner. The way she chooses will depend upon the nature of the request, the head nurse's age, experience, maturity, the trust the doctor has in her, whether she believes he would blame her or blame the system, how important the physician's approval is to the head nurse, her relationship with her department administrator and the nursing service. Problems of this kind face the head nurse because her relationship to the hospital administration is different from that of the medical practitioner.

It is necessary at this point to mention a type of conflict between medical orders and hospital policy that is becoming prevalent. Because of their

[4] The head nurse is in this instance in the unhappy position of being expected, at one and the same time, to take orders from and give orders to the doctor!

own increasing pressures, doctors are attempting to rid themselves of technical procedures which have become commonplace and which, therefore, consume a great deal of time. Administration of intravenous fluids falls into this category. (A solution to this problem was suggested in Chapter 4.) When the doctor requests that the head nurse and her staff take on responsibilities which are not theirs, it is important that the head nurse stand firmly on policy—to comply might mean breaking the state law. Likewise, the head nurse could be setting precedent by accepting responsibility which nursing service has been strongly resisting because the nursing staff already has more work than it can accomplish. Difficult as it may be for the head nurse to resist the doctor's request in this instance, it is imperative that she do so. She can deal with the request more easily if she understands and can accept the reason for the policy and especially if she has had a voice in making it. The problems which plague the head nurse because she is responsible for interpretation and enforcement of administrative policy, suggest that changes in roles and organizational patterns are needed.

POSSIBLE SOLUTIONS TO PROBLEMS RESULTING FROM PRESENT ORGANIZATION OF THE PATIENT CARE DIVISION

Is it possible within the present organizational structure of the division to effect changes which will lead to better patient care and a more satisfied staff, or will it be necessary to change the organization? The answer to this question is that *some* changes can be made although they will be palliative. However, it is too much to expect that every hospital can or will in the near future make the changes in organization which are needed if the head nurse is to achieve a new and more satisfying role and patients are to receive the care to which they are entitled.

What then can be done within the present framework to improve the situation on the patient care division and bring better care to patients? Possible solutions will be suggested.

Suggested Solutions to Problems Resulting from the Head Nurse's Dual Role

Frustration and tension, as we have seen, result from demands of the organization which require the head nurse to follow and enforce administrative policy made by persons remote from the place where action occurs and at the same time to carry out the medical care which is prescribed by many different doctors, each of whom sees his patients as all-important. Likewise, the demands of both administrator and physician may interfere with the nursing care of the patient. The head nurse is expected to exercise sound judgment and make decisions which will result in good patient care, satisfied patients and doctors, and contented staff, while at the same time she is expected to adhere to the rules of the institution.

Well-defined Nursing Objectives. Since nursing care should be the primary responsibility of the department of nursing, the first step in relieving the head nurse's frustration is for nursing service administration to make very clear the quality of nursing the head nurse is expected to provide. To do this, the director of nursing with the help of her assistants and the department administrators must think through the kind of nursing in which they believe and the extent to which they can expect this nursing to be done in their institution. The philosophy should be written and goals spelled out in specific terms to serve as a guide in selection and assignment of nursing personnel and in staff education. Objectives are formulated to be used, not written and then forgotten. Development of criteria for each objective makes them usable for supervision and evaluation (see Chapter 2). It cannot be overemphasized that objectives and criteria must be practical and attainable for the particular hospital since they are to be used as the standard for practice by the entire nursing staff. Delineated by the top level nursing service administrators, they should be studied by the head nurse and her staff with the department administrator and criteria specific for the individual service or division developed.

Plans for achieving objectives. Next, plans for the achievement of objectives are made—procedures, time tables, persons to be entrusted with responsibility, ways to prepare the staff members for their functions, procedures to be used in evaluating care of the individual patient, records to be kept. Again, it is important to be realistic in deciding on plans and procedures. They must be possible of achievement. The two steps indicated—development of objectives and criteria and a plan for their attainment—will necessitate that the entire nursing staff consider hospital and nursing policies—whether they are necessary, whether they can be followed, whether they are guides for action or rules. Those which are absolute rules (because of the law or a hospital board decision) should be made known by the hospital administrator to all doctors and nurses and the fact made clear that no exceptions are possible. These will be few in number. Many policies may become mere guides as a result of the study of goals and, hopefully, it will be decided that the head nurse, knowing the purpose of the policy, will be privileged to use her judgment in applying it in a given situation. Under such circumstances she would, of course, be accountable for the consequences of her decision. The freedom of the head nurse to use discrimination in applying policy would go a long way in preventing or resolving conflicts between medical and nursing staff over administrative directives.

This responsibility and authority would also give the head nurse greater satisfaction in her work. If she is not capable of such responsibility because of inexperience or immaturity, the head nurse would expect to consult the department administrator who would serve as a counselor helping the head nurse to see possible effects of different courses of action and supporting the head nurse if her convictions were in opposition to a physician's request. For example:

The family of a dying patient, who would ordinarily be transferred to a single room, requested that she be left with her friends in a four-bed unit, in the belief that if the patient were moved she would feel isolated and rejected, and frightened in her last hours. The other patients who were closely attached to the dying woman also expressed hope that she would stay in the room with them. They knew she was dying and although they realized it would be difficult to witness the death this would be preferable to not knowing what was happening. Since the patient was lucid and not suffering unusual pain, the head nurse decided she should remain in the multi-bed room.

However, the resident, in spite of the head nurse's explanation, decided the patient should be moved to a room by herself in accord with usual practice. The head nurse stood her ground and refused to follow the resident's order.[5] The head nurse in this situation was one with experience and clinical expertise who did not need the department administrator to counsel her. Instead the head nurse reported her decision and the reasons for it to the chief of service and received his support. Although the resident was angry and tried to make life miserable for the head nurse in other ways, the patient remained to die in her own room. Nurses supported the other patients through the experience. Although they freely admitted that it was more emotionally traumatizing than they had anticipated, each patient stated she was glad for the decision which had been made.

Although the head nurse, in this instance, did not need guidance in making the decision, a young head nurse would find this action exceedingly difficult if not impossible to take. She might not be sure she was right in her stand. She might very well feel too insecure to oppose the doctor and would fear to incur his wrath or even to displease him. Her feelings are under-

[5] Incidentally, allocation of patients to rooms is not a medical prerogative but an administrative one although it is within the province of the doctor to suggest changes. Even if placement of the patient were a medical privilege the head nurse in this instance was justified in ignoring the order because the best interests of the patient and her roommates so clearly demanded it.

standable and it is at times like this that the head nurse should be able to turn for help to a more experienced nurse, one with understanding of patients' needs, of interpersonal relationships, and a knowledge of administrative principles. The department administrator should be able to fill this role and help the head nurse make a decision—not make it for her. She should support the head nurse and help her handle any unpleasantness which results.

Establishment of priorities. In addition to setting objectives and making plans for their achievement, including a review of policies, a third way in which the head nurse's frustrations could be eased would be by the establishment of priorities to serve as guidelines for the head nurse. She needs an accepted guide to help her make decisions when a conflict arises between the demands of education and service, between the demands of medical or other health personnel and the patients' best interests, between the demands of the doctor and hospital administration, and between medical care and nursing care. The doctor's written order tends to take precedence over other patient care for the very reason that its accomplishment must be reported and charted. Is taking blood pressure every fifteen minutes, as ordered, more important than giving needed skin and mouth care? It is at times, but when vital signs are stabilized priority might be better given to nursing care. Many head nurses make such decisions. Many doctors expect them to do so. There is, however, no consistency in the matter. Therefore, guidelines, which are agreed upon in principle by top administration and which the head nurse is *expected* to use to protect the patient's welfare, would be of immeasurable help to her. She would still have problems but if she were held responsible for giving priority to the best interest of the patient and were supported by nursing service when she made a mistake in judgment, the head nurse's tensions would diminish. When such errors are made the head nurse needs help in analyzing the mistake. While her judgment may be criticized, the intent should be commended and the head nurse praised for taking the initiative in making the decision. Leadership in establishment of priorities must come from the nursing service administrator upon whom lies the responsibility for convincing the hospital administrator and the board of directors that priorities are essential.

When do nursing education and medical education take precedence over the best interests of the patient and when is the reverse true? For example, does the head nurse have the right—the responsibility—to decide that a patient's welfare might be jeopardized if a young inexperienced student nurse is assigned to his care, that the patient's well-being will be enhanced if the nurse who has already established a relationship with him continues to care for him on a particular day? Does the head nurse have a responsibility to the patient on whom a half dozen medical students wish to make pelvic examinations? When an intern keeps a patient and his family waiting because he has not written the discharge order, which takes precedence—the rights of the patient and his family or hospital policy or the convenience of the intern? What is the head nurse's responsibility when intravenous solution is infiltrating but the house officer fails to come and has given instructions that the needle is not to be pulled? Decisions relative to the head nurse's course of action under circumstances of this kind need to be made at top administrative levels after head nurses have submitted illustrations of the problems they encounter.

Thus far in the discussion we have considered possible ways, within present organizational structure, to lessen the head nurse's problems resulting from her dual responsibility—for delegated medical care and for the duties assigned her by hospital administration, namely nursing care and unit administration. Possible solutions to problems resulting from other causes pointed out earlier will be considered next.

Suggested Solution to the Problems Resulting from Centralization and Increased Administrative Load

The end result of the increase in clerical work, medical procedures, and coordinating activities which have descended upon the head nurse is a minimum of nursing care administration and a degeneration in the quality of nursing. At the same time, the centralization in other departments of many administrative activities, instituted to relieve the head nurse of nonnursing responsibilities, has increased unit traffic to such proportions that activity in the corridors and work rooms is incessant. The head nurse's desk has become the center for traffic control giving the impression of confusion whether or not it actually exists. The larger the patient care division the more this is true.

Again the question is raised: What can be done, in addition to suggestions made in Chapter 2, to alleviate these problems and relieve the overtaxed head nurse in order that she may have time for nursing responsibilities? Outside of complete reorganization of the division, the only answer to this question seems to be the employment of secretarial help for 14 to 16 hours a day, seven days a week. (Fewer hours may be adequate on a very small unit; 24 hour coverage may be necessary on a large unit.) The nursing service administrator must exert whatever pressure is necessary on the hospital administrator and board to procure this help for the head nurse and must see that salaries are adequate to attract competent persons. Leadership must come from the director of nursing, but she must make a clear case in terms of the benefits to patients if she is to be successful.

When this help has been authorized, head nurses and department administrators decide upon activities which a unit secretary can safely perform, and develop procedures to guide her. Someone other than the head nurse is employed to train the secretaries and supervise their practice until they are prepared to be useful. Only then are they turned over to the head nurse. The head nurse needs to know the duties of the secretary, and if she cannot, with a minimum of supervision from the head nurse, carry the responsibilities, the person who trained her is asked to give further help. Under no condition should the head nurse decide to perform any of the secretary's tasks. It is important too that the secretary not become a messenger. If messenger service is not presently provided, it should be instituted. Here again the director needs to have her facts, in order to be persuasive. Where centralized messenger service is inadequate or nonexistent, it is sometimes possible to employ a messenger-aide as part of the unit staff of a large division.

If the head nurse has a secretary to do most, if not all, of the clerical work, to maintain equipment and supplies, do whatever housekeeping supervision is now the responsibility of the head nurse, answer and make telephone calls, greet visitors and direct traffic, the head nurse will have time to spend with and in the interest of patients. How will she use this time? This is a very important question and it must be answered, or measures taken to free the head nurse's time will serve no useful purpose. The wise nursing administrator will foresee the need to help head nurses plan ways to use the time productively. It is very easy to let the extra minutes drift away, not to use them purposefully. Head nurses who for years have had no time to spend with patients frequently have lost the art of determining patients' needs and would find conferences or classes on interviewing beneficial. Likewise, under the leadership of the department administrator the head nurses as a group will find it rewarding to think through ways they can use their time to improve patient care (see Part 2).

SUMMARY

In this chapter the activities which go on in the patient care division have been considered and it can be seen that the head nurse has primary responsibility for most of them. The exceptions are medical care, dietary service, and housekeeping, and for these the head nurse shares responsibility. Not only have the activities of the head nurse increased in number and complexity during the past several years, but, as a result of this, the problems related to her dual responsibility—as representative of hospital administration and deputy of the physician—have been compounded. The head nurse, unless she has a secretary or clerk, spends most of her time in unit administration, traffic control, and coordination of both unit and patient care activities. Almost no time is left for nursing.

The head nurse of an active division will continue to have problems unless there is a change in organization of the division. However, since this change is not likely to come soon in most hospitals, palliative measures need to be taken to lighten the burden of the head nurse. Because nursing is the area which suffers most as a result of increased pressure, leadership by the nursing service administrator is needed to set attainable goals for nursing care and to establish priorities to guide the head nurse when conflicts in interest, which she must mediate, arise. The director of nursing must also take responsibility for convincing the administrator and, if necessary, the hospital board that if there is to be improvement in nursing care, the head nurse must have help, that competent secretarial assistance during days and evenings is part of the answer to the problem. Provisions must also be made to give the head nurse help in learning ways to utilize the released time for the benefit of patients.

In the next chapter, ideas for a new and more satisfying role for the head nurse will be presented together with the changes in organization which will be needed to bring about role change.

QUESTIONS FOR DISCUSSION

1. If the doctor and the head nurse believe a patient's welfare may be enhanced if his dog is permitted to visit him in the hospital, who in the institution makes the decision that this may happen? Is it enough for the doctor to write an order? Is a doctor's order necessary? If you were the head nurse how would you be expected to handle the situation in your hospital? Do you believe this is the best way to handle the patient's need? If not, how do you think the policy should be changed? What authority should the head nurse have in the matter? What should be the role of the department administrator? the nursing service director?
2. If the diet trays in your hospital are carried to patients by dietary aides do you approve of the system? Why? How could dietary service to patients in your hospital be improved? What responsibility does the head nurse have for improving it?

3. If your hospital already employs competent secretarial help for the nursing divisions what further activities now performed by head nurses would you not be willing to turn over to the secretary? Would this change give the head nurse more time for nursing care administration?

EXERCISES

1. Write your philosophy of nursing.
2. Prepare criteria for the evaluation of nursing care for a particular group of patients on your division, for example, patients with hemiplegia, mastectomy, or loss of hearing.
3. Recall or observe situations when the head nurse had to make a decision between following a doctor's request and adhering to hospital policy. Which way did she decide? What was the effect on the patient and others concerned? How would you have handled the situation? Where did priority lie in the head nurse's decision? in yours?
4. It is 3:00 PM. You, the head nurse, are due off at 3:30 PM. You cannot work late for you must make a plane. A patient has just been admitted in shock with a bleeding peptic ulcer (no intensive care unit in your hospital), a staff nurse is with him; the evening nurse has come on early to get the report and is waiting; a private physician is waiting to talk with you about plans for one of his patients who is going home; you have not counted the narcotics. What are the priorities for the head nurse in this situation?

REFERENCES

Anderson, Ruth M. Activity preferences and leadership behavior of head nurses: Part 1, Nurs. Res. Vol. 13 (Summer 1964), pp. 239-243.
Head nurses who preferred nursing care activities to personnel activities or coordinating activities were considered by their "subordinates" to be better leaders. This is interesting for in the study it had been otherwise hypothesized. The researcher gives a possible explanation.
Part II of this study (Vol. 13, Fall 1964, pp. 333-337) showed that the supervisors rated as the best leaders those head nurses who preferred coordinating activities. Thus: "—there is a decided difference in value judgments between the three levels in nursing hierarchy."

Argyris, Chris. Interpersonal Competence and Organizational Effectiveness, Homewood, Ill., The Dorsey Press Inc., Richard D. Irwin, Inc., pp. 15-27.

In order to understand interpersonal competence it is necessary to examine the nature of interpersonal relationships. The point of view of some scholars conducting research on interpersonal relationships is summarized here.

Bandman, Elsie, Wolpin, Sheila, and Rehm, Dorothy. The patient-relations nurse coordinator, Amer. J. Nurs., Vol. 64 (September 1964), pp. 133-135.
The nurse coordinator cuts across department lines and develops vertical as well as horizontal communications with and on behalf of the patient.

Barnes, Elizabeth. People in Hospital, London, Macmillan and Co. Ltd., 1961, Chapter 6, pp. 69-84.
Need for coordination in the care of patients given by all personnel, including paramedical workers, and ways to achieve it.

Cherescavich, Gertrude. The expanding role of the professional nurse in a hospital, Nurs. Forum, Vol. 3 (No. 4, 1964), pp. 8-20.
A nurse administrator describes the new role of the professional nurse as she sees her and suggests that the functions of the hospital school prepared nurse might be limited to caring for the patient's "living needs," ward management, and coordinating activities.

Donovan, Helen M. Determining priorities of nursing care, Nurs. Outlook, Vol. 11 (January 1963), pp. 44-45.
Many possibilities for setting priorities are listed. They must be determined in terms of the goal of nursing.

Erickson, Florence. The need for a specialist in modern pediatric nursing, Nurs. Forum, Vol. 4 (No. 4, 1965), pp. 24-31.
The modern pediatric nurse needs an understanding of child development and an ability to support the child and his parents. "She stands between child and hospital environment, interpreting to other disciplines how much each child can tolerate and the timing of additional stresses."

Hershey, Nathan. Question that drug order!—the court lays down the law, Amer. J. Nurs., Vol. 63 (January 1963), pp. 96-97.
A nurse was found guilty of negligence by the court for failure to question the prescribing physician about a drug order which she thought too large.

Hoffman, Frank O. How to promote right people right way, Mod. Hosp., Vol. 105 (October 1965), pp. 124-126.
Superior nurses are usually rewarded by promotion to supervisor with a salary increase whereas the nurse may have no supervisory skills. The writer suggests that 1) movement into supervision be considered a reassignment rather than a promotion; 2) supervisory skills be determined through trial tasks before appointment is made; 3) the salary scale for superior nurses be commensurate with that of supervisors.

Irwin, Patricia. The doctors are on our side now!, R.N., Vol. 29 (March 1963), pp. 69-72.
A supervisor (former head nurse) helped improve doctor-nurse relationships through trying to understand the house staff's problems.

Johnson, Betty Sue, and Campbell, Emily B. It's time to be realistic about the work load, Amer. J. Nurs., Vol. 66 (June 1966), pp. 1282-1285.
The authors suggest that it is often not possible to give individualized patient care and that the head nurse must decide at each period when such care can be given and when it must be routinized to accomplish even the necessities.

MacLeod, A. Isobel. The future role of nursing, Canad. Nurse, Vol. 61 (August 1965), pp. 611-613.

The summary of this article expresses well the trend in current thinking among nurse leaders.

Malone, Mary, Berkowitz, Norman H., and Klein, Malcolm W. Interpersonal conflict in the outpatient department. Reprinted from Am. J. Nursing, Vol. 62 (March 1962) in Skipper, James K. and Leonard, Robert C. Social Interaction and Patient Care, Philadelphia, J. B. Lippincott Company, 1965, pp. 356-365.
A study of nursing in the outpatient department showed that nurses are "rewarded" by both doctors and nursing supervisors for their administrative efficiency —not for teaching patients. Nurses will teach only if they are expected to do so, if their responsibility for admiistration is removed, and if institutional procedure is changed so that no patient leaves the clinic without first seeing a nurse.

Malone, Mary F. The dilemma of a professional in a bureaucracy, Nurs. Forum, Vol. 3 (No. 4, 1964), pp. 36-60.
The hospital is a bureaucracy of which nursing service administration is a part. "The individual nurse . . . stands at the bottom of three lines of authority . . . one stemming from administration, one from physicians, and one from the nursing department."

Mauksch, Hans O. The nurse: coordinator of patient care. In Social Interaction and Patient Care, Skipper, J. K. Jr., and Leonard, R. C., eds. Philadelphia, The J. B. Lippincott Company, 1965, pp. 251-265.
The patient care unit of which the head nurse is in charge has responsibility for continuity of time, space and function, for coordination within both the "care" and the "cure" structure and between the "care" and the "cure" structures.
The need for change in the head nurse role is very clear though not explicitly stated.

———— The organizational context of nursing practice. In The Nursing Profession: five sociological essays, Davis, F., ed. New York, John Wiley and Sons, Inc. 1966, pp. 109-137.
One of the most penetrating analyses yet made of the role of the head nurse, and discussion of the effect of the institution of a ward manager system.

Nursing service and nursing care, Nurs. Outlook, Vol. 10 (April 1962), p. 231.
An editorial describing the difference between nursing service and nursing care and questioning whether patient care services should be the responsibility of nursing.

Revans, R. W. Hospital internal communications, Part I, Keeping the recruits, Nurs. Times, Vol. 61 (August 6, 1965), pp. 1085-1086. Part II, Organic health and social vigour, Vol. 61 (August 13, 1965), pp. 1105-1106.
In hospitals from which 50 percent of the students withdrew for their own personal reasons the ward sisters' average length of stay was less than three years; where student attrition was only 10 percent, the average ward sister's stay was eight years. Is it not time to consider the places of work as possible causes for staff turnover?

Schufreider, Leonard A. A hospital fire safety program, Nurs. Outlook, Vol. 12 (January 1964), pp. 36-37.
A hospital safety program can prevent fires which may be costly in human life and in property.

Schulman, Sam. Basic fundamental roles in nursing: Mother surrogate and healer. In Patients, Physicians and Illness, Jaco, E. Gartly, ed., Glencoe, Ill., The Free Press, 1960, No. 54, pp. 528-537.
Traces the role of the nurse historically and decries what he considers to be the trend toward the nurse becoming the "healer" and nonprofessionals the "mother surrogates." The latter will still be nursing though done by others than the nurse.

Shetland, Margaret L. Teaching and learning in nursing, Amer. J. Nurs., Vol. 65 (September 1965) pp. 112-116.
A stimulating presentation of the writer's philosophy of nursing and teaching. Filled with helpful illustrations that provide challenge for even the most experienced teacher.

Snook, Irving D., Jr. Noise that annoys, Nurs. Outlook, Vol. 12 (July 1964), pp. 33-35.
Sources and effects of hospital noise and ways to curtail it.

Strauss, Anselm. The structure and ideology of American nursing: an interpretation. In The Nursing Profession: five sociological essays, Davis, F., ed. New York, John Wiley and Sons, Inc., 1966, pp. 60-108.
Changes in organization of nursing service will be "feeble" until the medical school faculty is convinced of the need for drastic change. Clinical innovation in nursing should be a deliberately guided process and research an institutionalized aspect of nursing. Research should be carried out in the hospital, not in the university, and should be in clinical nursing.

Stryker, Ruth P. Hospital study leads to vocational program, Nurs. Outlook, Vol. 14 (August 1966), pp. 43-44.
A study of the activities of the ward manager, ward secretary, and head nurse on two wards showed that the secretary did the major part of the managing. The manager by spending most of her time transcribing orders released the head nurse for more patient contact. A vocational school is now training secretaries.

————— What? no head nurse?, Nurs. Outlook, Vol. 14 (November 1966), pp. 36-37.
The head nurse in the situation described was replaced by two coordinators, one for each 24 patients. All unit administration was removed from nursing. Nursing personnel remain away from the nurses' station except for charting.

Ward sister's role in teaching hospitals: recommendations of Scottish Committee, Nurs. Mirror, Vol. 122 (July 3, 1966), p. 205.
Ward sisters (head nurses) are responsible for seeing that patients are not exploited for teaching purposes, according to this committee. Illustrations of need for nurse action are given.

chapter 6

A NEW ROLE FOR THE HEAD NURSE

In the preceding chapter, measures which would give the head nurse more time for nursing responsibilities within the present structure were suggested. It is probable that in the near future most hospitals will provide this type of relief for their head nurses. Many, however, will not wish or be able very soon to effect organizational changes which will make possible a new role for the head nurse. Indeed many nurses consider change in unit organization unnecessary, believing the head nurse should retain responsibility for management and coordination of the total system and be given whatever help she needs to do the work. Some hospitals which subscribe to this philosophy have gone a long way in relieving the head nurse of non-nursing functions. In addition to centralizing administrative activities (See Chapter 2) a secretary or unit manager has been assigned to the division to assist the head nurse with clerical and management duties. The unit manager is responsible either to the head nurse or to the central nursing administration. In the latter case he is a peer of the head nurse but her role may or may not be changed as a result of the manager's appointment. If the head nurse has to fill the gap when a disruption in unit management occurs, it is obvious that she retains some degree of responsibility for unit services, that her time is not completely free for nursing activities.

Despite the belief of some individuals that the head nurse should continue to be responsible for administration of the unit, an increasing number of nurse leaders foresee a major change in the organization of the patient care division wherein the management and coordination of unit functions will be assumed by hospital administration. Under this arrangement, unit management is a distinct department of hospital administration. It leaves to nursing the administration of nursing care and the coordination of patient care. Head nurse and unit manager are peers working side by side, with the manager assuming a great many of the functions which have always been associated with the head nurse role and which have in large part accounted for her status. The danger inherent in this pattern is that it might easily result in discontinuity of authority.[1] The system could break down if rela-

---

[1] Mauksch, *op. cit.,* p. 133.

94

tionships between head nurse and unit manager were not harmonious. Nevertheless division of responsibility along this line has been successfully made in some hospitals. At the same time in these places a new role for the head nurse has been created. The role varies from institution to institution but in each the head nurse has limited responsibility for unit functioning and greater responsibility for nursing care administration than the head nurse has customarily been able to assume. So different is the new role that in some hospitals the head nurse has been given a new title—senior nurse, senior team leader, service team leader, to name a few. Nurse administrators in none of these situations appear to believe that the best organizational arrangement has as yet been found. Although each has a vision of the roles of the head nurse and unit manager and of their relationship to one another, for various reasons, it has not been possible thus far to effect all the necessary changes.

It must be realized that no one head nurse role can be said to be "right" or "best." Different concepts need to be developed, tested, and evaluated. For purposes of discussion, however, the writer will present one concept of a new head nurse role and a model for the organization of a nursing care division in which the head nurse could effectively play this role. Observation of and conferences with head nurses, discussion with nursing service and departmental administrators and other colleagues, extensive reading together with experience in nursing service administration and in teaching, form the basis for this concept.

The head nurse as conceived is the administrator of nursing and of delegated medical care, partner of the physician and other members of the health team, coordinator of patient care, guardian of the patient's total welfare, staff counselor, supervisor and teacher, clinical practitioner, and investigator. Responsibilities in the first four areas are seen as relatively constant but the amount and kind of head nurse involvement in nursing practice, investigation, and supervision depends upon the degree of illness and number of patients for whom she is responsible and upon the quality of her staff. The head nurse as her role is visualized has full responsibility for the nursing care of a limited number of patients—perhaps 12 to 15— with a permanent 24 hour staff to assist her. She is autonomous in providing nursing care for her patients in the same way the attending physician or resident is autonomous in prescribing medical care. This means the head nurse knows each patient well through personal contact.

In addition to planning and administering nursing care for her group the head nurse gives care to selected patients. This she does for a number of reasons. *First,* the patient may be having special problems which require a highly skilled nurse practitioner for their diagnosis or alleviation. *Second,* by giving care to such patients the head nurse demonstrates quality nursing and is in a good position to counsel and supervise the staff. *Third,* by continuing to practice nursing the head nurse has opportunity to retain and further develop all facets of her nursing skill. *Fourth,* in nursing practice the head nurse is in a position to test ideas, to experiment with new ways of giving care and to carry out systematic nursing studies.

In her new role the head nurse and the doctor enjoy a close collaborative relationship, sharing information, conferring with patients, consulting other professional personnel when necessary, planning, and making decisions. Mutual trust and respect develop and a real partnership with all its interdependencies grows up between physician and head nurse. The doctor leaves many decisions regarding patient care to the head nurse's judgment. Fully cognizant of the therapeutic plan and expected results, the head nurse coordinates professional care, sees that all aspects of the medical and nursing regimen are integrated.

The nature of the head nurse's responsibilities necessitates her being free, not bound by a specific time schedule yet available for consultation at all times and on the division when needed. She has access to an experienced nurse to whom she may turn for consultation on nursing care, staff problems, or anything which pertains to the head nurse's responsibilities.[2] Decisions, however, are for the head nurse to make and she is legally and morally accountable for them.

The head nurse is employed by the nursing service administrator in consultation with a representative of hospital administration and the medical service chiefs with whom the head nurse will be collaborating. The head nurse is responsible to these persons for ethical practice and for results, that is, for good patient care, not for the manner in which she functions. General standards of conduct are established by the head nurses as a group and are enforced by the weight of peer group opinion.

The head nurse employs her own staff using the personnel department for recruitment and screening. By selecting the nurses and aides who will work with her she assumes responsibility for the care they give to patients.

In order that the head nurse may play this role, management of other services related to patient care is assumed by hospital administration. A unit manager, better called a unit director, is responsible for one or more patient care divisions. Prepared in hospital administration, he functions as

[2] The consultant might be the nursing service administrator, one of her associates, or a department administrator, depending on the size of the hospital. It is important that she be well versed in nursing and an able practitioner. Her responsibilities in addition to consultation include leadership in establishing and upholding standards for nursing care, development of head nurses, and, if she is also the director of nursing, liaison with hospital administration.

a junior executive starting at the unit level on his journey to top level posts. His position gives him status and incentive since it leads to advancement in his chosen career. The unit director coordinates with medicine and nursing the various patient care services,[3] and supervises the service personnel assigned to the division. A conceptual model depicting this administrative role is described in an unpublished document.[4] By permission the description and the organizational chart (Fig. 6) are reprinted here.

In essence, the preliminary conceptual model involved the centralization of responsibility for all inpatient services in the unit director. He would be the key figure, answering directly to administration of the institution, responsible for the coordination of all patient care activities on his unit. These would include nursing care, dietary, housekeeping, clerical, and supply and maintenance functions. Department heads would no longer supervise patient floor personnel directly; they would be utilized only as policy and consulting staffs, as can be seen in the accompanying diagram. The model, however, failed to establish a clear relationship between unit director and the medical staff; further study in this area is indicated.

In this model it is to be noted that while dietary, housekeeping, and nursing personnel assigned to the division are responsible to the unit director, no member of the medical staff has any direct relationship to him. It may be possible in this plan for the unit director, as deputy of the hospital administrator, to assume some of the administrator's responsibility for enforcing policies made by the medical staff and hospital board.

If the head nurse role which has been envisaged is considered in the light of this conceptual model of unit organization, a discrepancy will be noted, for the head nurse (unit chief nurse) in the model is in a different relationship to the unit director than is the doctor. This difference does not exist as the new head nurse role is pictured. If the concept of the head nurse and the model of the unit were to be coordinated either the head nurse, because she is visualized as having the same kind of professional autonomy enjoyed by the physician, would be removed from the organizational chart and be considered a part of an overall nursing staff, or the chart would show that both medicine and nursing have a responsibility to hospital administration for adhering to hospital policy. Physicians as well as the head nurse would appear in the line organization. See Figure 7

[3] Note that there is a difference between coordination of *patient care* and coordination of *patient care services*. The former is concerned with fitting together the various parts of the patient's care and assuming responsibility for the whole. The latter pertains to activities performed on the division by many departments and involves fitting these together so that administration functions smoothly, thereby benefiting patients.

[4] John D. Thompson and Barbara J. Lee. Progress report on unit manager system, New Haven, Department of Epidemiology and Public Health, Yale University School of Medicine, under U.S.P.H.S. Grant No. C.H.00037, 1963. Unpublished.

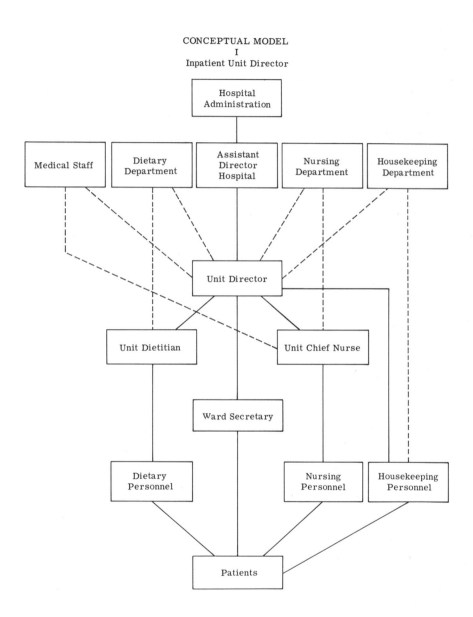

Fig. 6. Conceptual Model I—Inpatient Unit Director. Organizational pattern of a nursing care division in which the unit director is responsible for all services except the medical service. (Courtesy Thompson and Lee, *Ibid.*)

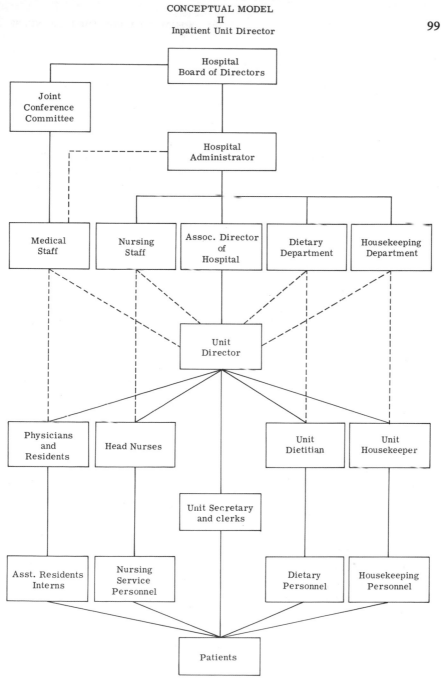

Fig. 7. Conceptual Model II—Inpatient Unit Director. Organization of patient care division modeled after Thompson and Lee's design (Figure 6) but with the unit director responsible for administration of all services. Solid lines show administrative relationships; dotted lines, advisory relationships; collaborative professional relationships are not shown.

which represents the second view. This arrangement substitutes the unit director as the line representative of hospital administration. The unit director instead of the head nurse acts as policeman in carrying out policy. Hospital policy as we have seen (Chapter 2) is established by the hospital board on recommendation of the medical staff. Although chiefs of staff and attending physicians might not be willing to accept this organizational plan for themselves it is possible they might be willing to do so for the resident and visiting staff.

FUNCTIONING OF THE REORGANIZED
PATIENT CARE DIVISION

In summary, responsibilities associated with the new head nurse role have been designated as administration of nursing care, coordination of patient care, nursing practice, scientific investigation, supervision, counselling and teaching. The unit director's role on the other hand is that of representative of hospital administration, administrator and coordinator of patient care services, supervisor of clerical, dietary and housekeeping personnel. The unit director may also be involved in development of his staff and in research.

In the unit organization scheme depicted (Fig. 7), activities are decentralized and the unit director placed in charge of all patient care services. The unit is thus administered as a small hospital within a large one with all the advantages of both. The head nurse and doctors are responsible to the unit director for abiding by the policies of the institution and for providing high quality professional care. The director does not determine what this quality shall be, but when he has doubts he has recourse through the hospital administrator to the medical staff and the nursing service administrator. The medical staff has ways of judging its members (through medical audit, for example). Although nursing has done only a little toward evaluation of its own practice some steps have been taken in this direction.[5]

The Unit Staff

It is suggested that the unit director be responsible for one to four patient care divisions totalling approximately sixty to seventy-five beds; that

[5] Maria C. Phaneuf. The nursing audit for evaluation of patient care, *Nurs. Outlook*, Vol. 14 (June 1966), pp. 51-54.

four to six head nurses have responsibility for the nursing care of the patients assigned to these units. The unit director would have one dietitian and perhaps a unit housekeeper in charge of these services. A 60 to 65 bed division needs a minimum of one secretary and one clerk during the day, a secretary and a clerk, or two clerks, during the evening, and one clerk at night. This number may not prove adequate and larger divisions undoubtedly will need more personnel. Demands of medicare have already enormously increased the clerical load on the divisions. On the other hand, use of the computer can be expected in the next few years to reduce the number of clerks which will be required. Clerical work of all kinds is exceedingly important from the point of view of patient care, unit and hospital administration. There should be enough clerical personnel to handle the exacting work safely and efficiently, but not so many persons that there are periods of inactivity.

Functions of the secretarial staff. The secretary assists the unit director and handles many administrative matters. Clerks usually work under the immediate supervision of the secretary but are responsible to the unit director. Duties are specifically delegated so that each person knows what is entailed in the job to which she is assigned.

The secretary with the help of the clerks receives and makes telephone calls and handles all clerical work. Written reports, work sheets, and requisitions are prepared, charts made up and closed, time and assignment sheets for nursing personnel made out according to a master plan. In addition, the secretary handles doctors' orders as they are received. She transmits them to other departments according to procedure, makes schedules of x-rays and operations, orders medications and diets, transcribes orders to the nursing cardex, and makes out medicine tickets if such is the procedure of the institution. Safeguards are established to prevent orders being carried out before the transcriptions have been checked and initialed by the head nurse. The cardex which contains a new order is flagged until the head nurse has approved it. Medicine tickets are put in a special slot for new unchecked cards or may be left clipped to the cardex. The system must be safe and sure. Never should the system of checking be permitted to break down, no matter how competent the secretary, because, regardless of her intelligence, her knowledge of medicine and nursing is highly limited.

The secretary or one of the clerks is always present at the central desk to greet and assist individuals who visit the unit. The all-important social amenities are her responsibility. She meets and greets the new patient and his family, calls and introduces the nurse who will admit him. She welcomes visitors, answers their questions, directs them to patients, greets doctors, and informs the head nurse of their presence. She receives representatives from other departments and special therapists. If the patient is to be administered an electrocardiogram, infusion, or special treatment, the patient's nurse is notified.

The individual at the central desk is not only a host but is a director of traffic. These should be her primary functions for upon her rests the responsibility for making patients, families, and visitors of all kinds feel that they and their needs are important and that their comfort, satisfaction, and time are of concern to the hospital. Needless to say, the person at the desk must be gracious, warm, helpful, as well as clear headed. In a very large active division, two or three hours at the desk is sufficient without a change in activity. Likewise, only if the responsibilities as host can be handled promptly and with serenity should the clerk be given additional duties such as answering the telephone or the intercom.

Responsibilities of the unit dietitian and unit housekeeper. The unit dietitian is in charge of the diet aides, but all are under the jurisdiction of the unit director. Housekeeping personnel assigned to the division may be supervised by the director if the division is too small to warrant a unit housekeeper.[6] Both dietary and housekeeping workers are trained by the central departments.

Composition of the Nursing Staff

The number of nurses and aides needed on the head nurse's staff, in general, is dependent on the amount and type of nursing and medical care the patients require. However, a few basic assumptions can be made when determining size and composition of the group. *First,* it is essential that each head nurse have a highly competent professional nurse on her staff. This nurse is appointed to a specific position and is responsible to the head nurse for handling the details of nursing care management and coordination. Having someone in this role is necessary in order that the head nurse may be free to spend uninterrupted time with a troubled patient or family, in conference with a physician, or in meeting with other head nurses. In other words although the head nurse is responsible for the nursing care of a group of patients, her constant presence on the division is precluded by her need for freedom to withdraw at times from the mainstream of activity. The head nurse, therefore, must have a strong assistant. Various titles have

[6] An alternative arrangement which has some advantages is the substitution of a general manager for the unit housekeeper. Responsible to this person is a group of workers who are assigned by him as needed to do housekeeping chores, set and carry diet trays, and the like. The general manager also handles all matters pertaining to supplies and equipment.

been given this nurse, one of the most appropriate being "service team leader." Her functions and the extent of her responsibility need to be stipulated. This nurse may be on call some nights in place of the head nurse although the latter is the final resource when she is available.

Second, at least one and usually more professional nurses are present and responsible for the patients every hour of every day. The need for stability and continuity in staff will be considered in Chapter 8.

Third, the number of practical nurses and aides depends in part upon the policy of the institution in regard to the functions of these groups (see Chapter 12).

Responsibilities of the Unit Director in the Reorganized Patient Care Division

Supervision. Just as the head nurse is responsible for patient care 24 hours a day, seven days a week, so is the unit director responsible for the administration of the unit at all times, and should be available when needed. Where he has qualified persons in charge as in nursing, medicine, and diet service, the unit director's supervision is more in the nature of administrative evaluation. On the other hand, he is immediately responsible for supervising the secretary, sometimes the clerks, and often the housekeeping staff.

Administration and coordination of patient care services. The objective of the unit director, in the envisaged organization of the patient care division, is to keep the activities functioning smoothly in order that medical and nursing care will be facilitated, not impeded. Equipment, linen, drugs, supplies of all kinds must be in ample quantity and ready for use at all times. So too must work space be kept clean and in order. If these goals are to be achieved, not only must there be a routine time for their accomplishment, but specific procedures for taking inventory, ordering, cleaning and the like must be devised, taught, and delegated, the work supervised and evaluated.

To help with these management functions, the unit director sometimes employs a unit helper. Stationed in the treatment or utility room, the helper keeps these units in order. She strips treatment trays as the nursing personnel bring them in, caring for used equipment and waste according to hospital procedure. The unit director is notified if supplies are not holding out. Unless provision of linen and other necessities is handled in entirety by the issuing department, the unit helper assists the director with preparation of daily and weekly requisitions. She washes, sterilizes, or sanitizes the bedside equipment on the discharge of patients unless this is the responsibility of the housekeeping department. Collecting, washing, and refilling water pitchers may be a task assigned to the unit helper. If it seems advisable to limit the number of individuals who go into the patient's room, the trays of fresh water may be obtained from a cart in the hall by the patient's own nurse or aide. It is probable that if there is enough to be done by a person in this position during the day period, there is also a need for the same type of service in the evening when there are fewer nurses. Each institution needs to determine its own requirements through activity studies.

The unit director, with the help of his clerical staff coordinates the work and movements of representatives of other departments. Laboratory reports and operative permits are assured for patients going to surgery. (The head nurse or doctor obtains the latter unless this is routinely done in the admitting office.) Discharge orders are procured, outdated narcotic orders called to the physician's attention. Plumbers and electricians come when needed and, except in an emergency, at a time when they will not interfere with patients' rest or the work of the professional staff. Nurses are informed of patient appointments in other departments so they may have their patients ready; the orderly who calls for the patient is told where to find him, a nurse informed of his arrival. The whereabouts of patients is known at all times through some kind of recording device. Addressograph plates may be flagged with different colors to indicate the department to which the patient has gone. Ambulatory patients may be asked to post their names when they leave the floor using a color code to indicate their location. The unit director sees that messages are delivered and keeps the machinery running smoothly. He makes no decisions relative to patient care; he notifies the head nurse of problems and irregularities which will affect patient welfare.

The unit director is responsible for the division budget, for employment of secretaries, clerks, and unit helpers. If the hospital has a program of systems management, the unit director helps with studies and recommends changes. He constantly strives to improve the administration of the unit, working closely with nurses and other personnel to solve problems of coordination and management.

Responsibilities of the Head Nurse in the Conceived Role

How does the head nurse operate in the role pictured? The way in which she carries her responsibility will be described in relation, first, to the unit director, second, to the patient, third, to her nursing staff, and, fourth, to the physician.

Responsibility in relation to the unit director. The head nurse must have a clear concept of her role and relationships and fully accept them. Fortunately, it is not as difficult to accept an entirely new role as it is merely to delegate a large number of her former responsibilities to a non-nurse. Under no circumstances must the head nurse usurp responsibilities that are no longer hers. In the beginning—right after role changes have been instituted—there will be minor delays because new appointees are not yet wholly familiar with routines. The head nurse will not be helpful if she steps in and performs a task herself or if she appears critical. This does not mean she fails to be helpful, but few persons like to have others perform their functions without first determining whether assistance is desired. In general, the sooner the head nurse divorces herself from activities which were formerly hers, the easier it is for all. Cooperation between the head nurse and unit director are essential to the success of the system. This relationship must stem from consideration, loyalty, and respect for one another. Once the two positions are established with this foundation, neither can function adequately without the other.

Responsibility in relation to the patient. The head nurse's responsibility for patient care administration will be discussed in detail in Part 2. Here we shall give an overview of the way in which she carries out her responsibility to the patient. It is important for her to know each patient sufficiently well to provide individualized care according to his needs as he sees them, as the doctor sees them, and as she, the nurse, sees them. The patient has needs affecting his immediate situation which he alone perceives. He also has needs which the doctor and nurse know about but he does not. It is up to the head nurse to discover those known only to the patient, to meet them when possible if the patient desires it, and to make the physician and members of the nursing staff aware of them if this seems advisable. It is also the head nurse's responsibility to help the patient understand health requirements, for example adhering to a special diet. It is one thing for the patient to understand a medical need, another to accept and act upon it. The head nurse, therefore, also tries to help the patient express the reason for his not accepting the prescription designed to meet the need.

To get acquainted with patients and establish a close relationship the head nurse interviews each one on admission. In addition to gathering information about his personal habits, interests, and family relationships which will help in formulation of a plan for his care, the head nurse attempts to find out how the patient feels about being in the hospital. She identifies major concerns and relieves them in so far as possible by clearing up misconceptions and letting the patient know what to expect. She learns the things of special importance to the patient and works out with him and his family ways in which these needs can be met. The head nurse observes the patient's clinical condition, his physical symptoms, any handicaps such as impaired sight and the adjustment he has made to them. Through direct contact with the patient the head nurse has knowledge of his personal needs and clinical state. This knowledge helps her determine who on the staff is capable of caring for the patient.[7] Daily, and in some instances much more frequently, the patient's condition is reassessed. As the head nurse deems necessary, changes are made in his plan for care and in the individual assigned to provide it.

Some patients appear to have problems which make acceptance of medical or nursing care difficult. With them the head nurse may need a longer contact than that provided by the initial interview and daily or twice daily rounds. Physical ministration increases the nurse's time with the patient. It also conveys her concern, thereby helping the patient decide whether he can safely reveal to her his doubts and fears. The head nurse, therefore, regularly assigns herself to care for patients who are having special problems. Ministering to a patient will give her opportunity to acquaint herself with his physical condition, to learn the causes of his behavior, to discover needs that are not being met, to allay unnecessary anxiety. By carrying a patient assignment the head nurse is also able to experiment with various nursing measures and to observe the effect of different approaches to the patient. Through giving care the head nurse is in a good position to interpret the patient's behavior and his needs to the staff and to guide them in establishing a plan for his care. Under the leadership of the head nurse, daily nursing staff conferences are held to share information, evaluate nursing care, and makes changes in plans for care.

Perhaps one of the most important services performed by the head nurse is that of guarding the patient's total welfare. This is more than mere coordination of patient care although the latter is involved. With all the different individuals and groups performing tasks at the patient's bedside, someone is needed to serve as the coordinating link between the various elements of his care, and to see that a unified therapeutic plan is developed. Someone is needed to interpret to and for the patient. Someone is needed to protect the patient from fatigue, interruption, boredom, the effects of unfavorable environment and exploitation. Noise including use of radio and television, visitors, prolonged treatments, all can sap vital energy. Frequent interruption of rest or meals for medications, tests, treatments and for nursing care are frustrating and annoying to some patients.

[7] Edmund Pellegrino. The changing role of the professional nurse in the hospital, *Hospitals,* Vol. 35 (December 16, 1961), pp. 56-62.

It is not possible to time perfectly every aspect of patient care when so many departments and services participate in it. However, the head nurse should consolidate and coordinate the elements of care so far as this is possible. Sometimes all that is necessary is a little thought and effort.

Some patients are bored with hospital life and should have help to find recreational outlets. (See Chapter 3.) Not only may the environment fail to provide interest but it may interfere with the patient's well-being in other ways. Inadequate light for reading, poor ventilation, drafts, inaccessible equipment can have ill effects. Improperly cleaned equipment, untidy surroundings, general disorder are a sure way to lose the confidence of the patient and the public. Broken equipment, matches in the possession of the irresponsible or in the presence of oxygen are positively hazardous. Although care of equipment and maintenance of a clean, orderly environment is the responsibility of the unit director, the head nurse as guardian of the patient's welfare is ever on the alert to make sure patient care is enhanced, and not jeopardized because of neglect, carelessness, or thoughtlessness on the part of anyone.

Many hospitals are involved in education of health personnel and in clinical research. Patients in these institutions expect to participate in the programs and usually appreciate their advantages. However, the patients are seldom in a position to know when educators, students, or researchers are taking advantage of them. An eager young student nurse may so prolong a patient's nursing care that he is worn out, or is upset because his visitors have been kept waiting an excessively long time. A medical student or intern may probe for a vein so many times that the patient has several ruined blood vessels. Many examples could be given, some more serious than these. The patient needs to be protected under such circumstances and someone must assume the responsibility for so doing. That someone in each of these situations is the head nurse. She knows the patient, his condition, alternative actions. She is the person best prepared to speak and act on behalf of the patient and must not shrink from so doing.

The question inevitably arises: With how many patients can the head nurse have sufficient contact to learn their needs? For how many can she provide quality care? The number varies with many factors, including the depth of social, emotional, and physical problems usually experienced by patients and their families as a result of the diagnosis, condition, or type of therapy. Also, the quality and number of the nursing staff, the type and number of medical and paramedical personnel involved in the patients' care, the number and type of medical tests and treatments performed; the type of equipment provided; the way in which procedures are carried out; and the geography of the unit are all determining factors. Exprimentation is necessary to determine the optimum number of patients assigned to one head nurse, but 12 to 15 medical or surgical patients in acute divisions seems a reasonable number to consider. Thus, a thirty bed division would have two "head nurses," a forty bed unit, three "head nurses."

Responsibility in Relation to her staff. The division staff looks to the head nurse for leadership. A generally accepted definition of leadership according to Hagen and Wolff[8] is "the ability to influence the behavior of others in order to accomplish the task of a group or to achieve the goals of a group while, at the same time, maintaining the integrity and morale of the group." The head nurse, accordingly, has two responsibilities or aims as the leader of her staff: *First,* helping them to attain their goal—presumably the best possible care for their patients—and *second,* maintaining their morale and keeping them working together as a unified group. These aims are interdependent. Achievement of one contributes to the achievement of the other.

As leader of her staff, the head nurse assists the group to formulate its objectives and stimulates members to learn and grow. Through her teaching, supervising, and counselling, she keeps staff members challenged. Many of them expect the head nurse to help them function at their best. Good administration contributes to this end, and the head nurse is obligated to adhere to sound administrative practices. (See Chapter 7.) In less tangible ways also the head nurse exerts her leadership. Staff members anticipate that she will help maintain morale by giving encouragement and promoting harmony. They want her to be understanding, kindly, considerate, sincere, and impartial, but they also want her to be firm, to uphold high standards of care, to maintain professional relationships, and to live by the rules with which she expects the staff to comply. In other words, the staff expects the head nurse to be a role model in her personal and professional behavior. They also expect her to be their role model as a practitioner. They believe she should not only be willing to participate in direct patient care but able to demonstrate a particular nursing approach or an unusual procedure.

In addition to being the leader of her staff, the head nurse, in a few hospitals thus far, is also their employer. If the head nurse employs her own staff, she not only becomes accountable for their work but has the corollary responsibility of terminating employment when a staff member's work is not satisfactory. In assuming this responsibility, the head nurse dare not waver for upon her rests the legal obligation to safeguard the wel-

[8] Elizabeth Hagen and Luverne Wolff. *Nursing Leadership Behavior in General Hospitals,* New York, Institute of Research and Service in Nursing Education, Teachers College, Columbia University, 1961, p. 19.

fare of her patients. She is also obligated to protect a staff member from the detrimental outcomes which might result from her own incompetent practice.

Responsibility in relation to the physician. In her new role the head nurse is collaborator and partner of the physician from the chief of staff to the intern. This partnership involves much more than the head nurse having the approval of the medical staff because she gives good care to patients, keeps the doctors informed, is courteous and deferent. Partnership is much more than the doctor saying, "Ask the head nurse" or "What do you think, Miss ———?" or having the doctor tell the head nurse to use her own judgment. In a real partnership a common goal is accepted, each member is an expert in his own field and has a special contribution to make. He is able to speak the language of his partners, understands the nature of their work, and the relationships between all specialties in achieving the goal. He has respect for his partners and appreciates their contributions.

Not many nurses up to the present time have achieved a partnership with the physician. The reason is twofold. The *first* reason, discussed at length earlier in this text (Chapter 2), results from the difference between the doctor's and the nurse's relationship with hospital administration. The *second* factor, the difference in their education, is responsible for a master-handmaid relationship rather than a partnership between physician and nurse. Although this situation has been changing in recent years, many nurses educated at graduate levels are not prepared in clinical nursing, and those who are do not return to the patient's bedside where the partnership with the clinical medical practitioner must be cultivated. The head nurse who fulfills the partnership role is an expert clinical practitioner, a specialist in the field of nursing in which she is functioning. She is thoroughly grounded in the biological, medical, and social sciences, and because she is able to "talk the language of the sciences," she can communicate with the doctor on his level.[9] The head nurse confidently and unhesitatingly raises questions and makes useful contributions in joint medical and nursing conferences and in informal discussions relative to patients. She keeps abreast of the latest medical and nursing research and other developments related to her specialty. When there is a partner relationship, doctor and head nurse have mutual trust and respect; they try to enhance the partner's relationships with others.

The head nurse helps maintain the confidence of the patient in his physician not only because doctors and nurses are helpless unless they work

[9] Pellegrino, *op. cit.*, p. 62.

as a team, but because the patient needs to have faith in his doctor if he is to have the peace of mind needed for recovery. The head nurse, therefore, in no way lowers the confidence of the nurses on her division in the integrity and ability of any member of the medical staff. She assumes the obligation to know that the nursing personnel are building the confidence of the patient in his physician. She recognizes that this is especially necessary when the doctor is not well known to the patient and when the patient is cared for by the house staff. As a rule, patients have great trust in the nurse's judgment. Doubt and question on the part of the nurse can be expressed in her manner as well as in the spoken word. It is just as true, of course, that the doctor, whether intern, resident, attending or private physician, is obligated to do all in his power to maintain the confidence of the patient, his family, and the general public in the head nurse and her staff. When a partnership exists, he realizes that people need to have confidence in the hospital to which they are entrusting their lives. The head nurse represents the hospital to the patient. Insinuations and criticism by doctors of the nurse or the nursing care not only cause fear and concern but lessen the effectiveness of the nurse in her relationship with his patients. Competence and consideration on the part of both nurse and physician go a long way in gaining the other's trust. Trust, in turn, makes complaint and destructive criticism unnecessary.

As in any partnership it is important to differentiate areas of responsibility. The doctor's responsibility is to diagnose disease and to prescribe for the patient; the nurse's to carry out the parts of medical therapy delegated to her by the doctor's orders and to do so safely and intelligently and in a way that will produce the desired effect. The head nurse, however, is primarily responsible for nursing and may need to interpret to the doctor that in this area she determines needs and prescribes care. When she assumes responsibility for care of skin, mouth, and eyes, for moving, positioning, and other nursing measures, the head nurse demonstrates nursing's contribution to the therapeutic plan, as well as to the patient's general comfort and well-being. The doctor comes to take good nursing care for granted and is less tempted to write prescriptions for nursing measures, which some physicians will do when nursing care is inadequate. The physician also depends on the head nurse for accurate clinical observation, reporting and recording of symptoms and results of treatments. Good judgment is expected in the use of p.r.n. medications and in calling the doctor about unusual happenings; in adhering to doctors' prescriptions or, if it seems appropriate, withholding action until she has consulted the physician. In addition to following the doctor's orders, the head nurse has the responsibility to bring about, to the highest possible degree, the patient's physical and mental comfort and thus help create a "therapeutic environment." (This responsibility will be fully considered in Part 2.)

A sociological study by Johnson and Martin compares the roles of the doctor and nurse.[10] The authors point out that because the doctor prescribes tests and treatments he is responsible for the things done to the patient, things that sometimes hurt and frighten. These activities of the doctor are tension-producing to the patient even when they are understood. The nurse, on the other hand, comforts, explains, reassures, supports, and ministers to the patient's physical needs. Even though she performs technical procedures which are painful or unpleasant, she shows by her attitude that she cares. The nurse's physical ministrations to the patient are primarily significant as a reflection of her attitudes toward him. "By caring for the patient she shows that she cares about him."[11] This is not to say that the doctor does not care or try to prevent stress, but due to the nature of the two roles the nurse is in a better position to comfort.

Thus, according to the study, patient care activities of the doctor and the nurse complement one another. Each is a specialist in his own right. The nurse's role is that of an expert in relieving tensions produced by the doctor in his role as therapist. It is suggested that this role of the nurse, rather than one as technical assistant, will prompt the doctor to accept her as an associate or partner rather than as a handmaiden.

How does a partnership between head nurse and physician function? First, each recognizes that the other has knowledge which will help in understanding the patient. Following the head nurse's admission interview with the patient and the history taking and physical examination by the doctor, the two discuss the physician's plans for diagnostic tests and therapy. The head nurse suggests the nursing emphasis which appears advisable. Together they talk with the patient, bringing him into the planning. Sessions of this kind occur frequently, offering opportunity for the doctor and head nurse to share what they know, to discuss problems, and to confer with the patient about changes in his plan for care. In each instance, the head nurse interprets for the patient who more often than not is unable to do so for himself.

Although the head nurse is in a partnership relationship with every member of the medical staff, the manner in which the doctor and head nurse work together depends upon the position of the physician, that is,

[10] Miriam M. Johnson and Harry W. Martin. A sociological analysis of the nurse's role, *Amer. J. Nurs.*, Vol. 58 (March 1958), pp. 373-377.
[11] *Ibid.*, p. 314.

whether he is a visiting or an attending physician,[12] a member of the house staff, or the chief of service.

The visiting physician may have as few as one patient in the group cared for by the head nurse. The head nurse may have as many as fifteen private doctors with whom to consult. Exchange of information with visiting physicians is on a one to one basis. If the patient's doctor is his family physician, he will know family problems and relationships and the effect of the illness on home life which if shared with the head nurse may help her in understanding the patient's needs. On the other hand, the patient may express fears and worries to the head nurse which he is hesitant to tell his doctor and which may influence the plan for his care. Sharing information is of such importance that the head nurse makes herself available to as many visiting physicians as possible, each day. There are some that she especially needs to see in order to gain or to give information or to discuss plans for the patient's care. For others she leaves a message and sees them that day only if they have need to confer or she is free at the time of their visits. Another nurse gives the doctor a report and whatever assistance he needs. Although the physician likes to have the head nurse accompany him to see his patients and appreciates having the opportunity for a direct report from her, he usually understands that she has obligation to others than himself. He is, therefore, satisfied if he receives his share of her time and can always see her when it is necessary. Under any circumstance the doctor knows the head nurse is fully aware of his patient's needs and that she provides the thread of continuity between all facets of his care.

In contrast to the visiting physicians, members of the resident staff (except surgeons) are on the unit a good share of the day. The head nurse regularly makes rounds with the resident and interns. She has already visited all the patients, usually with a member of her nursing staff, and is ready with a report on each patient. During or following rounds may be the most suitable time for exchange of information on the patient's condition, his reaction to treatment, problems. It is also the best opportunity for making changes in medical orders and plans for care. Perhaps it is with members of the house staff who are learners and who work under very great stress that the head nurse needs to be most aware that she interprets

---

[12] As seen in Chapter 2 the attending physician is responsible for the care of the medically indigent patients. In a teaching hospital he is a member of the medical school faculty and conducts teaching rounds which the head nurse attends when possible. The resident, under the supervision of the attending physician, often carries the immediate responsibility for planning and prescribing medical care for those patients. The head nurse, therefore, except for rounds, frequently has more contact with the resident than with the attending physician.

for the patient and guards his total welfare. In so doing, she calls into play her greatest powers of human understanding and all the interpersonal skill she can muster. She is not only considering the patient but is helping the young intern or resident to become a better doctor.

In a teaching hospital, where house officers are found in large numbers, interchange of ideas is often provided through regular conferences in which other professional groups, such as social workers, special therapists, and the chaplain, participate. Usually the nurses on the staff are encouraged to attend. This team of health workers discusses plans for the patient and problems in their implementation. The resident is the leader of the group. Shared thinking results in a broad plan of action in which many participate.

The house staff of a hospital rotates regularly—residents annually, interns every few months. They cannot expect the routine of the division or program of the nursing staff to be modified for every newcomer. However, the house officer does need to understand the routine and the program, and the way in which he can fit into it.

The unit director and the head nurse plan conferences with new house staff members to work out a cooperative program for medical and nursing care which can be coordinated with patient care services. Unless this is done many young doctors have little appreciation of the problems involved in managing a unit and giving nursing care. They cannot be expected to know these things unless thay have been told or unless they are unusually discerning. It is likewise true that some nurses have little conception of the responsibilities that engage a doctor's time and the problems which he encounters in trying to accomplish his work within a reasonable period of time.

New interns and residents are told of the organization of the patient's day, the times when meals are served, and when rest hours are observed. They need to understand that in so far as possible these hours are not to be interrupted for medical rounds, examinations, treatments, or dressings because the patients should be undisturbed. Outside these periods the doctor decides with the head nurse the best time for medical activities in relation to nursing care and patient comfort. If he cannot conveniently adjust his schedule to nursing and unit activities the division program, if possible, is adjusted. The important point is that understanding and agreement be reached.

When mutual decisions have been made both the medical and nursing groups should cooperate in carrying out their parts of the understanding. If the intern has agreed to notify the head nurse beforehand regarding the treatments he wishes to perform then she is obligated to see that the patient is ready, equipment at hand. If necessary, a nurse is assigned to assist him. Except in emergencies or when a patient's need requires a treatment at that time the house doctor cannot expect the same preparation and assistance if he arrives at an unscheduled hour. Nor should he expect all other activity to be halted in order to assist him at whatever time of day he happens to arrive. On the other hand, the head nurse can hardly expect a busy resident or intern, especially in the surgical or obstetric service, to maintain a rigid schedule. Both will find that cooperation is infinitely easier if they understand one another's problems, if each is reasonable in his demands on the other, and if both keep the best interest of the patient in mind.

The unit director wisely makes it a point to talk over hospital and ward policy with house officers who are new to the service. For example, it is helpful if he is told the policy for writing his orders and for handling emergencies. He should know that the secretary needs to use the patients' charts at certain hours of the day and that at all other times they are available for his use. He should be told the policy in regard to supplies and equipment and the need for economy.

In a teaching hospital the intern carries out many procedures without the help of the nurse. The head nurse or unit director should impress upon him his responsibility for removing equipment to the treatment room after use and for putting nondisposable syringes to soak if they have been used for withdrawing blood. The importance of protecting bedding and floor from soiling should be explained also. When team work exists, no group member adds to another's problems by the manner in which he performs his own tasks.

The third group of physicians with which the head nurse has association is the chiefs of services. There will usually be one or at most two chiefs responsible for the medical care of patients of whose nursing care the head nurse is in charge. When a partnership exists, the chief of service and the head nurse are indispensible to one another. The chief is dependent on the head nurse's intelligent observation based on understanding of normal and pathologic physiology, her perceptiveness of the patient's psychological needs and problems. He counts on her sound judgment in implementing delegated portions of the medical care plan and in providing nursing care which will complement medical care in bringing about optimum results. The chief appreciates especially the head nurse overseeing the patient's care as a whole, and providing continuity in the welter of procedures performed on the patient. He depends on her alertness to any interference with the patient's well being, her ideas for increasing his understanding, satisfaction, and progress. A chief who can rely on the head nurse and her staff for this type of care can rest comfortably in the knowledge that his work is being consistently enhanced, its effectiveness not blocked or reduced by an unknowing nursing staff.

The head nurse in her partnership role has a staunch supporter in the chief of service to whom she has made herself indispensable. He is the final medical authority, and in both regularly scheduled and impromptu conferences the head nurse has opportunity to talk over with him some of her nursing plans which might become controversial. (See example, p. 85.) The chief is, and is likely to remain, the most powerful figure in the institution. The head nurse in working with young house staff members, especially, may need the authority of the chief in safeguarding patients' rights and interests. Without his backing she would at times be powerless, for she would have to depend entirely upon interpersonal relationships and the force of her personality to win her point. Unless the chief recognizes the head nurse's authority in certain defined areas and requires cooperation from visiting physicians and house staff, the idea of a partnership will be nothing but a myth. The success of the new head nurse role thus is dependent, in part, on the chief of service.

IMPLEMENTATION OF THE NEW HEAD NURSE ROLE

Next we need to turn our attention to ways of gaining the support of the chiefs of medical services and of others for a new role for the head nurse. In other words, once this new role has been envisioned how is it to be implemented?

Changes in neither the head nurse role nor in unit organization can be accomplished quickly or easily. Before the hospital attempts any change in these areas, the ground must be carefully laid. Preliminary steps include determination of the quality of care which is desired and ways in which it now falls short, problems causing the shortcomings, conceptualization of unit organization which would solve the problems and of the roles of persons involved. Each of these points has been discussed and may serve as a guide to individual hospitals in making their own studies and decisions suitable to their particular situations. Following this preliminary work in relation to role change, the second step is to gain understanding and acceptance of the new roles. The third step in making changes is to try out the new roles and evaluate results.

Gaining Acceptance of the New Roles

The idea for a new head nurse role will probably come from nursing administration. More than likely the director of nursing will be the one to visualize the new role and promote necessary changes. Very early she will wish to capitalize on the ideas of her associates in the nursing department including head nurses. Likewise in the early stages of the director's thinking, the hospital administrator and other key persons must be involved. The role of the head nurse cannot be changed unless unit organization is modified, and with this the entire hospital is concerned. Key members of the medical staff should be brought into the beginning discussion, and, before any changes are made, chiefs of medical services must concur and be ready to support them wholeheartedly. Without full acceptance by the hospital administrator and the chiefs of medical services the new system is doomed to failure. To quote again from the study of the unit manager system by John Thompson and Barbara Lee:[13]

Basic to success in any project of this sort is the active involvement of key personnel, to begin at the planning stage and continue through each step. Neither administration, nursing, nor medicine can afford to give lip service only—this warning is particularly apt for medicine. . . . among doctors above all, enforcement must come from the head man. Chiefs of staff cannot support the program verbally but look the other way while physicians and house staff fail to carry it through. Heads of the various medical services must not only be in full accord with the new system but recommend it vigorously to subordinates, and be ready to exert force if necessary. Without full support from all three branches of the hospital, medical, nursing, and administrative, a unit manager program might just as well never be attempted, for it cannot succeed.

Experimental Unit

It is often easier to institute change if it is done on an experimental basis. The document quoted above strongly recommends that a project involving the addition of a unit director to the patient care division be undertaken as a research study to determine the effect of the change on the quality of patient care. Measures of quality are needed and when developed should be applied to the care given, both prior to and following the

13 Thompson and Lee, *op. cit.*, pp. 21-22.

institution of change in unit organization and the head nurse role.[14-17] If one nursing department administrator and the medical chief on the service are particularly interested and imaginative, making changes on one or two divisions of that service is advisable provided qualified head nurses are available or can be procured. The head nurse is a key figure in the success of the experiment. She must be in agreement with the concept of the role and have freedom to develop it. A unit director and clerical staff who meet requirements and are clear about their roles and responsibilities are also essential to a successful experiment. Although everything must be in readiness before a beginning is made, details of the unit director's responsibilities may not become clear cut until the experiment is underway. Counsellors for the head nurse and for the unit director are essential.

Procuring Head Nurses for the New Role

Where can enough nurses who are qualified to fill the new head nurse role be found? We have said the head nurse must be an expert nurse practitioner, highly prepared in biological, medical, and social sciences. Also essential are communication and interpersonal skills, dedication to nursing, leadership, and administrative ability. An inquiring mind and interest in scientific investigation are important if the head nurse is to exert influence toward improvement of nursing practice. Do we have nurses so qualified? Yes, some, and more are completing graduate programs every year. Instead of becoming involved in nursing practice, however, they become administrators and teachers. In these capacities it is not infrequent that they very soon lose their nursing expertise. No one will question the need for qualified nurses in teaching and administration but should not the road to both be through service in the head nurse role? Would there not be less need for

[14] Researchers are attempting to develop measures of nursing care. See: Myrtle Kitchell Aydelotte. The use of patient welfare as a criterion measure, *Nurs. Res.*, Vol. 11 (Winter 1962), pp. 10-14.

[15] Robert H. Edgecumbe. How C.A.S.H. helps nurses improve care, *Mod. Hosp.*, Vol. 106 (May 1966), pp. 97-99.

[16] Jean E. Johnson and James M. Dabbs, Jr. Enumeration of active sweat glands: a simple physiological indicator of psychological changes, *Nurs. Res.*, Vol. 16 (Summer 1967), pp. 273-276.

[17] Howard Leventhal and Elizabeth Sharp. Facial expressions as indicators of distress, In *Affect, Cognition, and Personality, Empirical Studies,* Tomkins, Silvan J., and Izard, Carroll E., eds. New York, Springer Publishing Company, Inc., 1965, Chap. 10.

nursing administrators at all levels if the head nurse were the clinical expert she needs to be and were given full responsibility for the nursing of her patients and for coordination of their care? Are not nursing decisions more appropriately made by the nurse who is intimately acquainted with the patient? Is a head nurseship not the most important as well as the most satisfying role for the well-prepared clinical nurse?

If nursing care were of high quality and the opportunity for satisfactory practice greater, would not nurses remain at the bedside? Would not some who have left be attracted to return? Could not a greater number of promising young women and men be attracted to the profession under these circumstances? The shortage of nurses is real, but need it remain so? Would a better utilization of nurse power not help solve the problem? The need for associate nursing directors and department administrators would be less if head nurses were autonomous. Clinical counselors for head nurses would be needed, but their number would not equal the number presently occupying administrative posts in nursing. Teachers must, of course, have sound clinical knowledge and skill. Would present numbers be able to handle an increased enrollment if the head nurse were once more to assume some responsibility for clinical education, if the nursing practice which students witnessed and in which they participated were of excellent quality?

If hospitals decided in the near future to move toward a new head nurse role which demanded the qualifications outlined, are there enough prepared nurses to provide the suggested ratio of one nurse to twelve or fifteen patients? No, but they could be developed. In this, university hospitals and university schools of nursing must take the lead. A few schools throughout the country might develop basic programs for the college graduate. If these were geared to preparing nurse clinicians, their graduates after a brief period of practice should be ready for head nurse positions.[18] No one knows how many college graduates are lost to nursing because at present there is only one school of nursing[19] designed especially for them. Outstanding baccalaureate graduates should be encouraged to have at least one year of carefully planned and guided experience and then to continue their education in clinical nursing. Those who, without special preparation, have already had such experience as staff nurses in hospital or public health agency, as head nurses, department administrators, or assistant directors of nursing need to be strongly urged to return to school. An attractive position as a head nurse for whom an entirely new, richly rewarding role has been

[18] Frances K. Reiter, The clinical nursing approach, *Nurs. Forum,* Vol. 5, No. 1, 1966, pp. 39-44.
[19] The Graduate School of Nursing, New York Medical College, New York, New York.

developed can be held out as a reward. Salaries must be commensurate with preparation, experience, and competency. These the hospital will be better able to afford because fewer high paying nursing administrative posts will be needed. To emphasize the difference between the old and new head nurse roles and to aid in recruitment, many hospitals will consider changing the head nurse's title to one which better describes her new responsibilities.

Another resource for head nurses is the recent graduate of a master's program who may be holding an administrative position in the hospital. If this nurse has not kept up to date she may need to refresh or further develop her clinical competence. Likewise, nurses with advanced clinical preparation who are coming out of graduate programs should be encouraged to become head nurses. If given status and proper remuneration, some may very well wish to continue in that role. Following experience, others will prefer to become administrator-counselors, or teachers. All nurses who are to stay in the mainstream of nursing will find it essential to continue to strengthen their nursing competence through direct patient care. No doctor expects to retain his skill unless he continues to practice medicine. Is there reason to believe a nurse can retain hers without practice? It has been suggested by a nurse leader that each nurse should assume a special interest in one small area of nursing which she would study deeply and in which she would add to knowledge through experimentation. In this area, the nurse would be an authority and could become an expert consultant to other nurses and to the health team.

Alternative Methods of Implementation

It is doubtful that the head nurse role as here conceived could be fulfilled if the head nurse were responsible for many more than 15 patients. However, experimentation may prove otherwise for some services of some institutions. When a sufficient number of prepared nurses is not available, hospitals may be tempted to compromise in one of two ways: *first,* give the head nurse charge over more patients than she can be responsible for and still carry out the role, or *second,* employ head nurses who do not have the necessary qualifications. In neither case will the conceived role be entirely fulfilled. Each hospital must decide for itself whether, for them, it is preferable to adhere strictly to the role concept of the head nurse and the desired model for the patient care division, or whether it would be better to make a start by instituting whatever changes in role are possible with personnel obtainable. In the first instance, as prepared persons become available one unit at a time would be changed in accord with concepts and models. In the second instance, as prepared head nurses and unit directors could be obtained they would replace those who were unprepared, or the number of patients delegated to the head nurse would be reduced. The system would be expected to develop gradually into one considered desirable. Some hospitals have already decided in favor of changing the organizational pattern of the division and giving the head nurse a new role even though they recognize she does not meet the qualifications they someday hope to require. As an interim step outstanding graduates of collegiate schools are appointed to head nurse positions and are helped to fulfill the desired role in so far as possible. Universities which conduct schools of nursing might well consider proposing that their top-ranking clinical faculty members be given dual appointments on the hospital staff and serve as consultants to young inexperienced head nurses. Likewise, clinically prepared department administrators or associate directors could also serve in this capacity.

An alternative to either of the two above possibilities for instituting change is the employment by the hospital of one or more clinical nurse experts, not as head nurses but as nurse clinicians free to plan and implement care for a few selected patients. (See Chapter 3, p. 48.) In situations where this type of plan is being used the head nurse continues to be responsible for nursing care administration but does not have the time needed for intimate patient contact. Where such programs are in operation it should be possible, as the number of clinical nurse experts increases, for the two roles to merge, with each nurse clinician becoming a head nurse responsible for the number of patients which study and experience has shown to be feasible. When this occurs, the title of the head nurse will unquestionably be changed.[20]

Enough experimentation with the head nurse role has taken place to convince some leaders in nursing that role change along the line of that described earlier in this chapter is necessary and will in time be achieved. During the next few years, before enough qualified head nurses can be procured, certain steps can and should be taken. Experimentation with various roles and models should be carried out utilizing head nurses and unit directors who are qualified. Those hospitals which decide to make a start toward a new head nurse role, despite lack of nurses who are prepared, need to select those who have a sound basic education and potential for graduate study, as well as the necessary personal characteristics. Effort should be made to send promising nurses for graduate study in clinical nursing. One of the most important immediate steps for the profession is the examination of all

[20] Frances Reiter describes a nurse clinician functioning in somewhat the same way that we have described the head nurse. See: The Nurse-clinician, *Amer. J. Nurs.,* Vol. 66 (February 1966), pp. 274-280.

forms of nursing education in light of new demands made upon nurses and a determination of the type of education needed to prepare the nurse for new roles which are emerging.

SUMMARY

Many hospitals in the near future will find ways to relieve head nurses of nonnursing functions. Some will make radical changes both in the head nurse role and in unit organization. For several years, nurse leaders have been promoting the concept of a nurse free from unit administrative responsibilities who would utilize her time for nursing. Some institutions have employed nurse clinicians who function in different ways in the various hospitals. In this chapter a concept of the nurse clinician functioning in the role of head nurse has been presented. She is pictured as responsible for the nursing and delegated medical care of a small group (12 to 15) of patients. Free to plan her own time, to come and go as she feels necessary, the head nurse is available at any time she is needed. She employs a competent staff to work under her supervision. Although decisions relative to nursing care are the head nurse's to make, she has a nurse consultant to whom she may turn for guidance. Since in this concept head nurses have greater responsibility, fewer top level administrative personnel are needed. In this new role the head nurse is envisaged as a practitioner, administrator of nursing care, coordinator of patient care, guardian of the patient's total welfare, partner of the physician, supervisor and developer of her staff, and researcher. Each of these roles, within the total role, requires that the head nurse be a clinical expert, a specialist in her field of nursing, well grounded in the sciences; that she be able to talk with physicians in their own language, be self-confident, skilled in communication and interpersonal relationships, and have the personal qualities which command trust and respect and portray warmth and friendliness.

The new head nurse role requires that management of the unit become the responsibility of someone other than the head nurse. A plan currently being promoted makes unit management a department of hospital administration. Most often the head nurse and the unit manager are peers. Some hospitals will try other patterns. One which has been visualized employs a qualified unit director responsible to hospital administration who would administer and coordinate all patient care services—clerical, dietary, housekeeping—with nursing and medical services. Nurses and doctors would be responsible to him for abiding by hospital policy. In professional practice the head nurse and the doctor would be autonomous except for the restrictions imposed upon them by their colleagues in their own professions.

A sufficient number of qualified head nurses will not quickly be available. In the beginning some hospitals will open experiental units, hopefully undertaking controlled research. Others may feel it wiser to place capable nurses who have a sound though limited scientific background in head nursing and provide them with strong counselling. At such times as they could be replaced by fully prepared clinicians, these head nurses would be encouraged to continue their own education. Clinically prepared department and associate administrators in nursing might be placed in head nurse positions, their salary and status remaining unchanged. Nurses completing graduate programs with preparation in clinical nursing could be placed in head nurse positions which well might become required experience for those who wish to go into teaching, clinical consultation, or administration. It is anticipated that the rewards would be so great that most would prefer to remain head nurses where they would have the satisfaction of close patient contact and medical collaboration together with the opportunity to carry out clinical research. Unquestionably, the title, head nurse, would be changed to one which more clearly describes her responsibilities.

When a hospital is considering changes in role or in unit organization it is imperative that the hospital administrator and chiefs of medical services or other key members of the medical staff be involved in the early planning. Without the wholehearted support of both the administrator and the medical chiefs important changes are impossible. Head nurses have a great deal to contribute in defining their new role. They can choose either to participate, or to resist the inevitable tides of change. If they choose the latter course, they will simply be bypassed because the momentum for change has already begun.

QUESTIONS FOR DISCUSSION

1. Should nurses be employed as unit managers if they so desire? Give reasons for your answer.
2. What specific reactions do you anticipate head nurses would have to being responsible to a unit director?
3. If major changes in unit organization and the head nurse role, such as those depicted in this chapter, were to be proposed for the hospital with which you are associated, how would nurses (staff nurses and head nurses) react? Would they support the change or resist it? What do you foresee

as the outcome of their behavior, be it for or against change? How can nursing service administration aid in the development of favorable responses?

4. What fears does the head nurse have when the transcription of medical orders is transferred to a nonnurse? To what extent are these fears legitimate?
5. A patient, in spite of special back care, is showing signs of a beginning decubitus. What is the head nurse's responsibility? What part should the doctor play?
6. How do you feel about the head nurse being a practitioner, a partner of the physician, a clinical expert, her own "boss" responsible for all decisions pertaining to nursing and prescribed medical care?
7. Give illustrations of questions and problems now referred to nursing administration for decision which would be handled by the head nurse if she were autonomous in relation to nursing care for the individual patient.
8. Do you believe the day should sometime come when the professional nurse would be an independent practitioner responsible to her professional colleagues for upholding recognized standards? What are the arguments for and against this idea?

EXERCISES

1. At a busy time of day, stand for fifteen minutes in a strategic place near the room of a very ill or uncomfortable patient. Make note of all the noises you hear, classifying them as "inside" or "outside." Analyze your findings. Which are harmful to the patient either because they are annoying to him or because they add to fatigue? Which are preventable? As a head nurse which would you feel responsible for reducing? How would you go about doing so in the present head nurse role? in the new role described?
2. Observe the activities of nursing personnel for an hour on one floor of a hospital. The hour preceding the transfer report to the evening nurse is sometimes a revealing one. Briefly note the general situation on the division, that is, what is happening, number of nurses, L.P.N.'s, aides, and others on duty. Make note of the things the head nurse does, what she appears to want to do but cannot find the time, jobs she delegates to others and who the "others" are, things you believe a head nurse should do but this one, perhaps for good reason, does not do. Analyze your findings.

Make a list of all the activities you have noted. Number them in order of priority for a head nurse herself to perform. On what basis did you make this decision?

3. Determine how a group of patients who have been hospitalized for three to ten days feel about the number of individuals who do things to and for them. Perhaps those patients who are able will keep track of this number, making a record of the category of personnel and the activity each performs. Try to find out why the patient reacts as he does. Compare findings with continuity of nursing care for each patient as determined by the assignment sheet. Do those patients who have been assigned to the same nurse for the preceding three or more days react in a different way from those for whom there has been no consistency? What "hunches" do you have relative to the problem of many persons coming and going in the patient's room?

4. Make a list of the information the doctor needs from the nurse and one of the information the nurse needs from the physician. Observe yourself, if you are a head nurse, or a head nurse if you are a staff nurse or student and make note of information pertaining to four or five new patients which is transmitted between doctor and nurse. Compare your notes with your two lists. Are there items which should be added to your list? Was any information consistently omitted? Which information transmitted was given as a report, and which in answer to questions? Was the information given freely or grudgingly? What are your impressions of the professional relationship between the doctor and nurse who were exchanging information?

5. Make a plan whereby the head nurse in your hospital can reassess her role. If you are a head nurse, it is suggested you collaborate with one or two of your head nurse colleagues and implement your plan of assessment. Results might be presented to a class or other group for discussion.

REFERENCES

Aasterud, Margaret. Explanation to the patient, Nurs. Forum, Vol. 2 (No. 4, 1963), pp. 36-44.
   Explanations to patients cannot be based on blanket rules but "rather they should be based upon knowledge of how people behave under stress, of how anxiety affects a person's ability to communicate, and of the influence of socio-cultural factors, and, in addition, on an assessment by the nurse of her own expectations."

Alfano, Genrose. Administration means working with nurses, Amer. J. Nurs., Vol. 64 (June 1964), pp. 83-85.
A companion article of two others in this issue on Loeb Center. Here a nurse administrator describes satisfactory functioning of staff nurses in the center and reasons for staff satisfaction in working there.

Anderson, Louise C. The clinical nurse expert, Nurs. Outlook, Vol. 14 (July 1966), pp. 62-64.
Annotation in Chapter 3 reference.

Aydelotte, Myrtle Kitchell The use of patient welfare as a criterion measure, Nurs. Res., Vol. 11 (Winter 1962), pp. 10-14.
Report on the so-called "Iowa Study" which "tested the validity of a speculation often heard in the nursing profession, namely that increases in the amount or quality of nursing care will produce improvements in patient welfare." This was found to be not true. The measures used in testing patient welfare are described and are defended as valid. The head nurse will find the criteria useful as she attempts to evaluate patient care.

Barnes, Elizabeth. People in Hospital, London, Macmillan and Co. Ltd., 1961, Ch. 4, pp. 37-53.
An excellent chapter describing the demands on nurses by patients; the satisfaction the nurse gains from being needed. The special demands on the head nurse are portrayed and the need for changes in the hospital setting before relief for the head nurse can be achieved.

Bates, Barbara. Nurse-physician teamwork, Med. Care, Vol. 4 (April-June 1965), pp. 69-80.
"An attempt is made to define the critical requirements in behaviour of physician and nurse in order to achieve effective nurse-physician teamwork in patient care." Thought-provoking and very worthy of study.

Bernardin, Estelle. Loeb Center—as the staff nurse sees it, Amer. J. Nurs., Vol. 64 (June 1964), pp. 85-86.
One of three articles on Loeb Center described in this issue. A staff nurse tells of her experience in learning the reflective technique, its value in helping patients, and her satisfactions in working at the center.

Bigham, Gloria D. To communicate with negro patients, Amer. J. Nurs. Vol. 64 (September 1964), pp. 113-115.
A negro nurse beautifully describes the negro's feelings and the causes for his behavior. She tells the ways in which negro patients are discriminated against in hospitals and the role of the head nurse in influencing attitudes of her staff.

Bressler, Bernard. The psychotherapeutic nurse, Amer. J. Nurs., Vol. 62 (May 1962), pp. 87-90.
Annotation in Chapter 3 reference.

Brown, Esther Lucile. The nurse must know—the nurse must speak, Nurs. Forum, Vol. 5 (No. 1, 1966), pp. 10-21.
Importance of two roles for the nurse are emphasized: 1) the nurse as manager of the patient's environment and representative of his interests and welfare and 2) the nurse as citizen in working for the improvement of community health services. A challenge for nurse and nursing!

Campbell, Emily B., Cheetham, Evonna, Bautch, Judy, and Roberts, Sara. Not education, not service, but nursing, Amer. J. Nurs., Vol. 67 (May 1967), pp. 990-997.
A teacher-supervisor describes her attempts to bridge the gap between education and practice—to discover whether nurses could give the kind of nursing they were

taught. This is a fascinating story of the results of her experiment. The head nurse and team leaders tell their part in the experience.

Christman, Luther P. Nurse-physician communications in the hospital, J.A.M.A., Vol. 194 (November 1, 1965), pp. 539-544.
Inadequate communication between doctor and nurse interferes with the quality of patient care. The reasons for failure to communicate are analyzed and corrective measures suggested. Busyness is a symptom rather than a cause of breakdown in communications.

Dean, D. J. The staff ward meeting, Nurs. Times, Vol. 61 (September 3, 1965), pp. 1221-1223.
The values in terms of better relationships, increased productivity, and staff growth of a weekly ward staff meeting are described.

Dumas, Rhetaugh G. and Leonard, Robert C. The effect of nursing on the incidence of postoperative vomiting, Nurs. Res., Vol. 12 (Winter 1963), pp. 12-15.
Patients whose preoperative care involves a special nursing approach designed to relieve distress had much less postoperative vomiting than a similar group of patients who did not have this approach. Every nurse can find a lesson in the results of this study.

Edgecumbe, Robert H. How C.A.S.H. helps nurses improve care, Mod. Hosp., Vol. 106 (May 1966), pp. 97-99.
The letters C.A.S.H. stand for Commission for Administrative Services in Hospitals, an organization which has helped hospitals devise a plan for continuing measurement of quality nursing care and a resulting guide for staffing. Forms are shown. This is an interesting system. Nurse administrators should study it. Head nurses will find the forms a useful tool in evaluating care.

Fagin, Claire M. The clinical specialist as supervisor, Nurs. Outlook, Vol. 15 (January 1967), pp. 34-36.
The clinical nurse specialist can function in many capacities one of which is a supervisor. Five sub-roles are described. Only the fifth function—evaluator-assessor —distinguishes the supervisor specialist from any other clinical specialist. The writer raises the interesting question: "does the specialist need this authority role to achieve positive change in nursing practice?"

Gray, June W. Liaison nurses bridge the care gap, Nurs. Outlook, Vol. 15 (May 1967), pp. 28-31.
Eight liaison nurses assume responsibility for the nursing care of high-risk maternity patients being followed in the clinic of a large hospital. The nurses coordinate the care of the patients between clinic, hospital, and home in an effort to reduce morbidity and mortality in both mothers and their babies.

Gunter, Laurie M. Research techniques applied to nursing, Nurs. Res., Vol. 13 (Summer 1964), pp. 230-232.
An article which will help the head nurse see the value of nursing research and the importance of the practitioner being research minded.

Hagen, Elizabeth, and Wolff, Luverne. Nursing Leadership Behavior in General Hospitals, New York, Institute of Research and Service in Nursing Education, Teachers College, Columbia University, 1961.
Report of a fascinating study using the critical incident technique, of the leadership characteristics of directors of nursing service, supervisors, and head nurses. Effective and ineffective behavior as reported by different levels of personnel are depicted. The head nurse will find "her" section both interesting and helpful. The leadership potential of the head nurse role is summarized on page 137.

Harrell, George T. Trends in Education, practice, and organization of health services, J.A.M.A., Vol. 196 (April 25, 1966), pp. 334-338.

Dr. Harrell presented this paper at the A.M.A.-A.N.A. Conference, "Nurse-Physician Collaboration Toward Improved Patient Care." He discusses the changing role of the nurse, her relationship to the doctor, the place of the emerging paramedical personnel, the institutional framework needed to bring about necessary collaboration among the health services.

Heckman, Mary K. What if it were I?, Amer. J. Nurs., Vol. 66 (April 1966), pp. 768-769.
The human qualities of helping, caring, staying, touching, and listening are illustrated in incidents described in this thoughtful paper.

Henderson, Cynthia. Can nursing care hasten recovery?, Amer. J. Nurs., Vol. 64 (June 1964), pp. 80-83.
An assistant editor of the Journal describes the unique plan for nursing care carried out at Loeb Center. Here, selected patients at a point of illness when their medical treatment is underway and "professional nursing can help them enter into the healing process," are cared for by professional nurses. Patients participate in planning their nursing care. Doctors and other health personnel are used as consultants.

——— Freeing the nurse to nurse, Amer. J. Nurs., Vol. 64 (March 1964), pp. 72-77.
Miss Henderson, assistant Journal editor, reports on her visits to several hospitals which have instituted the unit manager system. She answers such questions as: What does a unit manager do? Who is a unit manager? What is the relationship of the head nurse and unit manager? Does unit management, in fact, free nurses to nurse? What are the reactions of those involved to the system?

Henderson, Virginia. ICN Basic Principles of Nursing Care, London, ICN House, 1960.
Translated into many foreign languages this small booklet is a guide for nurses everywhere in their attempt to come to grips with the full meaning of nursing.

——— The nature of nursing, Amer. J. Nurs., Vol. 64 (August 1964), pp. 62-68. This is a condensed version of the paperback pamphlet published by the Macmillan Company, New York, 1966.
This renowned nurse and nurse educator describes her concept of nursing and the experiences from which she has formulated it. She also describes the implications of the concept for nursing practice, research, and education.

Johnson, Dorothy E. Competence in practice: technical and professional, Nurs. Outlook, Vol. 14 (October 1966), pp. 30-33.
The writer describes the difference in the kind and degree of knowledge and skill developed by the graduates of diploma and associate degree programs compared with graduates of baccalaureate programs.

——— Consequences for patients and personnel, Amer. J. Nurs., Vol. 62 (May 1962), pp. 96-100.
Job dissatisfaction and the less-than-good quality of nursing care which results from discontinuity in nurse-patient and nurse-other relations arise from the social system of the hospital and nursing service. A clinical nurse specialist may be the answer to the problem. Ways in which she would function are described.

Johnson, Jean E., and Dabbs, James M., Jr. Enumeration of active sweat glands: a simple physiological indicator of psychological changes, Nurs. Res., Vol. 16 (Summer 1967), pp. 273-276.
The number of active sweat glands on the palmer surface of a finger tip has been used by these researchers to test its effect as an indicator of psychological changes. The test shows promise.

Johnson, Miriam M. and Martin, Harry W. A sociological analysis of the nurse role, Amer. J. Nurs., Vol. 58 (March 1958), pp. 373-377.

In sociological terms the authors clearly describe the chief function of the nurse as one of releasing tension for the patient and maintaining a harmonious relationship between doctor, patient, and nurse. A stimulating and highly valuable article.

Kern, M. Sue. Organizing a new nursing service—a responsibility and opportunity for innovation, Int. J. Nurs. Studies, Vol. 2 (July 1965) pp. 163-169.
A description of the way the nursing service in a new university hospital has been organized to permit the nurse to nurse and the patient to receive continuity in his care.

Lambertsen, Eleanor C. Patient service will improve if nurse-doctor communications do, Mod. Hosp., Vol. 105 (December 1965), p. 108.
Nurses must do more than study independently the problem of the individual patient or groups of patients if today's problems are to be solved. Joint medical and nursing committees for evaluation of patient care and patient care rounds by physician and nurse together are ways suggested by Miss Lambertsen for breaking down artificial barriers.

Leventhal, Howard, and Sharp, Elizabeth. Facial expressions as indicators of distress, In Affect, Cognition, and Personality, Empirical Studies, Tomkins, Silvan J. and Izard, Carroll E., eds. New York, Springer Publishing Company, Inc., 1965. Ch. 10.
Forehead, brow, and eyelid behavior were found to be significant indicators of comfort and distress levels in women in labor.

Little, Dolores. The nurse specialist, Amer. J. Nurs., Vol. 67 (March 1967), pp. 552-556.
Report of two and a half year study at the University of Washington to determine whether the nurse specialist can favorably affect the course of the patient's illness. The objectives, the methods used, the role and the problems encountered are presented in a clear interesting way.

Martin, Harry W., and Prange, Arthur J. The stages of illness—psychosocial approach, Nurs. Outlook, Vol. 10 (March 1962), pp. 168-171.
Three stages of illness are described—transition to illness, acceptance, and convalescence. "The nurse has a clearly defined role in each stage of illness, and a responsibility for learning more about the psychological aspects of illness. . . ."

McBeth, Max A., and Carpenter, Douglas C., Jr. Seven-year appraisal of a ward manager system, Hospitals, Vol. 40 (March 16, 1966), pp. 79-86.
Hospital administrators tell about the organization, institution, values and success of the ward manager system in a 300 bed county hospital. There are several unique features about this program.

Melber, Ruth. The maternity nurse specialist in a hospital clinic setting, Nurs. Res., Vol. 16 (Winter 1967), pp. 68-71.
This study showed that a maternity nurse specialist identified more health needs, suggested a wider variety of actions, and saw the need for emotional care and counselling more often than other members of the health team in the clinic setting studied.

Mercadante, Lucille T. An organizational plan for nursing service, Nurs. Outlook, Vol. 10 (May 1962), pp. 305-306.
A description of the organization of the well-known and respected nursing service of the University of Florida Teaching Hospital. This was one of the first institutions to free nurses for nursing.

Meyers, Mary E. The effect of types of communication on patients' reactions to stress, Nurs. Res., Vol. 13 (Spring 1964), pp. 126-131.
In a mildly stressful situation less tension is created when the patient is given

specific information relative to what is to happen, than when distracting conversation is used or no explanation given. These conclusions were based on a questionnaire to patients who experienced one of these three approaches.

Myers, Robert S. Lack of liaison in hospital can impair the quality of patient care, Mod. Hosp., Vol. 106 (February 1966), p. 122.
"There is a distressing lack of liaison among physicians, nurses, and technicians in seeing to it that what must be done gets done at the proper time and that the patient is duly informed." So writes a doctor who documents the effects on patients of failure to assume such responsibility.

Norris, Catherine M. Administration for creative nursing, Nurs. Forum, Vol. 1 (Summer 1962), pp. 88-117.
A psychiatric hospital nursing service administrator describes the role of the nurse and the responsibility of the nurse administrator in fulfillment of the role expectations. The philosophy of nursing of the institution is included in the appendix.

Notter, Lucille. Nursing research is every nurse's business, Nurs. Outlook, Vol. 11 (January 1963), pp. 49-51.
Miss Notter discusses research in understandable terms and indicates that nurses should be able to use the guidelines listed to determine the worthiness of a research study.

Nursing service and nursing care, Nurs. Outlook, Vol. 10 (April 1962), p. 231.
A differentiation is made between nursing care and nursing service. Questions are raised as to the real meaning of nursing service.

O'Connor, Doris, and Hagan, Faye. Liaison nurse, Amer. J. Nurs., Vol. 64 (June 1964), pp. 101-103.
Annotation in Chapter 3 reference.

Pellegrino, Edmund D. Communication crisis in nursing and medical education, Nurs. Forum, Vol. 5 (No. 1, 1966), pp. 45-53.
If the patient is to receive good care in this present day, doctors and nurses must communicate better. Several suggestions are given including a joint committee on patient care and clinical teaching. As usual, Dr. Pellegrino has much helpful counsel for nursing.

—————— The ethical implications in changing practice, Amer. J. Nurs., Vol. 64 (September 1964), pp. 110-112.
". . . the cooperative activity of physicians, nurses, and other health professionals is a patent necessity today in optimum care." Nurses who foresee the need for a new relationship with medical personnel will receive a great deal of help from this article.

—————— The changing role of the professional nurse in the hospital, Hospitals, Vol. 35 (December 16, 1961), pp. 56-62.
A well-known physician describes his concept of the role of the nurse and her relationship to the doctor. Every nurse should read this article.

—————— The ethical implications of changing patterns of medical care, North Carolina Med. J., Vol. 26 (February 1965), pp. 73-76.
Dr. Pellegrino finds nothing in medical or nursing professional codes to countermand changes in patterns of medical care. Both codes insist on good patient care thus making it mandatory "to explore fully every possible avenue for improving service even when this means yielding professional prerogatives." An inspiring article!

Peplau, Hildegard E. Nurse-doctor relationships, Nurs. Forum, Vol. 5 (No. 1, 1966), pp. 60-75.
Annotation in Chapter 3 reference.

———— Specialization in professional nursing, Nurs. Science, Vol. 3 (August 1965), pp. 268-287.
Possible specialty areas for nursing are presented. A clinical specialist provides a model for expert, up-to-date nursing practice. Her knowledge is greater and more recent than that of the general practitioner. She has greater freedom to exercise judgment.

———— The heart of nursing: interpersonal relations, Canad. Nurse, Vol. 61 (April 1965), pp. 273-275.
If we accept that interpersonal relations are the heart of nursing "we shall be forced to look at our relationships not only with patients but with other disciplines." Through such relationships nursing will grow.

Phaneuf, Maria C. The nursing audit for evaluation of patient care, Nurs. Outlook, Vol. 14 (June 1966), pp. 51-54.
Nurses in hospitals and public health nursing agencies are beginning to use the formal audit of nursing service records for evaluation of nursing care. The list of 50 components and descriptive statements for use in appraisal would be very useful for any nursing service.

Pratt, Henry. The doctor's view of the changing nurse-physician relationship, J. Med. Educ., Vol. 40 (August 1965), pp. 767-771.
Rapid changes in medical science and practice have necessitated a change in doctor-nurse relationships. The fact that the nurse is becoming more a partner to the doctor is advantageous. The fact that the complexity of the head nurse's job makes communication difficult, creates problems. It is good to have a doctor's sympathetic understanding view of the nursing dilemma.

Reiter, Frances. The nurse-clinician, Amer. J. Nurs., Vol. 66 (February 1966), pp. 274-280.
Clearly and forcibly Miss Reiter describes her concept of the nurse-clinician, her competencies, and her preparation. An article no nurse should fail to read.

———— The clinical nursing approach, Nurs. Forum, Vol. 5 (No. 1, 1966), pp. 39-44.
". . . the only colleges of nursing that can prepare beginning nurse-clinicians are those in which there is a clinical faculty of nursing composed of nurse-clinicians engaged in clinical practice and clinical research as well as in the teaching of students."

Schwartz, Doris R. Planning the telephone call, Nurs. Outlook, Vol. 13 (January 1965), pp. 44-45.
A controlled experiment showed that careful analysis of the family situation and planning of reports by the visiting nurse to the doctor resulted in reevaluation of the case while the usual factual report of the nurse's observations did not. Many implications for the hospital head nurse.

Scully, Nancy Rae. The clinical nursing specialist: practicing nurse, Nurs. Outlook, Vol. 13 (August 1965), pp. 28-30.
Annotation in Chapter 3 reference.

Sheps, Cecile G., and Bachar, Miriam E. Emerging patterns of practice, Amer. J. Nurs., Vol. 64 (September 1964), pp. 107-109.
Nursing and medical functions are no longer clear cut. Procedures and judgments are on a continuum with overlapping gray areas in the middle. This necessitates a different relationship between physician and nurse who must both exercise judgment regarding the degree of mutual involvement.

Sherman, Robert T. Total patient care from a surgeon's point of view, Nurs. Forum, Vol. 4 (No. 3, 1965), pp. 27-32.
A surgeon strongly advocates many of the changes which nurse leaders are promoting as necessary if the nursing profession is to fulfill its responsibility.

Simms, Laura L. The clinical nursing specialist, J.A.M.A., Vol. 198 (November 7, 1966), pp. 675-677.
Miss Simms lists three changes in present-day nursing service patterns which appear to be indicated in order to make use of clinically prepared nurses.

——— The clinical nursing specialist: an experiment, Nurs. Outlook, Vol. 13 (August 1965), pp. 26-28.
Annotation in Chapter 3 reference.

Sister Charles Marie, Nursing needs more freedom, Amer. J. Nurs., Vol. 62 (July 1962), pp. 53-55.
Lack of freedom still characterizes nursing. Nurses need to be allowed freedom to assess patients' needs and plan their care. But there is concern that nurses may not know how to use freedom. They should be prepared for it.

Sister Mary Mercita. Rehabilitation—bridge to a useful and happy life, Nurs. Outlook, Vol. 10 (September 1962), pp. 580-583.
The nurse's role in rehabilitation is one of leadership, coordination, and teaching. Prevention of physical deformities and pressure sores, maintenance of elimination, and motivation for recovery are other ways by which the nurse contributes to rehabilitation.

Skipper, James K., Jr., and Leonard, Robert C. Communication and patient care, Canad. Nurse, Vol. 61 (July 1965), pp. 562F-562H.
A brief but interesting illustrated discussion of the inadequacies in nurses' responses to patients. Some barriers to effective communication are enumerated by these sociologists.

Smith, Sidney. The psychology of illness, Nurs. Forum, Vol. 3 (No. 1, 1964), pp. 34-37.
A psychologist discusses the symbolic meaning and the threat of illness to the sick individual, and calls upon the nurse to help him maintain his independence, emotionally prepare him for what is to take place, to try to understand the patient's behavior and her own emotional responses to the patient.

Stillar, Edith M. Continuity of care, Nurs. Outlook, Vol. 10 (September 1962), pp. 584-585.
One of a series, the article in this issue stresses the nurse's role as coordinator of the rehabilitation team, the great importance of early planning, and the need to involve families in the teaching program for patients.

The Surgeon-General looks at nursing, Amer. J. Nursing, Vol. 67 (January 1967), pp. 64-67.
In an interview with the Journal, Dr. William H. Stewart, the chief of the U. S. Public Health Service, discusses problems in the nursing profession and gives his view of the solutions and the groups responsible for participating in them. He stresses the need for the nurse to be a partner with the physician.

Thompson, John D., and Lee, Barbara J. Progress report on unit manager system, New Haven, Dept. of Epidemiology and Public Health, Yale University School of Medicine, under U.S.P.H.S. Grant No. CH 00037, 1963. Unpublished.
Several hospitals having unit manager systems are compared with a conceptual model.

Thornton, Thelma N., and Leonard, Robert C. Experimental comparison of effectiveness and efficiency of three nursing approaches, Nursing Research, Vol. 13 (Spring 1964), pp. 122-125.
A nursing approach which focused on the purpose of an interaction and on exploration of the patient's reactions was more effective and less time consuming (hence more efficient) than other approaches which did not so focus.

Validating a theory of nursing practice, Amer. J. Nurs., Vol. 63 (August 1963), pp.
        52-59.
    Article 1: Dumas, Rhetaugh Graves. Psychological preparation for surgery,
    pp. 52-55.
    Exploration with a preoperative patient to determine causes of distress reduced
    postoperative vomiting.
    Article 2: Dye, Mary C. Clarifying patients' communications, pp. 56-59.
    By exploring the cause of the patient's behavior or complaints, patient's tensions
    and discomforts were relieved. Validation by the patient that he does feel relieved
    is essential.
    On p. 54 will be found Ida Jean Orlando's theory of nursing practice on
    which these two studies were based and on p. 59 quotations from her book (The
    Dynamic Nurse Patient Relationship) on the Meaning and Purpose of Nursing.

Wald, Florence S. Emerging Nursing Practice, Amer. J. Public Health, Vol. 56
        (August 1966), pp. 1252-1260.
    A very clear description of the problems facing nursing today, their challenge to
    nursing education and to the profession. No nurse will be umoved by this article.

Walker, Virginia H., and Hawkins, James L. Management: a factor in clinical nursing,
        Nurs. Outlook, Vol. 13 (February 1965), pp. 57-58.
    A nurse may transfer unit management functions to nonnurses but she still needs
    managerial skills to diagnose patient needs and plan care, to organize patient
    care, delegate responsibility, communicate.

Wiedenbach, Ernestine. The helping art of nursing, Amer. J. Nurs., Vol. 63 (Novem-
        ber 1963), pp. 54-57.
    Here Miss Wiedenbach relates her philosophy of nursing, the purpose of nursing
    and the nurse's use of her thoughts and feelings in achieving her purpose.

Yokes, Jean A. The clinical specialist in cardiovascular nursing, Amer. J. Nurs., Vol.
        66 (December 1966), pp. 2667-2670.
    A description of the way in which the clinical specialist functions in one medical
    center.

chapter 7

PRINCIPLES OF ADMINISTRATION AND THEIR APPLICATION BY THE HEAD NURSE

In the preceding chapter it has been seen that both the head nurse and the unit director are administrators and coordinators. The head nurse is in charge of nursing and patient care while the unit director is responsible for the division and of patient care services. Principles of administration apply to the responsibilities of both individuals. In this chapter we shall consider these principles and their application to activities which occur on the nursing care division of every hospital. In present organizational patterns, head nurses are responsible for most of these activities. In hospitals where a unit manager is employed some are in his province. Because the majority of head nurses are involved directly or indirectly in these activities, important aspects of their handling will be considered in this and the next chapter.

A statement of the principles of administration will be followed with a discussion of their application by the head nurse and unit manager in the patient care division. The next chapter will concentrate on four administrative procedures with which the head nurse is especially concerned.

PRINCIPLES OF ADMINISTRATION

One can find many lists of principles of administration, management organization, and coordination. Those which follow are most pertinent to the effective management of patient care and patient care services.

1) Responsibility for decision making is clearly designated.
2) Responsibility is clearly delegated. Implicit in the delegation is authority to carry the responsibility.
3) Each individual in the organization knows the limits of his responsibility, to whom he is responsible, to whom he may go for counsel or appeal. He also knows who is responsible to him and for what.
4) Coordination and cooperation are facilitated by:
   a) organization of work
   b) an effective system of communication

133

c) development of routines for frequently-performed technical activities

d) advance planning

e) voluntary effort

5) The development of personnel, supervision of work, and evaluation of outcomes are functions of administration.

Responsibility for Decision-Making Is Clearly Designated

This responsibility may be vested in a group or in an individual depending on the question to be decided. In democratic administrations, members of the organization who will be affected by the decision have opportunity to express their views. Some matters the group may decide. Where policy is involved, however, the deciding voice is usually that of one person—the one who has responsibility for the consequences. This executive—which may be the hospital administrator, the director of nursing, or the head nurse—if he functions in a democratic manner, takes into account the desires and opinions of the group but is obligated to act in accord with his own best judgment. It should be clear to the group *before* the subject is opened for discussion whether or not the members are to have a voice in the decision and why. If the final decision is made by the executive and the wishes of the group are not followed, members need a frank presentation of the thinking which determined the decision. More often than not final decision will rest with the administrator at the level where responsibility has been given and accepted. If the head nurse has been made fully responsible for the nursing care of a group of patients (as new roles suggest), she may discuss alternative actions with her staff, the doctor, her consultant, but in the final analysis the decision is hers. She and everyone else should know this, for the responsibility is great.

Responsibility Is Clearly Delegated. Implicit in the Responsibility Is Authority to Carry the Responsibility

This principle has been considered above in relation to decision making, but responsibility for other functions as well is inherent in this principle. Every worker must know his responsibilities. The unit director, for example, needs to know whether he or the dietary department is responsible for patients receiving their food in palatable condition; whether he or the nurse or the admitting office decides to which rooms patients shall be assigned;

whether he or the head nurse arranges for private duty nurses. If the unit director is responsible for patients' satisfaction with their diet trays, he has authority to fire the unit dietition should she be the source of the trouble; or he has the authority to go directly to the associate administrator in charge of food service for the hospital if the problem seems to be centered there.

The head nurse is responsible for all nursing functions carried out by her staff. She delegates tasks and enough responsibility and authority for the nurse or aid to function, but she does not forfeit accountability (see Chapter 2). The staff member will have greater satisfaction in her work if she is given responsibility for a job and permitted to carry it out in her own way, provided of course she understands the objectives and has guidelines, such as a nursing procedure to follow. For example, a staff nurse is likely to be more interested in her work if she is given responsibility for a group of patients—for planning their nursing care and the way it will be given— and is held responsible for meeting the patients' nursing needs. So too, an aide, who is assigned to make beds and straighten the units of up-patients, will be more content, more productive if she is allowed to organize her work but knows that the objective is to coordinate with the nurse giving the patient's care and to keep no patient waiting to have his unit put in order. Again, if the head nurse decides to make the collecting, cleaning, filling, and distributing of water pitchers a function of the aide she will make sure the aide understands this fact, when it is to be done, ways to prevent error, and the like. Thereafter, the head nurse will observe to see whether the task is being done well, give further instruction as needed, continue to observe that patients' needs for water are being met. She has delegated the job to the aide and expects her to carry it through. If for any reason a nurse or aide is unable to meet the obligation delegated to her the head nurse should be informed and her help solicited.

Delegation of responsibility for nursing care will be considered in Chapter 12.

Each Individual in the Organization Knows the Limits of His Responsibility, to Whom He Is Responsible, to Whom He May Go for Counsel or Appeal. He also Knows Who Is Responsible to Him and for What

In the above illustration the aide knows that she is responsible to the head nurse (or her relief). She knows she may not give drinking water to any new patient without permission of the head nurse. The aide also is aware that she may appeal to the department administrator if she feels the head nurse is hypercritical of her. The staff nurse knows she is responsible to the head nurse; that the aide and practical nurse are responsible to her only if she is their team leader, is the assistant head nurse, or is relieving the head nurse. This all sounds very formal, but it illustrates the principle. However, we remember that every institution has an informal organization as well as a formal one. If relationships are good among the staff, the aide will feel free to turn to any staff nurse for advice or the answer to a question, and the staff nurse, if she is sure of her information, will not hesitate to give the answer.

The functions to be performed by the holder of a job, his obligations, and the person or persons to whom he is responsible should be clearly set down in a job description. These descriptions are customarily prepared by the employer and serve as a form of contractual agreement. Both employer and employee know what is expected. The head nurse should be familiar with the job descriptions for the positions filled by persons on her staff. If the head nurse employs her own staff she prepares the job descriptions listing the functions of each person responsible to her—the professional nurse, practical nurse, aide, and orderly. There should be descriptions of the activities and responsibilities of the assistant head nurse, evening and night nurses. Included also is the person to whom the nurse is responsible and to whom she should turn for help in the absence of the head nurse. It is advisable to work out with the clinical instructor a statement of the student's responsibilities to the head nurse. It must be clear that the head nurse is responsible for the care of all patients. She or the team leader if nursing teams are in use are, therefore, to be consulted about a change in nursing method, kept informed of the patient's condition, and given a report when the student goes off duty. It is not enough that a student report to her instructor.

Coordination and Cooperation Are Facilitated by:

Organization of work. Organization is essential to the efficient accomplishment of even the simplest task. To organize nursing care effectively, it is necessary that the head nurse be thoroughly familiar with all activities which must be performed in the care of the patient including those for which a unit manager or unit director may be responsible. Nursing is planned around the schedules of other departments, but the head nurse should endeavor to have the schedule planned with the individual patient and readjusted when this will be to his benefit. The entire nursing staff needs to be familiar with the regular routine for patient care services. Diets are served at a fairly definite time. Patients go to the operating room and return to the division between certain hours. In general, doctors are on the floor about the same time each day. Nonemergency admissions usually take place during specified hours. Knowing the schedule, the head nurse is able to plan the day's program.

Each day's work should be planned in advance and proper assignments made. Since a nurse can care for a patient more quickly when she is acquainted, through personal experience, with his individual preferences and with the details of his care, it is well for her to keep the same assignment of patients indefinitely except when a change is necessary for educational or other reasons. The staff members should be encouraged to read and plan their work for the next day before leaving the floor. The day then begins with each individual knowing what she is to do. Adjustments, of course, may have to be made due to changes which have occurred over-night such as admissions, discharges, new treatments. For this reason the head nurse will probably wish to come on duty a few minutes before the day is to begin. This gives her time to note need for change in plans and minimizes delay for her staff in starting the day's work. The night nurse or clerk should prepare a list of patients who will leave the division for various tests or treatments, mothers who are to attend baby bath or formula dem-onstrations, patients to have breakfast held, those to be fed, patients for discharge.

The program for the day is reviewed by the head nurse with the staff at which time each member is expected to consider her assignment in re-lation to the time she has in which to complete it. She is also expected to make a mental plan for organizing her day's work. Organization is necessary for activities of every kind even if all the time one could desire were avail-able to achieve a purpose. Everyone has had the experience of being late to an event because, though he had plenty of time to get ready, he failed to organize it. On the other hand when time is at a premium, some of the most important items may be omitted unless a plan is made for their in-clusion. Having a plan gives each staff member confidence, encouragement, and the satisfaction of accomplishment. A great deal of time need not be taken for the organization of activities contributing to the patients' care provided the head nurse is well acquainted with the patients, their nursing needs, and medical prescriptions. The establishment of priorities and budgeting of time is necessary. When services must be cut back, it is often very useful to do this planning as a group, especially if some members are inexperienced, unfamiliar with the patients, or if others than professional nurses are assigned to care for some of the patients. Even though the day may be starting uneventfully, the situation can quickly change. If every staff member is aware of priorities the most important elements of patient care will be accomplished. However, the head nurse must, in addition, be alert to the needs of individual staff members for help in budgeting time.

What are some of the priorities in patient care situations which need to be established and for which time should be budgeted? Patients must get to the operating room and to other departments to undergo the tests and treatments for which they have been hospitalized. Therapeutic measures including certain medications may be the chief means by which the objectives of hospitalization will be reached and must therefore receive high priority. However, there are situations in which it would appear that priorities need to be set in favor of nursing activities in order best to meet the patient's needs. For instance, can certain medications be delayed to allow time for some more important measure such as a back rub, a treatment, or a chance for the patient to talk? Do those things which nurses are expected to record *always* have to take precedence over others? Should the head nurse not have the professional judgment to make decisions of this kind? Should not her staff raise such questions with the head nurse? Which patients need close observation for their safety? Are there some who do not need to have the morning temperature taken? For whom are mouth care, skin care, fluids, exercise, turning, ambulation, or other aspects of care vital to achieve progress, to maintain homeostasis, or to prevent complications? Are there some patients for whom bath and bed change could be omitted that day? Are there some patients or families in despair or weighted down with worry whom the head nurse must make time to see? In considering priorities, time for a thorough transfer report (see p. 157) must be high on the list. Without it the oncoming group is greatly handicapped in providing quality care. This is not to say that the report may not sometimes be given with greater dispatch and more meaning than frequently is the case.

In establishing priorities, the head nurse may well remind the staff that patients feel staff pressures, that well-organized work reduces feelings of frustration and pressure among personnel. It helps also for nurses to remember that keeping patients satisfied reduces the work load for they then make fewer demands or requests. On the busiest days, then, anticipation of patients' needs, answering calls promptly and cheerfully, showing interest, being sympathetic with complaints, and handling them promptly —all these attempts to keep patients content and happy—are an integral part of the daily plan of work for a patient care division.

Four other key factors in effectively organizing work will be mentioned. Every nurse has been familiar with the first two since her early days in the school of nursing. One is the time saved by putting things in order as she goes along—rinsing a syringe, placing soiled linen in a bag as it is removed, putting away equipment such as soap, comb, powder immediately after use, arranging the patient's unit for his convenience, and surveying the whole before she leaves the room. This first point is closely allied to the second which is an integral part of good organization—working in an orderly environment. Good organization involves maintenance of surroundings which are conducive to clear thinking and free from distractions which interfere with the achievement of the goal. It disorder exists, time will probably be saved if the situation is rearranged before undertaking the work of the day. For example, there are occasions when the night nurse is delayed by an emergency during the last hours of the early morning which prevents her completing her work. The head nurse quickly realizes that the night nurse cannot finish without remaining overtime and that the entire morning's schedule will be upset unless the night work is completed promptly. She also knows that many of the day's activities should not start until those of the night have been finished. With the assistance of the night nurse she should divide the remaining tasks among the day staff and see that they are completed before the regular program of the day begins. If the spirit of the staff is cooperative and there is no attitude of blame or criticism, the delay in the day's activities probably will be minimal. If the head nurse fails to step into the breach and adjust the assignments or if she adjusts them grudgingly, the entire day's program may well be thrown out of balance.

If delays in the work of the night nurse occur frequently, the head nurse needs to look for the causes. Perhaps the night nurse needs help in planning her program. Perhaps there needs to be a reorganization of the activities which constitute the night nurse's work. It may be that if all duties are to be properly performed the night nurse needs more assistance. These are problems for serious consideration. The head nurse needs the help of the night nurse and the night nurse administrator in solving them.

The third additional factor contributing to good organization is starting the day's work promptly, that is, beginning the day on time. Every nurse should be expected to be on the floor at the hour assigned. The night nurse, whether or not all her work is completed, should be prepared to give the night report at the designated time. The head nurse who comes to work early must not become so involved that she fails to start the day promptly. Casualness in this matter on the part of the head nurse is apt to influence the members of the staff to arrive a few minutes late. The head nurse will find also that it is possible to begin each new day more promptly if she has left her desk clear the night before. It is difficult to work in confusion. If the early part of the day is spent gathering up loose ends from the preceding day much valuable time is lost.

The fourth facilitator of organization is prevention of interruption. Since time is wasted in going from one activity to another, good management requires avoidance of interference with continuity of work whenever possible. This is true for all personnel including the head nurse. Changes in assignments of patients and of time should be kept to a minimum although they are impossible to avoid altogether, since new patients are admitted and emergencies arise. One nurse, however, may be assigned to care for new patients and the rest of her assignment arranged accordingly. This will save interruptions for those with heavier loads. Some head nurses admit patients and conduct the initial interview.

The head nurse who has a clerk or unit manager to answer the telephone and deal with questions finds it easier to prevent interruptions. She should, as far as possible, complete one activity before beginning another. If she can finish making patient rounds with only minor interruptions, she will then be free for other duties such as spending time with a patient who needs to talk or a new nurse who wishes help.

During periods of the day when the head nurse has reports to write, progress notes to read, and medicine tickets to check, she should make every effort to arrange her time so she will be uninterrupted. Although the head nurse should always be accessible, thoughtfulness on the part of the nursing and medical staffs can often save her from many needless interruptions. A private office is a great help to the head nurse, and it may be possible, at certain periods, to leave some other nurse in charge of the division for a short period while she completes an important piece of work such as planning time or assignments.

An effective system of communication. Communication is more than exchange of information and ideas; it also involves the receiving of the intended message. Language, culture, education, bias, emotions, preoccupation, and other factors may preclude hearing that which was said or intended. When this happens the individuals are not communicating.

This chapter in speaking of a system of communication, considers planned means by which information is transmitted as well as unplanned exchange of information and ideas. Examples of unplanned communication are asking for opinion, informal teaching, expressing appreciation. This type of communication aids the functioning of a hospital in so far as the exchange builds morale, facilitates getting the work done, makes a good impression on others within or without the organization. It is interesting to note in a study of the general hospital,[1] that coordination was found to be better in those hospitals where it is easier for personnel to meet and exchange information and ideas about their work, and that coordination is also better where supervisory and administrative practices which foster subordinate communication on work-relevant matters are more prevalent.

Planned communication in the hospital is frequently in the form of written orders, reports, or records. Common also is oral communication which occurs between individuals, in small groups, in conferences, classes, and meetings of all kinds. Communication may consist of a report, discussion, lecture, or a combination of methods. The head nurse is primarily concerned about three types of planned communication: medical orders, reports, and records, each of which will be discussed in the next chapter.

Development of routines for frequently performed activities. One of the most important factors in achieving the coordination essential to good administration is standardization of frequently performed activities. This is accomplished by establishing procedures and routines, by timing and sequencing activities. Patient care does not lend itself to routinization but certain aspects of its management do. When a system is established for day to day tasks, time is available for handling the unusual occurrence. A definite routine for giving transfer reports, a specific system for assigning new patients, a carefully worked out procedure for preparing patients for meals permit these daily activities to be accomplished regardless of emergencies which arise. A systematized service functions well whether or not the head nurse is present.

Time will be saved and greater accuracy will result if routines are outlined in detail and placed in a guide book. Likewise, a nursing procedure book is invaluable when it contains a description of procedures specific for the division. Some head nurses prefer to write the procedure outline on cards which are then placed in an indexed file box. The advantage of the latter is that individual cards are more easily handled than a book. The life of the cards may be prolonged by covering them with washed x-ray film. The preparation of a policy book and special procedures where none exist is an interesting and worthwhile undertaking for the nursing staff.

Each head nurse should be aware of problems and situations on her division which interfere with good nursing and those which cause interruption, delays, and frustration. Consultation with staff nurses and with other nursing personnel, if they are involved, brings to light problems and suggestions for their solution. Often the establishment of a division routine or

[1] Basil S. Georgopoulos and Floyd C. Mann. *The Community General Hospital,* New York, The Macmillan Company 1962, pp. 599-600.

the changing of one which exists makes a marked improvement in the care of patients or results in a saving of time for the personnel.

For example, the patient who goes to the operating room must have complete preparation which includes many points for which the nurse is usually responsible—clean skin and mouth, operative area free from hair, empty bladder, removal of jewelry, dentures, nail polish, hair pins of all kinds, and presence of identification band. Time may be at a premium especially early in the morning when the first patients are called to the operating room. The inexperienced nurse often has difficulty remembering all the details of preparation. The head nurse, unless she has delegated this responsibility to another nurse, should observe the patient to assure herself that he has been properly prepared. She may find that considerable time can be saved and that omissions may be avoided if a check list is prepared which itemizes the points necessary to proper preparedness of the patient. Upon this sheet the names of all patients scheduled for surgery are listed and after the nurse has completed her preparation of the patient she checks the list and finishes any parts of the care which she may have omitted (Fig. 8). The head nurse finds the check list useful in making her final observation. Check lists for this and other matters may be posted on bulletin boards in convenient places. They not only save time and effort, but they are often safeguards against injury due to oversight.

No system can be constructed to meet all the needs that arise on a busy hospital division. In fact care must be taken that the system does not detract from good patient care rather than contribute to it. A schedule which requires that a nurse adhere to it regardless of a patient's personal needs, or a system for serving diet trays that does not consider individual preferences for food or permit a patient to be served out of turn in order that he may eat with his neighbors, may be worse than no routine. Schedules and routines are valuable in so far as they serve to provide better nursing care. Never should the system become more important than the individuals who are affected by it, that is, the patients and the members of the staff. A system which is so inflexible that it permits no initiative or originality on the part of the nurses is demoralizing. So, too, efficiency can be carried so far as to be noneducational and uninteresting.

The head nurse is not entirely free to establish routines on her floor, for the hospital has set up certain procedures around which the unit system must be built. Meal hours, admission and discharge procedures, methods for handling valuables, perhaps the use of the patient or team method of assignment are practices which are established by the hospital and cannot be changed by individual head nurses. Routine for the division usually must be established within the existing pattern. The head nurse may be

GRACE-NEW HAVEN COMMUNITY HOSPITAL

DIVISION
OR
CLINIC
W I

NAME... *Jones, John* .... *00-00-00* UNIT NO.
ADDRESS... *14 South St. New Haven* ....
BIRTH DATE ...*9-1-18 New Haven WM 1 Ward* ...ACCOMMODATION

CHECK LIST FOR PRE-OPERATIVE PREPARATION
Check each item as it has been completed in the Pre-Operative preparation of the patient.

OPERATIVE PERMIT (F.89): SIGNED BY PATIENT ✓ HUSBAND___ PARENT___ GUARDIAN___

DATED *Jan. 5, 1962* WITNESSED *B Barrell*

SKIN PREPARATION: DONE BY *Dr. Parkchie* CHECKED BY *B Barrell*

SURGICAL BED PREPARED:_____ PATIENT VOIDED *8 45 AM*

MEDICATION GIVEN *Seconal 100 mgm Atropine 0.4 mg* TIME GIVEN *8 45 AM* TIME GIVEN CHARTING COMPLETE ✓

FORMS PLACED ON CHART: ON ✓ DOCTOR'S ORDER SHEET (F.677-B)
✓ ANESTHESIA SHEET (F.667)

PATIENT'S ADDRESSOGRAPH PLATE ✓

FOLLOWING REMOVED: JEWELRY *NONE* HAIRPINS, ETC. *NONE*

NAILPOLISH AND LIPSTICK ✓ CLOTHING OTHER THAN HOSPITAL GOWN ✓

DENTURES REMOVED & PLACED IN DENTURE CUP *No Dentures*

WEDDING RING ~~TIED~~: *TAPED*

REMARKS:

F.1165 (REV. 10-61)

SIGNATURE *B Barrell*
NURSE

Fig. 8. Check list, filled out by the nurse preparing the patient for surgery, is signed by the head nurse and sent in the patient's chart to the operating room (Courtesy Yale-New Haven Hospital.)

influential in having the pattern changed, however, if she can present evidence in a clear and convincing way that the existing system is inefficient, uneconomical, impractical, or detrimental to the best interests of the patients or staff. She must have facts to substantiate her statements. No head nurse should disregard a hospital policy nor should she complacently accept it if it is interfering with the smooth management of patient care or putting an apparently unnecessary burden on the nursing staff. Ideally, there are few inflexible policies. Instead guide lines assist the head nurse in making decisions. However, when a definite policy does exist which the head nurse considers detrimental, she should feel obligated to present the facts of the situation, together with her suggestions for changes, through the department administrator, to the director of the nursing service. Written statements are usually more effective than oral reports because they can be studied at leisure. Brevity and conciseness are important. The forward-looking director of nursing will welcome suggestions from head nurses who have insight and initiative enough to make factual studies of this type.

Advance planning. Organizing each day's activities is essential to coordination. Important as such planning is, however, it deals only with the present and goes little beyond the needs of the day or week. For administration to be highly effective and for coordination to reach a significant level of proficiency, advance planning to achieve long-range goals is essential. For the head nurse this planning might involve evaluating nursing care including the development of measures. It could lead to experiments to determine the results of different nursing methods and approaches; studies to improve nursing practice. It might concentrate on ways to motivate, challenge, and develop the staff; the determination of staff problems which interfere with quality patient care. Staffing patterns and time planning markedly affect continuity in patient care and satisfaction of staff. Long-range planning in these areas should try to find answers to problems. These are a few examples of subjects yet to be discussed in this text in which advance planning by head nurses is needed.

Voluntary effort. Coordination, one of the key requirements for good administration, determines the extent to which an organization runs as a well-regulated machine. It depends not only on routines and the other facilitating factors described above but also relies on voluntary efforts. Common understandings, shared attitudes and goals among those who work together result in appreciation of others' problems and willingness to help one another. These are powerful forces essential to coordination of those activities which cannot be completely routinized.[2] Chapter 2 has discussed

---

[2] Georgopoulos and Mann, *op. cit.,* pp. 597-598.

the strength which resides in small groups. Chapter 8 will consider the head nurse's leadership role in building morale.

The Development of Personnel, Supervision of Work, and Evaluation of Outcomes Are Functions of Administration

This principle will be elaborated later in the text (Part 3 and Chapter 13). Suffice it to say here: unless administration assumes responsi biltiy for the quality of output and provides necessary supervision of the worker and the work, it will fail; unless it constantly strives to develop the potential of all workers, administration is at best doomed to mediocrity.

EVIDENCE OF GOOD NURSING CARE ADMINISTRATION

Before completing this chapter it will be useful to consider the evidence which indicates that management pertaining to nursing care is well carried out, that principles have been fulfilled. In so doing it is being assumed that good nursing care administration helps bring about patient care of high quality. However, since other factors also contribute to good care, it cannot be used as a criterion measure solely of good administration. What, then, are the criteria for judging the quality of nursing care administration? Nursing care can usually be judged to be well administered when work is accomplished with a minimum of tension; staff members work well together, and there is willingness to help those in other roles, shifts and divisions; take-over between tours of duty is smooth—a full report is given, no work is left over for the next shift. (Time for *nursing care* should, of course, always remain flexible in relation to patients' needs.) Evidence points to positive correlation between organizational coordination, a component of effective administration, and 1) conformity to policy; 2) a small amount of absenteeism among professional nurses; 3) work-relevant conversation among the staff; and 4) freedom to discuss work across peer levels—staff nurse and aide with department administrator, for example.[3] One would, therefore, infer that these four points could be used as criteria to evaluate nursing care administration. Good administration of nursing care is also in evidence when there is order in work areas; when

[3] Georgopoulos and Mann, *op. cit.,* p. 600.

the staff members use their time productively and do not spend an excess amount in the rest room, at coffee or meals; do not congregate in the office but keep busy in acivities related to patients. Quality of administration is also judged by the ability of the head nurse and her staff to find solutions to their own problems and not always call for help. Does the head nurse adjust to inevitable situations without complaint, and help her staff to do so by her manner and encouraging words? Does the head nurse analyze a situation, make a decision with despatch and take prompt action when these are called for, involving the staff when time permits but not at the expense of assuming responsibility for decision when this is needed promptly? Other criteria for judging the administrative effectiveness of the head nurse are the satisfaction of patients and families with the care they receive, the satisfaction of the physicians, and the enthusiastic spirit of the nursing staff. The problem of judging by these means is that valid measures of satisfaction are as yet practically nonexistent. It is recognized, too, that satisfaction with nursing care is dependent upon factors other than administration.

SUMMARY

The principles of administration are applicable to any organization. The head nurse, as administrator of nursing care and coordinator of patient care, needs to be familiar with the principles and the ways in which they apply to her and her work. It is especially important that she know she has both professional and administrative responsibility. She, as is every nurse, is responsible for professional nursing practice in whatever role she is cast. As long as she remains in the administrative line of the hospital she will also have administrative responsibility to someone on a higher level. As long as she remains a head nurse she will be administratively responsible for work carried out by others. She will be the person to delegate that work, together with sufficient responsibility to accomplish it. The accountability remains hers. The supervision of personnel is also the head nurse's responsibility as an administrator, as is decision-making, short and long range planning, communication, and coordination.

The effectiveness of the head nurse's administration is evident in the smoothness with which nursing activities are achieved, the degree of freedom from tension, the purposefulness, and dependability of the staff; the satisfaction with care expressed by patients, families, doctors, and nursing staff to name but a few criteria.

QUESTIONS FOR DISCUSSION

1. How well do you keep the environment cleaned up as you proceed with your work? arrange materials convenient for use? Do you succeed in avoiding *unnecessary* interruptions such as having to obtain a forgotten item of equipment or stopping one activity and taking up another? Would you accomplish more if you organized your time and work space more efficiently? Why? Illustrate.
2. How would you compare the effectiveness of "voluntary effort" and of "planned activities" (routines, organization, etc.) in achieving coordination on the division where you are working?

EXERCISES

1. Select one of the principles of administration listed, and on one division over a period of several days observe the way nursing care is administered in relation to the principle. Briefly describe instances in which the head nurse adheres to the principle and ways in which her administration could have been improved in this regard.
2. If you are a head nurse who does not hold regular daily conferences with your staff to establish priorities, and budget time, try doing so on an especially busy day. Preliminary planning on your part will be essential to success. For your first attempt, you might prefer to plan with practical nurses and aides only.
3. Using the "Evidences of Good Nursing Care Administration" and a three-point scale evaluate on each point the administration of the division where you are working. Substantiate each judgment with an illustration or explanation.
4. Plan your day's work, whatever it may be. To what activities are you giving top priority? At the end of the day review your activities. Did you have to budget your time to accomplish everything you needed to do? Did you succeed in accomplishing these things? Did you do everything on the priority list? Did it have to be augmented? Did you complete the augmented list? How did you feel about your day's accomplishments? Did planning help? Did it frustrate? If the latter, try again.

REFERENCES

Argyris, Chris. Personality and Organization, New York, Harper and Brothers, 1957, pp. 61-63.
"Chain of command," an organizational principle which is discussed here, pictures the situation from which nursing service administrators, in some centers, are endeavoring to remove their head nurses.

Babnew, David, Jr. The "whys" of wise delegation, Hospitals, Vol. 59 (July 16, 1965), pp. 62-64.
Delegation is an art essential to an administrator. Guides for effective delegating are given as well as illustrations of results of failure to delegate.

Fischer, Frank E. A new look at management communication. In Readings in Management, Koontz, H., and O'Donnell, C., eds. New York, McGraw-Hill Book Company, Inc., 1959, pp. 210-219.
Describes the communication process and ways to achieve effective communication. Hospitals could learn from this discussion in relation to business.

Georgopoulos, Basil S., and Mann, Floyd C. The Community General Hospital, New York, The Macmillan Company, 1962, Ch. 6, pp. 265-304, Ch. 7, pp. 305-364, Summary and Conclusions, pp. 596-605.
Organizational coordination is defined and described. Both programmed and general coordination are essential to the effectiveness of the hospital in meeting its patient care objective. Report of a research study.

Mooney, James D. The coordinative principle. In Readings in Management, Koontz, H., and O'Donnell, C., eds. New York, McGraw-Hill Book Company, Inc., 1959, pp. 7-12.
Coordination is the all-inclusive principle of organization and must be based on a community of interest in the attainment of an objective which is well understood by all concerned. The result of coordination is team work. It can only be attained by self-discipline.

Strauss, George, and Sayles, Leonard R. The Human Problems of Management, Englewood Cliffs, New Jersey, Prentice-Hall, Inc., 1960.
Administrative principles are clearly presented throughout this interesting book. The importance of advance planning is stressed on pages 277-282.

chapter 8

ADMINISTRATIVE ACTIVITIES
WITH WHICH THE HEAD NURSE IS CONCERNED

The administration of four activities which markedly affect nursing care and may, therefore, be considered part of its administration will be discussed in turn: 1) medical orders or prescriptions, 2) reports, 3) records, 4) staffing and time planning.

MEDICAL ORDERS

By means of medical orders the physician communicates to the nurse the prescriptions which he expects her to carry out and thereby gives her legal right to do so. Clear, specific orders for medical therapy are necessary to safeguard the patient's welfare. They help to prevent errors and thus they protect the doctor, the nurse, and the hospital. Confusion and waste of time can be avoided in many instances by well-written orders. No head nurse can afford to consider them lightly.

Requisites for Doctors' Orders

The nurse can be sued for the practice of medicine without a license if she performs treatments and gives medications without the doctor's order. Therefore, for her protection *all orders are written and accompanied by the signature of the physician.* Without a written, signed order the nurse has no proof that she was directed to treat the patient. A graduate nurse who accepts a verbal order assumes the risk of being accused of illegal practice. The student nurse is unlicensed and is permitted to practice nursing only because she is working under close supervision. If an error is made by a student, the responsibility may rest with the hospital. Some institutions which are lax in permitting graduate nurses to take verbal orders are strict in not allowing students to do so.

The doctor's written order, although primarily a protection for the nurse, also serves to safeguard the patient, the hospital, and the doctor. There is less likelihood of error in understanding and carrying out an order if it is in writing. The patient may thus be saved from the result of an incorrect drug or dosage or a wrong treatment. Oral instructions may be forgotten or misinterpreted. Harm to a patient resulting from a misunderstood order may reflect on medical care and the doctor has no proof of what he ordered for the patient unless the order is written and signed.

The doctor's orders effectively serve their purpose only if they are *clear, specific, complete, and written legibly.* Sufficient information is necessary to indicate the physician's intentions. Orders for moist applications need to specify the part to be treated, the type of solution to be used, and the frequency of the application. When a nursing procedure which has been approved by a joint nursing care committee composed of nurses and doctors gives specific directions for duration of a procedure, the extent of the area to be treated, or the solution to be used, the individual order of the physician need not include this information. Any variation from the usual method should, however, be given in writing. Nurses are familiar with the accepted methods of the institution and are likewise expected to know the indications for sterility, desirable and safe temperatures for solutions and hot water bags. This common knowledge, which is based on scientific principles, is an essential part of every nurse's education.

Orders are *reviewed periodically* by the doctor to assure that drugs and treatments are not being given beyond the time they are necessary or advisable. Some sure way of limiting the time an order is in effect is essential. An acceptable way to discontinue an order is to limit it in the original writing, as

q.4 h. for 6 doses
t.i.d. for 2 days

or a separate order for discontinuance of running orders may be written, dated, and signed. Some orders automatically supersede previous ones, as, for example, a regular diet order replaces an earlier one for liquid or soft foods; an order to get the patient up cancels one previously written for bed rest; operation or the transfer of a patient from one service to another automatically cancels all previous orders. Hospital policy often stipulates that narcotic orders are valid for 48 hours only. If the drug is to be continued, a new order is written at the end of that period. In some teaching hospitals all drug and treatment orders are invalidated after a 48-hour period thus necessitating their review. It is important that the doctor not fail to rewrite orders he wishes carried out. The secretary flags order sheets of patients whose orders are outdated.

Ways to Limit Verbal Orders

In hospitals where the administrator and the chiefs of service are firm in their conviction that verbal orders are hazardous, there is little or no problem in this area. In some institutions, unfortunately, it is left to the head nurse to enforce the regulation. If a unit director is employed this is his responsibility as representative of hospital administration. In still other hospitals, there seems to be little concern whether or not orders are written. As a result doctors have lost the habit of doing so. It has been previously indicated that it is the nurse, primarily, who is protected by the written, signed order. Therefore it is to her advantage to initiate measures for the control of verbal orders when she, not a unit director, has responsibility for enforcement of the policy. What can she do?

Her *first* step is to seek a clear understanding with the doctors on her service. Friendly talks between the head nurse and the resident or intern or, if necessary, with each individual doctor will do a great deal to gain mutual understanding. If her approach is reasonable and considerate it is rare that a head nurse is unable to win the cooperation and good will of the doctors with whom she works. Established policy concerning orders is discussed with new interns to give them an understanding of its purpose. The head nurse sees that facilities are provided to make the writing of orders convenient.

Second, to be workable, policy must provide for systematic functioning. Every nurse and clerk on the division as well as the unit manager needs to be familiar with its details. *Third,* once an agreement has been reached, all personnel are expected to adhere to it. If the head nurse herself does not waver in her compliance with the policy, the clerks, staff, and student nurses will have very little difficulty in declining to take verbal orders.

Telephone orders are harder to control than other verbal orders, but they should be avoided whenever possible. Orders for a newly admitted patient are often telephoned in by the physician or his office nurse. Ways have been found to eliminate calls for this purpose. The doctor who anticipates his patient's hospitalization writes his orders and leaves them in the admitting office when he makes his morning visit to the hospital. The patient who is sent in from the doctor's office brings with him, in a sealed envelope, the medical orders written by the physician on the hospital order sheet. Doctors have a supply of forms for this purpose. In instances where these methods are not feasible, the intern who is given the orders on the telephone writes them on the order sheet.

Telephone orders are also given when the doctor is tied up in the operating room, delivery room, or elsewhere and cannot leave to write an order. Because the patient is in need of a narcotic, analgesic, or diet order, the head nurse takes the order on the telephone. However, orders for relief of pain as well as for diet, enemas, cathartics, and sedatives are rather easily anticipated. A patient's need can be foreseen to some degree, at least, and a telephone order thus averted. Although the doctor should provide for his patient's comfort by anticipating his needs, the head nurse is also responsible for thinking through the contingencies when a p.r.n. order might be necessary. A notation of questions relative to orders for his patient may be clipped to the chart where the doctor will see it on his next visit. A brightly colored printed form headed "Dear Doctor"[1] may be used for many kinds of messages. The head nurse will also wish to be present, if possible, to confer with the doctor when he visits the division. With foresight, telephone orders can be held to a minimum.

On the few occasions when a telephone order is unavoidable the nurse in charge should take it. She writes the order on the patient's order sheet, signs the doctor's name per her own, and leaves a note on the front of the chart that the order is to be signed the next time the physician is on the division.

In an emergency, a telephone order may save a life. The order is written as dictated on a pad of paper which is kept near the telephone at all times. The charge nurse who receives the order reads it back for verification. She must never fail to know from whom the order is received. Before carrying it out she considers whether it is reasonable, whether it is the usual dosage of medication for the age and size of the patient, whether it is the type of treatment that is likely to be ordered under the present circumstances. It is safer to question before administering a drug than after it has been given. Taking time to think may prevent a serious error. As with any other telephone order the emergency order is written by the nurse and signed later by the doctor.

The same safeguards should be used if it is necessary in an emergency to take a verbal order from a doctor who is examining or treating a patient. Before administering the drug the nurse should get the physician's attention and tell him the drug and dose she has prepared. If these are reasonable for the age, size, and condition of the patient the nurse may feel safe in giving the drug before the order is written. If they do not seem to her to be safe or suitable she must remember that the doctor is under stress and suggest a possible alternative. "Is it cocaine or novocaine you wish?" or, "This child is seven years old. Did you say he is to have a sixteenth or a sixth?" Under no circumstances should she prepare or give a medication

---

[1] Dorothy Merrell. Dear Doctor, *Nurs. Outlook,* Vol. 8 (April 1960), pp. 218-221.

which she knows to be unsafe. Lives have been lost in this way. Nurses, doctors, and hospitals have been sued for malpractice and negligence. If, through courteous handling, she cannot get the doctor to recognize an error in speaking, she had best take to the bedside the equipment, the drug he ordered and the one she believes he intended to order and have the doctor prepare and give the medication himself. He will without doubt select the correct drug, give the nurse the proper order, and be forever grateful to her.

Standing Orders

Standing orders are in common use by some private physicians. Especially is this true when the care is fairly routine for his patients. An obstetrician usually has similar postpartal orders for all mothers whom he has delivered. So too, the ear, nose, and throat specialist has routine postoperative orders for patients on whom he has performed tonsillectomies. Standing orders save time for the doctor, but in hospitals where interns are learning to prescribe they are seldom used.

When standing orders are inappropriate for a patient, it is the doctor's responsibility to alter them. As a protection for the patient and nurse, the individual patient should have an order from his physician that standing orders are to be followed. There are two ways in which this may be managed. In one method the physician writes on the patient's order sheet, "Follow routine tonsillectomy orders," and affixes his signature. Any exceptions are indicated. When this method is used the standing orders have been previously typed, dated, and signed by the physician. The sheet is placed on a bulletin board where it can be easily seen by all. The second method is easier for the nurse. Orders are printed or, if brief, placed on a rubber stamp. When their use is anticipated, the clerk places the printed sheet in the front of the patient's chart or stamps the orders on the order sheet. There is space for the patient's name and the doctor's signature without which the orders are not in effect. On the printed sheet the doctor crosses out items he does not wish to order and, in spaces provided, writes any additions he wishes to make.

Limitations on Doctors in Writing Orders

It has been stated earlier that doctors are limited in writing orders by the administrative policy of the hospital. Some hospitals do not permit the use of electric heating pads; some do not allow hot water bags to be filled with water over a certain degree of temperature even if it is so ordered by a physician. Such policies are recommended or concurred in by the Joint Conference Committee of the hospital (see Chapter 2). They are adopted to prevent injury to patients which would reflect not only on the doctor but on the hospital.

Policies of this nature are best put in writing and either posted on a bulletin board or placed in a hospital routine or policy book. They should be included in the teaching of every nurse and medical student and should be called to the attention of new interns, residents, and attending physicians (by the unit director or manager, or by the nurse, if necessary) before the occasion arises when the information is needed. If the doctor feels that an exception should be made for one of his patients, he should be encouraged to consult with the hospital administrator. If the unit director is empowered to make such exceptions, he should consult the head nurse.

Methods by which Orders Are Handled

Specific procedures for the handling of orders vary, but certain principles are important. A systematic check of order sheets is essential to discover new orders promptly. Since it is not practical for the secretary or head nurse to make a frequent search of charts or a doctor's order book for new orders, a quick method of check is needed. Each hospital has its own established procedure. When the order sheet is kept in the patient's record, the chart containing a new order is placed in a separate rack, left on top of the chart desk, or flagged so that the order can be handled promptly. If order sheets for all patients are kept in a loose-leaf book, a sheet is fastened to the front on which the doctor writes the name of the patient for whom he has written a new order. Failure to comply with the policy means that the order may not be discovered immediately and that the patient will fail to receive the prescribed therapy. All order sheets are routinely checked for new orders several times a day but this does not assure an order being carried out as early as the doctor desires.

A definite routine for handling new orders is a necessity so that there may be no question about their having been noted and carried out. Taking care of a new diet order includes making a new diet card, destroying the old one, perhaps notifying the dietary department, and changing the diet order on the plan for patient care or on the diet list. Not until all aspects have been cared for is the order book signed. It is safer if only one member of the clerical staff handles new orders, and only the charge nurse checks and approves them. There should be a specific method to designate that an order for a single dose of medication or a single treatment has been carried out. The nurse who administers the medication or performs the treatment is usually the one to sign the order indicating that it has been completed.

To prevent error and avoid confusion, policy with relation to orders should be the same throughout the institution especially if nurses transfer from unit to unit. Matters of this kind can be handled by group consultation and joint discussion among the persons responsible; that is, the unit directors or the head nurses, whichever group deals with medical orders.

Obligations of the Nurse and the Doctor in Regard to Orders

Communication of medical orders implies certain obligations between the nurse and the doctor. The nurse should expect to be taken into the doctor's full confidence concerning his purpose and expectations in writing an order. On the other hand the nurse is obligated to the doctor, *first* to understand the order completely and not to assume that she knows what is meant. *Second,* the doctor expects that she will report promptly any inability to comply with his orders such as unavailability of a medication or lack of facilities to perform a treatment. *Third,* he depends on her to carry out his orders safely and effectively and to report and record results of treatments and their effects on the patient so that he will be able to judge the therapeutic value and know when to discontinue the procedure. *Fourth,* the doctor expects the nurse to use good judgment in the administration of drugs and treatments and to let him know if circumstances appear to contraindicate their use. *Fifth,* he depends upon her to determine how much he wants the patient to know about the purpose of his tests and treatments and to interpret them to the patient accordingly. On the other hand the head nurse should anticipate that the physician would expect her to use her judgment in discerning a patient's need and in answering a direct question. *Sixth,* he expects that the nurse will report any difficulty relative to the performance of the treatment, that is, an unfavorable psychological or physical reaction in the patient. For example, the patient may strenuously object to the treatment even after a careful explanation by the nurse, or catheterization may have been omitted because severe pain was produced by the attempted passage of the catheter. If the head nurse is unable to discover the reason and eliminate the patient's objection or the anxiety which may be causing the pain, the doctor is informed.

REPORTS

Importance of Reports

Probably no other single factor is more vital to good administration than prompt, complete reports. They save duplication of effort and eliminate the need for investigation to learn the facts in a situation. Patients receive better care when reports are thorough and give all pertinent data. When they are inadequate it is possible for medications or treatments to be duplicated or omitted. Reports may also save embarrassment due to ignorance of a situation. If complete, they give a sense of security which comes from knowing all factors in the situation.

Intradivision Reports

Reports between nursing staff members. Formal and informal reporting goes on continuously in the hospital division. The head nurse or the nurse in charge looks to her staff to keep her informed throughout the day of changes in the condition of patients and results of treatments if they are unusual or significant. She expects staff members to let her know whether they have insufficient or too much time to carry out their assignments. She also expects to be told of problems in relation to patients, such as the nurse's inability to give the care ordered, patients' complaints or their difficulties in adjustment.

The head nurse should expect a report from each nurse and aide at the end of her day's work and when the staff member leaves the division for a class or meeting. When team nursing is practiced, members report on their patients to the team. The head nurse should be a regular attendant at these conferences. In divisions which are not organized into nursing teams, the individual nurse reports to the head nurse briefly and concisely on each patient and on any unfulfilled assignments. At this time the head nurse has an opportunity to help the nurse learn what is important to report and how to do it in the most economical way. It is an excellent practice to have nurses, particularly students and new staff nurses, bring to the head nurse for her review the nurses' notes for the day, the records of treatments and medications which have been given, and summaries of fluid intake and elimination. In this way questions are raised in the mind of the head nurse and can be cleared before the nurse leaves the floor. It also gives her an excellent opportunity to discuss with the nurse the completeness and form of her charting, the significance of symptoms, needs of the patient for health teaching, to suggest methods of approach to patients and ways of helping them utilize the information. The nurse is reminded of problems which she wishes to talk over with the head nurse. If this method of reporting is used not as mere inspection for completeness but as the simplest way to transmit information and avoid omissions in recording and reporting, staff nurses and senior students as well as younger students welcome and do not resent it.

Transfer reports. A report is given at any time that responsibility for patient care management is turned over to another person. The nurse giving the report may be the head nurse, the evening or night nurse, or a team leader. On occasion a one-to-one report is given, but more often one nurse (head nurse or team leader, who may be the same individual) reports to a group, having previously learned about the patients from the staff members who are going off duty. When the head nurse is on the division, she participates in transfer reports. The group receiving the report may be a nursing team or the entire day, evening, or night staff. All may include practical nurses and aides and sometimes students. There are always some in the group who have been absent for a day or more. The report therefore needs to be full enough to bring them up-to-date.

The transferring nurse uses the cardex from which to report. She and the nurse who is to be in charge together look at each patient's card which contains his current medical orders, nursing orders, and the plan for his care (see Chapter 10). In this way the nurse who is giving the report will be reminded of information which should be transmitted and questions can be answered. Members of the group should be encouraged to comment and ask questions. Not only is it a waste of time but it is discourteous as well for the nurse who is reporting to disregard the group and speak in a low voice to the oncoming charge nurse only. Every one present should be included in the report and each has an obligation to listen and to comprehend it. For the staff member to participate, the report must be given so she can hear it, interesting enough to hold her attention, and sufficiently detailed to have meaning.

A good transfer report is unhurried. It is well to set aside a block of time to be kept for report purposes. It should be a firm policy that reports are not to be interrupted except in an emergency, for if continuity is broken important points may be easily forgotten. The importance of giving reports on time cannot be overemphasized. Delays waste the time of nurses who are coming on duty. Unfinished work can be completed following the report. In some institutions the night nurse records her report on tape an hour or so before she is to go off duty. Undistracted, she tends to organize her report better and does not digress. She may remain on the division until the report has been played to the day staff, in case there are questions. A recorded report is a decided advantage to the head nurse when staff members start the day at different hours, some at 7:00 AM, others at 8, 9, or 10:00 AM. It is advisable for the nurse who is to take charge of the division to accompany the departing charge nurse on rounds to see the patients. If there are further questions they usually arise at this time.

Between the head nurse and her assistant, reporting goes on informally almost continuously as each tries to keep the other informed. The assistant head nurse should know everything pertinent to the administration of patient care on the unit even though she may never be concerned with parts of the information. She is expected to take over the supervision of patient care in the event of the enforced absence of the head nurse. There can be a great deal of confusion if the head nurse possesses important information which she has failed to tell to her assistant because she expected to handle the situation herself. The assistant or nurse who is to be in charge needs to be fully informed also when the head nurse is away from the division for a few hours or for her weekly days off.

The well-informed assistant head nurse knows the condition of all patients, the treatment they are receiving, observations which are to be made, problems of staffing and the plans for meeting them, expected admissions, discharges, and treatments, plans for a new nurse's experience, changes in routine. In other words she has all the information she needs to insure good patient care and prevent waste of time.

When the head nurse returns after hours or days of absence, the assistant head nurse reports to her all changes in the situation including the condition of patients and the happenings during her absence. Adequate reporting between the head nurse and her assistant can be achieved only if they have time together prior to the transfer of responsibility. Consecutive days off for the head nurse and the person who is to be in charge in her absence do not permit proper briefing.

It is advisable for the head nurse and her assistant to keep, in a notebook or on a note pad, memoranda of information which they plan to report. This saves the effort of trying to remember an infinite amount of detail. Prior to giving the report, time is taken to organize the material in a logical sequence. The notes are used as a reminder in making the report. **Reports between head nurse and unit director or manager.**[2] These two individuals because of their close working relationship need to communicate frequently. Much of their communication takes place informally, but time should be set aside daily for the head nurse and director to report to one another on a more formal, organized basis. The unit director will need a brief report on patients. The amount and kind of information which he needs and should receive concerning patients depends on the director's role. If he is administrator of the unit, he should be well informed about the patient's condition, though he need not know details of pathology or clinical state. Nor should he be told about patients' personal problems except as they are related to hospital services. A unit manager who has no responsibility in relation to the individual patient, needs less information but should know enough about his diagnosis, therapy, and condition to be understanding of the family's needs and the environmental conditions which are of special importance to the particular patient. The unit manager has full access to the patient's chart and can obtain from that source any information he needs or desires. In other words in deciding the content of a report to the unit manager the purpose is not to conceal but to discriminate that information which the manager needs in order to do his job intelligently. Only experience can determine this content and it is a subject worthy of study. Regardless of what may be learned, however, the policy should be flexible. If the unit manager is to be interested in patients' welfare he must be interested in the patient. If he is interested in the patient, he will want and need to have information about him. The manager should feel free to ask questions and in most instances to have them answered. It is one thing for the head nurse to answer questions and another to feel that a complete clinical report needs to be given.

The report to the unit director should also include problems which nursing is having in providing needed care. Again, content of the report will depend on the role and responsibilities of the director or manager. If the unit director's function is to provide a coordinated, smoothly functioning service which will make it possible for nurses and doctors to function at their professional best, then anything which will either promote or interfere

[2] In this volume, *unit director* refers to a representative of hospital administration who has administrative responsibility for one or more patient care divisions as portrayed in the conceptual model (p. 99). Unit manager refers to an individual with considerably less authority who is either a peer of the head nurse or is responsible to her. In referring to either of the two, both titles—unit director and unit manager—may be used, but when this is awkward and the meaning seems clear, one or the other is used.

with unit administration should be brought up for discussion. In any given situation, the head nurse and the unit director or manager need to think through information each needs to have about the program, plans, and problems of the other and to transmit this information systematically and regularly.

Reports between the physician and head nurse. The interchange of information between the doctor and the head nurse and the type of information each needs to receive from the other was discussed in Chapter 6 and on pages 155-156.

Reports to the Administrator of the Department and the Nursing Service

When the head nurse is professionally responsible for a group of patients, as in the visualized role, she makes no report to nursing service administration but only to members of her own staff who will be carrying responsibility in her absence. However, when the head nurse is responsible to a department administrator, the administrator needs to receive from the head nurse an overview of the situation on the division. The amount of detail she wishes depends on many factors including the competency of the head nurse to plan and supervise patient care, the total number of patients for whom she has administrative resopnsibility, and the other activities in which she is involved. She should be told about complaints of patients, visitors, doctors, and members of the nursing staff as well as about accidents and mistakes. It is important also that she know of personnel problems involving congeniality, cooperation, adjustment and growth; problems in relationships with other departments and those concerned with hospital routine.

In small hospitals in which there is no department administrator the head nurse reports directly to the nursing service administrator or to one of her assistants. In this case the information reported is much the same as that described above. It is very stimulating for the head nurse when the nursing administrator makes rounds and can be given a direct report. The administrator usually wishes to receive a general picture of the division, to learn the condition of the sickest patients, to be told of new and interesting treatments, the difficulties in giving nursing care, including problems of staffing. In large institutions it is impossible for the nursing administrator or even for her assistants to be in such close contact with patients. They must depend on the written report from the division for most of their information.

The day, evening, and night report. This report serves as a ready reference for nurse administrators and lets them know at the beginning of every transfer period the trouble spots where help may be needed. Prepared by the charge nurse with the help of the clerk, this report may list all patients or just the sickest ones. In either case only that information which is necessary to give a general picture of the division needs to be included such as the census, the names, diagnoses, and general condition of patients, the patients admitted, operated, or discharged. Hospital and nursing service administrators usually wish information about certain patients whose accident or illness is reported by the press and those who undergo unusual surgery or other therapy.

Sometimes the same report sheet is used to include all three reports, day, evening, and night, thus making it necessary for the clerk to write the patient's name only once in a 24-hour period. This saves considerable time. Self-duplicating or carbon paper is used and as many copies are made as are necessary. This type of report is particularly useful when all patients are included, not just a few. Time is also saved if report forms are devised so that names can be printed by the addressograph. Some hospitals have special departments to prepare addressographed lists of patients, which can be used for many purposes throughout the hospital.

Evaluation reports. An evaluation report on each nursing staff member is usually required by nursing service when personnel is centrally employed. A full discussion will be found in Chapter 18.

Reports Pertaining to Hospital Administration

Interdepartmental reports. Reports from the division to administrative departments are usually the responsibility of a unit manager or secretary. Reports on census, patients to be discharged, and patients' conditions are sent daily on a special form to the departments and offices which need this information. Promptness and accuracy in transmitting them are essential if the work of each department is to function smoothly.

Legal reports. Incident reports and reports on accidents, mistakes, and complaints are legal in nature. There are times when a hospital is criticized for what is claimed to be negligence or poor care because of a condition which resulted in discomfort and perhaps serious harm to a patient. Conditions which have been known to induce severe criticism are breaks in the skin including pressure sores, reactions to treatments such as transfusions and infusions, pediculosis, and badly snarled or matted hair. To be sure, some of these conditions may result from poor nursing or medical care but sometimes they are present when the patient is admitted or they may have occurred in spite of efforts to prevent them. Whatever the explanation, it is often considered advisable to have on file a report of any situation which might raise a question relative to the quality of nursing or medical care. Reports of this type, often called *Incident Reports,* also aid the head nurse or nursing service administrator in evaluating the work for which she is responsible. To be accurate the report should be written by the persons directly involved and at the time when the details of causes, preventive measures, and treatment are fresh in their minds.

A report of this nature includes complete identifying data—date of the report, name of the patient and his diagnosis, date of admission, and the division. Then follows a description of the condition, when and under what circumstances it was first noted, to whom it was reported, what had been done to prevent the condition, how it was treated and the results of treatment, the names of all individuals involved and the signature of the person writing the report.

In such a report the content is stated briefly and objectively giving all pertinent information. Facts are given from first-hand observation. The report is written either by the individual who first observed and reported the condition, the person who was responsible for it, the head nurse, or by all three. If the condition seems to be of a serious nature or if it in any way involves medical treatment the nurse's statement is accompanied by a note written and signed by the doctor. He gives his interpretation of the cause and a description of the treatment instituted. The report is sent to the nursing office after having been seen by the department administrator.

Reports on mistakes and accidents are also essential. If the hospital is decentralized (according to the conceptual model) such reports would be given to the unit director. Errors and accidents are usually due to carelessness of individuals and sometimes occur in spite of elaborate precautions taken to prevent them. A hospital, as are other institutions, is obligated to use every means in its power to guard the welfare of those on its property. Each employee is responsible for using every known precaution to prevent injury to a patient or hospital visitor. This necessitates knowledge of and adherence to the regulations and the safeguards established by the institution whether or not the reason for their existence is clear.

When an accident or mistake occurs it is important to know how it happened in order that a repetition may be avoided. For several reasons it is advisable for a report of this nature to be in writing—it must be accurate, it must be understood, it needs to be studied, it may be needed for legal purposes. The report indicates whether due care was taken. In other words was there a "Caution" sign in use to show that the floor was being waxed? Was the patient strapped on the narrow stretcher or were side rails used while he was being transported to the x-ray department? Answers to these questions indicate whether the hospital or the individual was negligent. If the individual failed to follow regulations what was the reason?

Did the nurse who gave the wrong medication comply with the established procedure of the institution? If she did not, was it because she had not been properly instructed, because it was impractical or impossible to do so, because she was pressed for time, or because she did not consider it necessary? In writing the report, the nurse may discover the loophole in her procedure which led to the accident or mistake. The report thus becomes a teaching device.

To serve the purposes which have been indicated, reports must contain all the facts. The exact hour, the day, and the date are important as is the name of the patient, the visitor, or the employee, and the name and position of the nurse who made the mistake or witnessed the incident. Included also are the name of the division, place of occurrence, and any unusual condition which prevailed such as the presence of many visitors on the unit, the existence of an emergency which tied up most of the staff, or the fact that all but two nurses were off the floor to luncheon.

Never should any individual be made to feel that the writing of a report is a punitive measure. It is a device to help prevent similar incidents or it is an instrument to help individuals analyze their shortcomings with a view to overcoming them. Nursing instructors and administrators including the head nurse lose an opportunity to determine the inadequacies in their teaching and the impracticability of the procedures which they have established if they fail to study the reports on errors and accidents which are made by personnel.

Certain criticisms of the institution, its personnel or service are also reported. If the complaint of a patient or visitor is of such serious nature that it cannot be easily resolved by the division personnel to the satisfaction of the individuals concerned, it is wise to make a written report which should be filed in the office of the hospital administrator, nurse administrator, or unit director according to the hospital's organization. Serious complaints if not well handled may result in embarrassment for the hospital. Untold harm can be done by lowering the confidence of the public in an institution in which it is highly important that it have faith. When a report of this nature is written it should include an objective statement of the complaint, the justification for it as seen by the nurse, measures taken to overcome the dissatisfaction, the results, and the names of the people involved. As with all other reports it is dated and signed.

RECORDS

Every organization keeps some kind of records. The hospital is no exception. Records are important for historical purposes and they serve as data for research and evidence in substantiating verbal statements and requests. Every department in the hospital has its own records. There is a tendency in many organizations to add a new record without careful study to determine its usefulness. Since keeping records is time consuming, it is important that their number be kept to a minimum. The use of each one should be reviewed periodically to see whether it is fulfilling its purpose or whether it could be eliminated.

The head nurse might well review the records she is keeping. Is the information being used? If not and if it is a record for division use only, she should discuss the advisability of its discontinuance with her staff and the department administrator. If general agreement is reached that the original purpose of the record no longer exists, it should be discontinued. Sometimes records are kept for short periods when a special study is being made by the division staff or the nursing service. When the study is complete the records are filed or destroyed after the data are tabulated. Records requested by hospital or nursing service administration may not be discontinued by the head nurse. If she sees no purpose in a record she has been asked to keep, she should question the department administrator. Perhaps the record has outlived its usefulness.

The Patient's Clinical Record

The patient's clinical chart is the record with which the head nurse is most concerned. It's importance is evidenced by the fact that the approval of a hospital for the teaching of interns is granted only if it has a satisfactory clinical record system. The value of the record is both scientific and legal. It serves as evidence to the patient that his care is being intelligently managed. As a record of illness and treatment it saves duplication of effort in future care and aids in prompt treatment. The record supplies material for medical and nursing research and hence aids in the promotion of health and the cure of disease. It serves as legal protection to the hospital, the doctor, and the nurse by making provision for the recording of symptoms and treatment of the patient at the time of their occurrence.

The head nurse with the unit manager is responsible for safeguarding the patient's record from loss or destruction. If it should become mislaid, immediate steps are instituted to locate it. No individual sheet is separated from the complete record unless the doctor's order sheet is kept in a special place where its safety is guarded. It is easy to lose or destroy parts of the patient's chart unless personnel adhere to this principle.

An even more difficult undertaking to which the unit staff is committed is the protection of the patient by guarding the content of his record. Charts are kept in a place not accessible to patients and visitors. No stranger is ever permitted to read records. Insurance doctors and lawyers may not read them without the permission of the patient which it is wise to procure in writing. The hospital administration usually has a procedure with which the head nurse and unit manager should be familiar for handling legal matters of this kind. The patient has a right to insist that his record be confidential. Hospitals are legally and ethically obligated to protect the information in his chart from the eyes of unauthorized individuals.

Only those individuals who have a legitimate purpose are permitted to read the patient's history. If a visiting doctor wishes to read a record, permission is obtained from the patient's physician. Only the nurses, social workers, and other professional people who are responsible for the care of the patient or are in need of information for study purposes should be free to read a patient's record. Curiosity about a friend or acquaintance is not a sufficient reason for a nurse or doctor to violate the right of the patient to have his record held in confidence. If hospital policy permits nurse's aides or clerks to read charts, the head nurse must make sure that the confidential nature of the record is fully understood. It is probably preferable for the head nurse or team leader to give aides and orderlies the information they need about patients rather than to encourage these workers to read any of the chart except the nurses' notes. If the need for and right to information about the patients for whom nonnurses are caring is recognized and satisfied and if the nonprofessional personnel realize that their integrity is respected, they will probably have, in most instances, little desire to read the technical aspects of the chart.

Methods vary widely for the recording of nurses' observations, medications, treatments, diet, and so forth. The form which has been established by the hospital should be adhered to by all nurses whether or not it accords with their previous experience. The head nurse is responsible for seeing that nurses who may be accustomed to other ways of charting are taught the accepted methods, that they understand and adhere to them.

Nurses' observations. Since the clinical record is a legal document it is essential that nurses' notes be accurate, clearly stated, and legible. All entries are signed by the individual who writes them. Eradications and erasures may invalidate the record for legal purposes and are therefore not acceptable. Errors are indicated by drawing a single line through the word or sentence. If an explanation is needed it should be made immediately in the body of the nurse's notes.[3] The nurse protects both the hospital and herself by recording accurate observations when symptoms develop which might be attributed to negligence. It is also a protection to record evidence of precautionary measures which are taken, such as the temperatures of solutions used to apply local heat, and measures instituted to protect a suicidal patient against self-inflicted injury. It has been said that it is possible to give good nursing without recording it but that it is not possible to write good records unless the nursing care has been of good quality.

Especially important from the legal point of view is the careful recording of any symptoms present on admission which are indicative of poor hygiene, poor care, or injury. The following are some of the more common points which are included in initial notes if any untoward symptoms are observed: condition of skin such as bedsores, burns, wounds, bruises; condition of mouth and teeth, presence of sordes, ulcers, or other lesions, visible caries, dentures; condition of hair including pediculi, nits, dandruff, uncleanliness, or matting.

Other observations to be recorded on admission are the physical symptoms which may or may not be related to the disorder from which the patient is suffering such as dyspnea, edema, cyanosis, and irregular pulse. Disabilities are noted, including impaired hearing or sight, as are the patient's emotional state, orientation, state of consciousness, and mood. Any condition which may influence the care of the patient should be included in the admission note of the nurse.

Daily notes of the nurse should describe the physical and emotional symptoms exhibited by the patient as well as lack of symptoms which might be expected in a particular condition and situation but which instead are absent. Their absence may be significant. To state that a patient was nauseated but that no vomiting occurred or that there is no evidence of rash when other symptoms of a drug reaction are present may be important observations. Treatments and medications from which results or effects are evident are briefly stated in the nurses' observations. Emphasis should be placed on the reason for giving them, the results, and their general effect

[3] Emanuel Hayt et al. *Law of Hospital and Nurse,* New York, Hospital Textbook Co., 1958, pp. 316-319.

on the patient rather than on the mere fact that the treatment was administered. It should be posssible to gain from the nurses' notes a picture of the physical and psychological progress of the patient from day to day. Clues to his personality and emotional state may be gained if the nurses' notes consistently, over a period of time, describe his physical activity and behavior and quote pertinent statements.

A meaningful record of nurses' observations is very helpful to the doctor and to other nurses. The excuse many nurses give for discontinuing the time-consuming task of writing nurses' notes is that "the doctor never reads them." However, notes on observations of the new patient, one in for diagnostic tests or for surgery who is unusually anxious, the emotionally disturbed individual, the patient with an obscure diagnosis, one who is acutely ill or newly operated *could* be made so worthwhile that the doctor *would* read them. The nurses' record of symptoms, when thoughtfully prepared, is an aid in medical diagnosis and in helping the doctor understand his patient's behavior. It is also a guide in his relationship with the patient.

Well-written nurses' notes have just as much value for the nurse as for the doctor. If they describe how the patient seems to feel, how he acts, the objective evidence of change in condition as well as the effects of medical treatments and nursing care, this information serves as a guide to the next nurse in observing the patient and planning his care. If today the nurses' notes indicate that the patient shows symptoms of edema, or confusion, or discouragement, the nurse who cares for him tonight and tomorrow and next week will know to observe the patient for these signs and in turn record her findings whether the symptoms be present or absent.

Nurses' observations, if well kept, also serve as an aid in making a nursing diagnosis. Notations made over a period of time on Mrs. Jones' chart, when looked at together, give a clue to her needs. For example, nurses' notes stating that she had her light on frequently for minor requests, that she used many excuses to keep the nurse in the room, that she was incontinent of urine although the nurse had been in her room five minutes earlier, that she complained the nurses do not like her, indicate that Mrs. Jones may feel lonely, frightened, or rejected. With this as a tentative nursing diagnosis it is possible to plan a program of "tender loving care" for the patient.

In a few hospitals, nurses and doctors record their observations of the patient sequentially in a joint report. This practice not only gives a consecutive picture of the patient but emphasizes that nurses as well as doctors have a contribution to make in describing the patient's daily progress. It has the added advantages of making it easy for the medical staff to read the nurses' notes and, more important, of impressing on nurses the need to be selective in determining content, as well as the need for clarity and conciseness in expression.

Record of therapy. Somewhere in the patient's permanent record the medications and treatments which were administered by the nurse on doctors' orders must be recorded. The method for doing so varies. Therapy administered several times daily may be recorded in the nurses' notes, on special sheets for treatments or medications, or on the graphic sheet where it can be seen in relation to the vital signs and other information such as intake and output, weight and diet. Time is saved if the name and dose of medication and the type of treatment is written on the sheet only once daily or, if possible, weekly and the hour added or checked and initialed by the nurse who carried out the order for that time. In general, forms for recording the fulfillment of doctors' orders should be simple to use, the data easy to interpret. The fewer pages in the chart on which nurses have to record information and the fewer places medical and nursing personnel have to look for it the more efficient the system. However, to prevent omissions and duplications and to protect the nurse legally, there must be some record to show that the doctor's orders have been carried out and by whom.

The head nurse's responsibility in relation to the patient's record. In addition to her responsibilities for safeguarding the record and for the accuracy and pertinency of the recording done by nurses, the head nurse has two educational opportunities. First, many nurses do not know how to write meaningful notes which give a clear picture of the patient. They can learn to do so only if they practice writing notes under supervision. The head nurse who knows all the patients is in a good position to give this assistance. Nurses new to the service need help in determining the observations which are important to record for disorders and type of therapy common to the service. For example, the nurse may need to become familiar with the observations which are of special significance following brain, chest, or ear surgery or for patients thought to have infectious hepatitis or Hodgkin's disease.

The second educational responsibility of the head nurse is to assist professional nurses on her staff in the interpretation of data on the chart. Some nurses will already have this ability. Others may need the help of the head nurse in understanding the significance of physical findings and laboratory reports and in seeing their relationship to the diagnosis and plan for medical care. By studying the chart the nurse gains new insight into the effect of clinical findings on nursing care, the significance of symptoms, the importance of accuracy in specimen collection and in recording observations. Nursing takes on new meaning as the staff nurse learns to use the clinical record to understand the scientific basis for the care the patient is receiving.

The head nurse who is interested in the development of her professional staff will expect the nurse to form the habit of following her patient's progress by reading his medical history and keeping up with progress notes and laboratory data. One method to encourage chart study is for the head nurse or the patient's nurse to follow the transfer report with a brief resume of findings which are of special interest or significance. If reports of this kind are made short and interesting they will do a great deal to stimulate the study of clinical records.

Records of Performance

Records which describe performance of staff members are indispensable to the head nurse who assumes responsibility for the development of her staff. Every individual should be helped to grow professionally. The head nurse is in a position to observe the work of her staff. Evaluation of their work and discussion with each individual are necessary for growth. If evaluation is to be helpful, it must be objective. Objectivity is more easily attained if anecdoted records are made at the time an important incident occurs. This subject will be discussed in detail in Chapter 18.

STAFFING

The term *staffing* pertains to the number and composition of personnel assigned to work on a division at a given time. The goal of those who are responsible for staffing a division is to provide an adequate amount of staff of the right mixture of personnel to give proper care to the patients housed on the division at that particular time. Staffing has two elements: 1) assignment of individuals to a division and 2) arranging the time these persons are to work. The second can negate the first. Staff placement is most often the responsibility of the nursing office or the department administrator and may be handled in part by a secretary or administrative assistant. When the head nurse employs her own personnel, staffing the unit is her responsibility although she is limited by budgetary considerations. Planning time is usually carried out by the head nurse. However, in small institutions this may be done in the central office while in very large hospitals time planning may be handled by the department administrator with the collaboration of the head nurses and sometimes the help of a computer. It is quite common for the time of evening and night staff to be centrally planned since many work these hours permanently and part-time relief is frequently used. Even when this is true the head nurse may plan the hours and days off for the day staff.

Assignment of Personnel

Basic staff. It is essential that every division have a basic staff of personnel qualified to carry out at least the minimum essentials of care. Nursing service administrators over the years have studied staffing needs to determine the requirements of different divisions under normal or average circumstances. Some have been able to analyze the needs and to arrive at a pattern for staffing each nursing unit. The number of professional nurses, practical nurses, and nurses' aides required for each period of the day as well as the amount of part-time help necessary for relief has been determined. During the past six or seven years considerable study and research on staffing has been undertaken in both the United States and England. Purpose of the studies has been to find a key or index to determine the quantity and composition of nursing staff needed for a division.[4] The basis used for judgment has been largely the degree to which patients are capable of meeting their own needs since this is considered a judicable indication of the degree of illness.[5] Being sought by many are formulas for classifying patients according to the amount of care they need such as self care, intermediate care, intensive care, and an index to determine the quantity and categories of staff required to meet the needs of patients on a unit at any particular time. (See reference list at end of chapter.) After the formulas and index have been developed a scientifically structured basic staff can be established. It may be based on maximum, average, or minimal needs. The first is unrealistic and uneconomical. If the staff is determined by average needs, members must expect to be moved during periods of lull. If it is

---

[4] A British study: Estimation of nurse staffing establishments: Newcastle RHB studies the problem, *Nurs. Times*, Vol. 61 (August 13, 1965), pp. 1099-1100, presents a formula for staffing the different nursing care divisions of hospitals in England and Wales. An American study: Harvey Wolfe and John P. Young. Staffing the nursing unit, *Nurs. Res.*, Vol. 14, Part I (Summer 1965), pp. 236-243; Part II (Fall 1965), pp. 299-303, develops a key for staffing adult units for a particular hospital. The method for developing the key is applicable in other hospitals.

[5] *Ibid.*, Summer 1965, pp. 237-238.

based on minimum or average requirements, personnel will need to be moved in when demands exceed the capabilities of the basic staff. At the same time that staffing patterns are established, therefore, provision must be made to augment the basic staff during the periods when it is inadequate. Once the key has been developed for determining staffing needs, the information can be collected daily or twice daily, tabulated and analyzed by a nurse administrator, a secretary, or an administrative assistant. In some hospitals this information is fed to a computer which quickly gives the number of staff needed and the best "mix"[6] of professional nurses, practical nurses, and aides. With this information available as a guide a wiser distribution of personnel is possible.

Methods of augmenting the basic nursing staff. A common method of augmenting the staff of a division is to borrow from floors which have the most, to help those who have too little. The trouble with this procedure is that seldom does a head nurse think she has an excess. Likewise, a staff member often resents being transferred the minute the situation eases, from a division where she has been working under great pressure, to one she knows will demand her maximum energy. A better way of managing the increased staffing needs which always exist somewhere is by formation of a float or p.r.n. staff whose members are assigned by the day or part of a day to divisions which are shorthanded. Nurses who like this type of assignment work well under pressure, adjust easily, do not feel the need to "belong" to any special unit group. A recent study[7] shows that in one hospital there are wide day to day fluctuations in staffing needs on individual units but that when the requirements of four floors are looked at together the total number of personnel needed is found to be fairly consistent. Other studies corroborate this finding and one[8] learned that the amount of day to day variation in volume of work diminished as patient care units grew in size. These studies might indicate the value of a float staff assigned by services who would be sent by the department administrator to the busiest divisions.

A question immediately comes to mind. What is to be done when the number of personnel is insufficient to staff the divisions adequately? All too frequently this is the case. Sometimes it is possible for a head nurse and her staff, with careful planning and a little greater effort, to absorb the extra load without jeopardizing the quality of care. There are limits to this solution, however. Many times priorities will need to be called into play and

---

[6] *Ibid.,* Fall 1965, p. 299.
[7] Robert J. Connor et al. Effective use of nursing resources: a research report, *Hospitals,* Vol. 35 (May 1, 1961), pp. 30-39.
[8] B. Bellaby. Hospital internal communications: operational research in nursing, *Nurs. Times,* Vol. 61 (September 10, 1965), pp. 1248-1249.

cutbacks made in the quality of care. (See Chapter 12.) Some hospitals are fortunate in having a pool of nurses—often interested alumnae of its school of nursing—who are willing to be on call for such eventualities. There are times when the situtaion is so serious that it is necessary to close one or more floors. All circumstances in which staff is seriously inadequate pose problems for which the nursing service administrator must assume responsibility. The head nurse is expected to make the best possible use of the staff available to her and *to keep those to whom she is responsible informed* when she is unable to provide the care which her patients need. (For further discussion of the head nurse's ways of handling poor staffing see Chapter 12.)

Permanent evening and night staff. Staffing weekends, evenings and nights is almost always a problem. Many times it is possible to employ permanent evening and night nurses and to relieve them consistently with the same part-time nurses. Married women with growing children may need to be home weekends with their families but are often happy to work weekday nights or evenings. Others who can give only two nights may prefer or be willing to work on Friday and Saturday or Saturday and Sunday. Students, widows with grown children, women whose husbands' employment includes weekends or nights often fall into this category. If each such two-night nurse is paired with a five-night nurse, who cannot work weekends, to give seven consecutive nights of care, staffing problems would be eased. One hospital is known to engage two or three part-time nurses for the same position. One nurse may work four nights (or days) the other three, or three nurses may work on a 3—2—2 day basis. They plan their time together so that one of them is on duty each of the seven nights. These nurses should not be placed in charge.

The head nurse's responsibility in staffing. The head nurse may wonder how staffing would be handled if she were functioning in the autonomous role conceived for her. Factors in the envisioned new role which affect staffing will be reviewed here:

1) The head nurse employs her own staff.
2) She has 12 to 15 patients for whose nursing care she is accountable. On a 40 to 50 bed division there are three head nurses; on a 60 bed unit, four or five head nurses. On a 20 bed unit there are one or two head nurses depending on the average nursing load.
3) One unit manager is responsible for the administration of the entire division.
4) The head nurse has no responsibility for unit administration.

With the trend toward building larger nursing care divisions which are considered more economical to administer the chances are good that three or four head nurses will function on the same division. Each will have her own geographic area with its assigned patients and her own staff. All will use the same facilities. It is convenient and natural for these head nurses to coordinate their staffing, and it is more than likely that the night staff, and perhaps evening personnel, can be shared. Likewise, the group could have common pools of p.r.n. and "on call" nurses. Joint planning would be essential. It is suggested that each head nurse determine the basic staff for her own team of personnel, that additional persons of various categories be employed full time to float among the teams as assigned in order to supplement the basic staffs. It is further suggested that each float staff member have a "home base"; that is, that she be a member of one head nurse's team with the understanding that she will frequently serve on the team of another head nurse in the same division.[9] Staff may be employed to function permanently as floats (or until a stationary job opens up), or all staff may be employed with the understanding that every few months they will take their turn in this role.

The following is conceived as a way the two, three, or more head nurses on one division or in one group would function: A master plan for staffing covering six to ten weeks is jointly developed. On the plan are the basic staff of each head nurse, as well as the evening, night, and p.r.n. staff which will be shared. Days off for each person are blocked in according to a scheme which adheres to principles of time planning (page 176) and which has been reviewed, revised as necessary, and accepted by the division nursing staff. (See pages 182-186, *Rotation schedule for time planning* for full discussion of scheme.) At least once daily the head nurses, or, if they are unable to be present, their representatives meet briefly to review the staffing situation and to plan ahead. During midafternoon, patients expected to be present next day are classified. Using the index or whatever guide has been developed, the staffing needs of each team for the next day are estimated. If a computer is used for this purpose, the head nurses see that information is given to the unit manager who procures the slate of staff which the data indicate is needed. When figures for all teams are available the head nurses meet to plan tentative placement of the p.r.n. staff for the next day. Early in the morning before the night staff leaves a new estimate is made. The night clerk notes the changes called for by the guide or computer, and a copy of the report is given to each head nurse

[9] The geography may be such that adjacent floors will need to be used to form a group for head nurse joint planning, but the same unit manager should be responsible for all floors used by the group. If at all possible, the patients on the cooperating divisions should have common nursing needs. A nurse should not be expected to care for children or obstetric patients one day and geriatric patients the next.

before she takes the night report. Each head nurse can see her own needs in relation to others, and a brief conference with the night nurse helps to verify the report. Change in the assignment of the p.r.n. staff may sometimes be made without waiting for a head nurse conference. If not, following transfer reports from the night nurses the head nurses meet to see if adjustments in staff can be made. When necessary, the head nurse who needs extra help calls someone from the pool. Each head nurse knows she is doing so in order that there will be no duplication of calls.

Coordination of staffing. It is possible that a coordinator will be needed to help with staffing problems especially if more than three head nurses share staff. If at night two nurses are assigned to care for the patients of three head nurses, there should be no problems in relation to patient care. Each night nurse is responsible to two head nurses but for different patients. She will at times have to set priorities, but if she is unable to meet the basic needs of any patient, she is obligated to call the appropriate head nurse for counsel. Head nurses have been known to return to the hospital under such circumstances if they could not suggest a satisfactory solution. The greatest problem which might result from the sharing of staff is in the designation of responsibility for replacing a member of the night or evening staff should she be ill or unable to come to work. As long as harmony exists among the head nurses, problems will be minimal. The group will decide which one can best make the replacement. However, it is not possible always to depend on full harmony, and someone must have responsibility for making a decision when three autonomous head nurses cannot agree on a matter of mutual concern. If a nurse from the central office were designated coordinator, she would have to have authority to act. This would place responsibility on someone not in direct touch with the situation. Another possibility might be for the head nurses in the group to elect one of their number as coordinator and agree to bow to her judgment if affairs came to an impasse. A decision could be made to rotate the coordinator responsibility. A third alternative and one which might be more feasible would be to assign each staff member, who has responsibility for patients in more than one team, to the staff of one head nurse as was suggested for the float staff. For example three head nurses may have 15 patients each, in adjoining corridors. At night there are two professional charge nurses each with a supporting staff. One is assigned the care of all patients in Corridor I and half in Corridor II. The second nurse has the other half of Corridor II and all of Corridor III. The first nurse is on the staff of Head Nurse I; the second, on the staff of Head Nurse III. This means each night nurse is employed, relieved, and replaced as necessary by the head nurse of whose staff she is considered a member. The other members of the night and evening staff are designated in the same way.

Perhaps the best possibility for a coordinator of staffing, which actually is largely an administrative function, is the unit director, that is, the unit director in our conceptual model to whom the head nurse is administratively responsible. No unit director or manager would be capable of making the professional judgment involved in decisions about staffing. However, when the day comes that the hospital has a formula for determining patients' nursing requirements and an index for determining the staffing needed to care for the patients on a division, and when staffing has become fairly well stabilized, it should not be necessary for a nurse to determine where p.r.n. staff should be placed. It is expected that head nurses would be consulted, that they would have access to the computerized reports, but that they need not be concerned with the details. There would be no reason for head nurses not to consult one another or to make suggestions to the unit manager.

Since the head nurse in the conceptualized situation is responsible for seeing that her patients receive prescribed medical care and needed nursing, when staff is inadequate, she must interpret this fact to the unit manager and the chief of service. It is within her province to suggest that no more patients be admitted or that some of the present patients be discharged. This is equivalent to the nursing service administrator instigating the closing of a patient care division when she does not have sufficient personnel to staff the institution.

Time Planning

Arranging the time the nursing staff is to work is the second aspect of staffing. The first was the assignment of individuals to divisions. The plan made for the days and hours which the personnel of the division are to spend on duty influences markedly the quality of patient care and the smoothness with which the organization functions. If the time is not carefully planned to provide personnel who have enough competence to meet the requirements for nursing activities and to furnish the assistance which is needed by the medical staff, there will be periods when the patients will suffer from insufficient care and the nurses will carry too heavy a load. Time planning, likewise, may affect the health and morale of the staff. Usually the head nurse has considerable freedom in the planning of time for nurses and aides, and this section will indicate to her some of the principles involved.

Objectives. The head nurse has three objectives in mind when planning time for her staff: 1) To staff the division adequately for good nursing care during the 24 hour period, 2) To provide the best possible experience for her staff, and 3) To comply with good personnel practices and maintain morale.

First objective: To staff the division adequately. The realization of this objective is not wholly under the control of the head nurse if she has only the nurses to staff her unit who are assigned by the department administrator or the director of nursing. If she employs her own staff, she does have control, provided personnel and adequate funds are available. The head nurse is responsible, in any case, for making the best use of the staff which is available. Two principal activities are involved, the distribution of nurses' time throughout the week and the distribution within the 24 hour period. These will be considered in turn.

1) Distribution of Time Throughout the Week. The days on which the members of the staff are to be off duty and the number of individuals who will be on duty to care for the patients are determined by the way in which the head nurse distributes the available nursing hours throughout the week. Planning must take into account the nursing load for each hour of the day, all days of the week. Time is arranged as equitably as possible to meet the demands of each period. There may be little danger that the division will be overstaffed by unequal distribution of hours but there is cause for concern when certain times, such as evenings and week ends, are completely understaffed. The latter frequently happens when the head nurse (or the nursing service administrator) considers it necessary for every member of the staff to be off every second weekend. There is generally less activity on Saturday and Sunday making it legitimate to have fewer hours of nursing time on these days. However, dividing the staff in half may be an unsafe practice unless part-time staff is available weekends.

In deciding which days off each individual shall be assigned, many factors need to be considered. Those pertaining primarily to staff morale will be considered later. The following practices are important to staffing the division for good nursing:

Days off are so planned that there is enough staff present each day and during each period of the day to provide essential care to patients.

At least two professional nurses are on duty during the day period, 7:00 or 8:00 am to 7:00 or 8:00 pm. This is essential to cover meal hours.

A day together between their days off is planned for the head nurse and the nurse who is to relieve her. This provides for adequate reporting.

A day off before and after a night on duty is given so the nurse may have proper rest. For the relief night nurse the following day is one of her free days for the week.

There is always at least one person to provide continuity for each evening and night period. Whenever possible a part-time relief charge nurse on an acute division has all other regular personnel with her when she has been off the division for a period of four or five days.

Example: A 28-bed division has a staff composed of professional nurses, practical nurses, and aides on all three tours. Evening and night staff are permanent, and regular "outside" relief is provided for the evening and night professional nurses. The evening practical nurse is relieved by the day staff. The evening and night aides, and the night practical nurse are not relieved. If the time were equitably divided between the seven days of the week, the schedule would be as follows:[10]

Staff	Number	Days off	Division of days off
Day			
R.N. (includes H.N.)	5	10 L.D.	{ 1 L.D. for 4 days { 2 L.D. for 3 days
L.P.N.	4	8 L.D.	{ 12 L.D. + 2 L.P.N. eve. relief = 14 =
Aide	2	4 L.D.	2 L.D. each of 7 days
Eve.			
R.N.	1	2 L.D.	Cover 7 eves.
R.N. relief (2 eves.)	1	5 L.D.	
L.P.N.	1	2 L.D. (relieved by day staff)	Cover 7 eves.
Aide	1	2 L.D. (no relief)	1 L.D. for 2 eves. 0 L.D. for 5 eves.
Night			
R.N.	1	2 L.D.	Cover 7 nights
R.N. relief (2 N)	1	5 L.D.	
L.P.N.	1	2 L.D. (no relief)	1 L.D. for 4 nights 0 L.D. for 3 nights
Aide	1	2 L.D. (no relief)	

Summary of Day Staff

5 R.N. On 4 days there will be 4 nurses = 16 days
On 3 days there will be 3 nurses = 9 days
25 days
(Total worked by 5 nurses)

4 L.P.N. }
2 Aide } On 7 days there will be 4 persons = 28 days
(Total worked by 6 persons minus 2 eve. relief)

Total 4 days = 8 staff members
3 days = 7 staff members

2) Distribution of Time Throughout the 24 Hour Period. The daily distribution of hours determines when the staff members shall work and

[10] Other factors than even distribution of days off need to be considered as we shall see in succeeding pages. This staff is used in the time plan (Fig. 9 on p. 183) which takes into account these other factors as well as the desirable practices listed above.

when they shall be off duty. Distribution is based on the nursing load at different hours of the day. This load cannot be definitely predicted since it is determined to a large extent by the needs of the patients present at any given time. However, certain basic activities occur regularly, and time to perform them can be predicted. It is important to find some kind of norm on which to base the requirements for staffing at various periods in the 24 hours. Every division has its times of peak activity. In units where infants and young children, cardiacs, or helpless individuals need to be fed, there is a heavy demand on nursing time at feeding or meal hours. Peaks are also reached at the time patients are returning from the operating or recovery room and at periods when patients are admitted. In making the daily time plan, the head nurse arranges for adequate staffing to handle the periods of heavy activity whenever they occur.

It is also important to plan the coverage of the division in relation to the experience of the individuals comprising the staff. The head nurse makes certain that the division is covered at all times with a sufficient number of experienced nurses to ensure the safety of the patients and to effect efficiency. This necessitates a professional nurse being in charge of the nursing service on the division every hour of the day and night [11] and seeing that the time of staff nurses, students, and aides is well balanced. Students are permitted to carry only that responsibility which is safe for the patient and educationally sound. For seniors this may include a short period of charge experience.

The head nurse makes sure that the unit is adequately staffed when an inexperienced person is in charge whether she be a graduate who is new to the division or a senior student. If there are shortages of staff at any period of the day, an experienced individual needs to be on hand to manage the situation. Also if there are two night nurses, time is planned so that both are not new on the same night, for neither would be familiar with the routine and perhaps not with the patients. Not only would efficiency by impaired but the quality of patient care would suffer.

Nursing service policy determines whether staff members shall work straight time or whether they may be assigned split hours for one or two days a week. Broken time is becoming much less common than formerly. It requires that the nurse work during two periods of heavy physical demand. In addition, middle hours can seldom be used to advantage unless the nurse lives near the hospital. When she resides some distance away the transportation cost is doubled if she goes home in the middle of the day. Time spent in changing the uniform and in travel may utilize a large part of her off

---

[11] An exception to this requirement is made in self care units where a practical nurse is frequently in charge at night.

duty hours giving her little chance to do anything constructive. On the other hand, split hours provide a greater number of staff members for patient care during times when the work is heaviest.

When a staff member has her hours divided her working time should fall within a 12 or 13 hour period. When middle hours are the accepted practice of an institution, one or two staff members are assigned hours off between 12:00 noon and 3:30 PM or 12:00 noon and 4:30 PM. In the latter instance, if the day begins at 7:00 AM, the nurse works from 7:00 AM to 12:00 noon and from 4:30 PM to 8:00 PM.

The usual working hours for the day staff are from 7:00 AM to 3:30 PM or from 8:00 AM to 4:30 PM. The evening and night hours are from 3:00 PM to 11:30 PM or 4:00 PM to 12:30 AM and from 11:15 PM to 7:15 AM or 12:15 AM to 8:15 AM, respectively. Time is planned to provide a 15 to 30 minute overlapping period for transfer reports. This encourages a thorough, unhurried report.

When all personnel are assigned straight time, the early afternoon hours, 1:00 to 3:00 or 4:00, may be more heavily staffed than any other time of day. Traditionally this has been the period of lightest activity in hospitals. Most patients are occupied with visitors. Some patients rest after the noon meal. Few treatments and medications are scheduled between 1:00 and 4:00 PM. Baths and general care have been given before noon. Afternoon care does not begin before 3:00 or 4:00 PM. It is obvious that if hours of nursing time are not to be lost to patients some reorganization of activities is necessary. What changes can be made to prevent this waste?

Early afternoon is often a good time to get to know the patients' families. It may not be appropriate for the nurse to take up the time of family members if they visit infrequently. However, some patients see their wives, husbands, parents, or children daily and are happy to have the nurse join them for awhile. This might be a time for consideration of plans for the future. There may also be questions which families wish to ask or problems to discuss when they find the nurse is in no hurry. There are many things she can observe about family relationships, needs for instruction, or for reassurance.

Some patients do not have visitors and may be lonely. This is a time which nurses can plan to spend with those who are her special responsibility. If she knows the patient is not expecting company, the nurse may make him comfortable in the morning and save his bath to give in the afternoon. The patient, of course, should be aware of and approve the plan. He may welcome having something to do when other patients are enjoying their friends. Although this arrangement is designed to relieve the work pressure in the morning, it has the added advantage of giving the nurse more time to talk with the patient.

The early afternoon hours are also a time to study records. The well-organized head nurse will plan a group conference for this period to discuss a specially interesting record or a nursing care plan for one of the patients. Unless something constructive is planned the time will slip by without being properly used.

If the number and category of personnel for the evening and night periods are not designated by nursing service policy or pattern, the head nurse must estimate very carefully the time needed to meet the nursing requirements of patients and to accomplish other tasks for which the staff is responsible. Staff nurses with experience during these hours should be consulted and should help in deciding the personnel needed. It would be very advantageous for the head nurse herself to spend a week on evenings and a week on nights. This would give her an even better picture of the nursing load.

In some services such as pediatrics and intensive care units the evening and night requirements for personnel are almost the same as for the day period. In most others, however, while the staff needs in the evening equal those of the day, night needs are somewhat less. The time between 4:00 and 6:00 PM or 4:00 and 9:00 PM, is very busy and requires more staff than the later hours. To cover this busy period the head nurse can assign a nurse or aide from 9:30 AM to 6:00 PM or from 1:00 PM to 9:30 PM depending on the comparative needs of the late morning (9:30 AM to 12:00 noon) and the early evening (6:00 to 9:30 PM). The staff member who is assigned to come to work at the later hour must be given a report. Since this repetition is time-consuming for the head nurse the staggering of hours for coming on duty is avoided as much as possible. A tape recorded night report helps to alleviate the problem.

Second objective: To provide the best possible experience for staff members. There is a close connection between time planning and assignment planning. Consecutive experience with the same patients or activities usually provides better learning than does interrupted experience. This is one reason for planning blocks of several weeks or months on evening or night duty. If this is not feasible, four to six consecutive nights give the nurse or aide a chance to organize and plan a program, to know the patients and their needs. An interrupted experience, that is, one or two nights a week, proves frustrating and defies efficiency unless the individual is experienced and knows the division. If possible, therefore, time is planned to permit a relief nurse or aide to spend four days on night or evening duty in one week and none the next, rather than working these hours on two days each week. This can often be managed by having her relieve two persons for their days off. For example, a practical nurse may relieve the evening practical nurse and the evening aide.

In an active division the turnover in patients is rapid. The new nurse learns very little in caring for a group of patients unfamiliar to her unless she spends four or five consecutive days with them. This is important to remember in planning her days off.

Third objective: To comply with good personnel practices and maintain morale. The nursing divisions of the hospital must be staffed during evenings, nights, and weekends as must many other organizations which serve the public. Nursing service administrators, recognizing the problems this creates for some persons, have experimented with plans used by industrial concerns which also must have staff on duty seven days and nights a week. Reports[12,13]on two hospital experiments indicate success in recruiting and holding nursing staff by a reorganization in arrangement of hours. Evening and night tours have been shortened while the staff member who works these hours receives no reduction in salary.

When traditional hours are still the policy, the nursing personnel on the division cannot have evenings and weekends free as often as they would like without the risk of jeopardizing patient care. However, the staff member, justifiably, expects to have her share of the desirable hours and days and the opportunity to plan her personal and family affairs.

A general pattern for time distribution is usually established centrally. Such a pattern[14] pertains to the following: 1) Frequency of weekends off. 2) Which days may be given in a weekend, that is, Saturday or Sunday only, or may Friday and Saturday or Sunday and Monday be substituted. 3) Number of days that may or shall be given consecutively over a weekend and how frequently, that is, two, three, or four days. 4) The maximum and minimum number of days permitted between days off. 5) Whether days off must be consecutive or may be split.

The staff should understand the possibilities and limitations in planning time and as a group be given opportunity to decide the overall plan. Seldom is it possible for each staff member to have an individual pattern designed in relation to the above points. Members must realize that the more frequently free weekends are scheduled the more irregularity there is in the time span between their days off. In other words there are some long stretches and some very short ones. To overcome this difficulty, in part, long days (days off) may be split. However, the short stretches of working time created by these two means tend to interrupt continuity in patient

---

[12] Julia Kriegel. Tampering with tradition, *Nurs. Outlook,* Vol. 5 (October 1957), pp. 578-579.

[13] Ann C. Deeds. The worker you save may be your own, *Nurs. Outlook,* Vol. 6 (January 1958), pp. 18-19.

[14] These examples assume the week begins on Monday. It may not. Sometimes time is more easily planned if Sunday or Tuesday is considered the first day. The system must be consistent within the institution.

care.[15] After weighing the alternatives, the staff usually has a choice of 1) every third weekend, a highly irregular time span between days off, and split long days, or 2) fewer free weekends and better spaced working time. **Rotation schedule for time planning.** When basic staffing patterns are well worked out they provide an excellent guide for long-range time planning, provided, of course, it is possible to staff the division with the full complement of personnel.

The head nurse who can count on a relatively stable staff, at least as it concerns the number and category of personnel, should plan days off and relief time for weeks in advance (Fig. 9) so that staff members can make good use of their free time. From this plan a rotation schedule may be devised (Fig. 10). This is a means by which a good design can be recorded for repeated use. Preparation of the weekly time sheet becomes a simple matter which can be handled by the secretary or unit manager. The schedule is available to all staff members who can see at a glance the time they will be assigned many weeks later. By study of the master time plan in Figure 9 and the rotation design in Figure 10, it will be seen that the practices important to staffing for good nursing listed on page 176 have been taken into account.

The staff tends to be stable in hospitals where a rotation schedule for days off is in use. Such a schedule contributes to a more satisfied staff because members can plan ahead for trips, dental appointments, meetings, and social affairs. Although each person recognizes that occasional adjustments in the schedule are necessary, days off should not be changed without consulting the individual involved since she or other persons might be inconvenienced by the proposed change. There is usually some member of the

Fig. 9. A master time plan for a six week period. From this plan the rotation schedule in Figure 10 was devised. The staff is that listed on page 177 but the time off is not distributed evenly (as there shown) due to the needs of members for frequent free weekends. The head nurse and her assistant in this plan have every second weekend free. All other staff members have every third weekend. Three- or four-day combinations have been planned once or twice for all but the head nurse, her assistant, and the evening nurse. Changes in this regard could be made with little difficulty if staff-determined policy so dictated. It is not suggested that this plan is ideal. Rather it is designed to show results of common practices in relation to weekends. Attempt has been made to adhere to the principles listed on page 176, especially the need for a day between the long days of the head nurse and assistant. Because of the frequency of free weekends the time between days off is very irregular. In no instance is this time more than eight days nor less than two. If the head nurse had two or more staff members who could relieve her for days off instead of only one as shown in this plan, the eight-day time span between long days could be reduced.

[15] Lack of continuity may interfere with the learning of a new staff member (see p. 181) and, without definite provision for communicating plans for nursing care, is likely to jeopardize quality nursing.

TIME PLAN

Day Staff	I M	I T	I W	I T	I F	I S	I S	II M	II T	II W	II T	II F	II S	II S	III M	III T	III W	III T	III F	III S	III S	IV M	IV T	IV W	IV T	IV F	IV S	IV S	V M	V T	V W	V T	V F	V S	V S	VI M	VI T	VI W	VI T	VI F	VI S	VI S
Head Nurse			X	X			X		X	X				X			X				X					X		X				X			X			X	X				X
Ass't Head Nurse	X	X				X	X						X	X					X	X					X	X				X	X			X	X			X		X	X	
Staff Nurse 1					X	X						X	X					X	X						X	X									X	X		X				
Staff Nurse 2	X				X	X					X	X						X	X							X	X						X	X						X	X	
Staff Nurse 3									X																			X						X	X	X				X		X
L.P.N.'s 1	X		X				X			X				X			X				X			X				X				X			X			X			X		X
L.P.N.'s 2						E	E		E	E			E	E		E	E	E		E	E		E				E	E		E	E	E			E				E		E	E
L.P.N.'s 3			X		X	X	X	X	X		X		X	X	X				X	X		X		X	X			X						X	X	X	X				X	X
L.P.N.'s 4	X						X	X		X		X	X				X				X			X	X			X		X				X		X	X		X				
Aides 1	X					X	X		X	X	X		X	X		X				X	X		X	X			X	X			X	X	X		X		X		X		X	X
Aides 2	X	X						X			X	X					X	X					X	X					X						X	X			X			
Day Staff off R.N.'s	1	1	1	1	2	2	2	1	1	1	1	2	2	2	1	1	1	1	2	2	2	1	1	1	1	2	2	2	1	1	1	1	2	2	2	1	1	1	1	2	2	2
L.P.N.'s	1	2	2	–	1	2	2	1	1	2	1	1	2	2	2	1	2	1	1	1	1	1	2	2	1	–	1	2	2	1	1	1	1	–	2	2	2	1	1	2	1	2
Aides	1	–	–	1	1	1	1	1	1	1	1	1	–	1	1	1	1	1	1	–	1	–	1	–	–	1	1	1	1	1	1	1	1	1	1	1	–	–	1	–	1	1
Total	3	3	3	2	5	5	5	3	3	4	3	4	4	5	4	3	4	3	4	3	4	2	3	3	2	3	4	5	4	3	3	3	3	3	4	4	3	3	4	4	4	4
Evening Staff R.N. Charge		X	X		X	X	X		X	X	X		X	X		X	X	X		X	X		X	X		X	X	X		X	X	X		X	X		X	X	X		X	X
R.N. Relief	X	E	E	X	E	E	E	X	X	E	E	E	E	E	X	X	E	E	E	E	E	X	E	E	X	E	E	E	X	X	E	E	X	E	E	X	X	E	E	E	E	E
L.P.N.	X	X						X							X	X						X			X				X	X			X			X	X					
Aide	X							X							X							X							X		X					X		X			X	X
Total	0	0	0	0	0	0	0	0	1	0	0	0	0	0	1	0	0	0	0	0	0	1	0	0	1	0	0	0	0	0	1	1	0	0	0	0	0	0	0	0	1	1
Night Staff R.N. Charge	X	X					X	X	X				X	X	X				X	X					X	X	X		X	N				X	N		N	N			X	X
R.N. Relief	X	X	N	N	X	X	N	X	X	N	N	X	X	N	X	X	N	N	X	X	N	X	X	N	N	X	X	N	N	N	N	X	X	N	N	X	N	N	X	X	X	X
L.P.N.	X	X			X	X			X	X		X	X			X			X			X	X										X	X								
Aide	X		X	X		X	X	X	X		X	X		X	X		X			X	X	X		X									X		X	X				X	X	
Total	1	1	0	1	1	1	0	0	0	1	1	1	1	1	1	0	0	1	0	0	1	1	1	1	1	0	0	0	0	0	0	1	1	1	0	1	0	0	0	0	0	1

ROTATION SCHEDULE - DAYS OFF

	Weeks	I	II	III	IV	V	VI	VII	VIII	IX
Day Staff										
R.N.'s	Head Nurse	S S	W Th	S S	W Th	S S	W Th	S S	W Th	S S
	Ass't. Head Nurse	W Th	S S	W Th	S S	W Th	S S	W Th	S S	W Th
	Staff Nurse 1	S S	M F	Tu F	S S	M F	Tu F	S S	M F	Tu F
	Staff Nurse 2	Tu F	S S	M F	Tu F	S S	M F	Tu F	S S	M F
	Staff Nurse 3	M F	Tu F	S S	M F	Tu F	S S	M F	Tu F	S S
L.P.N.'s	Practical Nurse 1	W Th	S S	M Tu ●	W Th	S S	M F	W Th	S S	M F ●
	Practical Nurse 2	M Tu ●	W Th ●	S S	M Tu	W Th	S S	M Tu	W Th	S S
	Practical Nurse 3	S S	M F	Th F	S S	M Tu	Tu F ●	S S	M Tu ●	Th F
	Practical Nurse 4	W Th	S S	M Tu	W Th ●	S S ●	M Tu	W Th	S S	M Tu
Aides	Nurses' Aide 1	S S	M Tu	W Th	S S	M F	W Th	S S	M Tu	Tu W
	Nurses' Aide 2	M Tu	W Th	S S	M F	W Th	S S	M F	Th F	S S
Evening Staff										
R.N.'s	Charge Nurse	Th F	S S	F S	Th F	S S	F S	Th F	S S	F S
	Relief Nurse	MTW S S	MTW Th F	MTW Th Su	MTW S S	MTW Th F	MTW Th Su	MTW S S	MTW Th F	MTW Th Su
L.P.N	Practical Nurse	S S	M Tu	W Th	S S	M Tu	W Th	S S	W Th	W Th
Aide	Nurses' Aide	Tu W	W Th	Tu Su	M Tu	W Th	S S	M Tu	Th F	S S
Night Staff										
R.N.'s	Charge Nurse	S S	M Tu	W Th	S S	M Tu	W Th	S S	M Tu	W Th
	Relief Nurse	MTW Th F	W Th F SS	MTuF S S	MTW Th F	W Th F SS	MTuF S S	MTW Th F	W Th F SS	MTuF S S
L.P.N.	Practical Nurse	M Tu	Th F	S S	M Tu	Th F	S S	M Tu	Th F	S S
Aide	Nurses' Aide	Th F	S S	M Tu	Th F	S S	M Tu	Th F	S S	M Tu

Fig. 10. **The rotation schedule for days off completes a cycle in six weeks for the professional staff, nine weeks for the practical nurses and aides after which the rotation starts again. Days off are indicated by letters, evening relief by a dot. For example, in the first week Practical Nurse 2 relieves the evening practical nurse on Saturday and Sunday, has her own days off the preceding Monday and Tuesday.**

staff who does not have special plans that week and is willing to adjust her time. Where the rotation system has been tried absenteeism is minimal as a result of high morale. Each staff member is cooperative and considerate because she knows what it will do to a co-worker if she does not fulfill her obligation. When the cycle of the rotation pattern has been completed and is to be started again, personnel should have a chance to choose which arrangement of time they wish for the next period. If the selection is made in conference the group takes care of duplicate requests.

When the evening and night staff is relieved by day personnel (rather than by permanent relief nurses as described on page 172), a rotation plan should, if possible, indicate the individuals scheduled for this relief each week. This practice helps the nurse in planning her family and social affairs. In making the plan or in assigning relief in the absence of a long-range plan, the head nurse avoids scheduling a member of the day staff for evening relief the night before her days off. However, when other important factors are considered also, this practice is often of less importance. The length of time off can sometimes be extended in the other direction by having the nurse or aide assigned to evening or night relief on the day she comes back to work. If a nurse for whom this arrangement is made is to be in charge of the division on her return, she should be assigned to come to work 30 minutes early in order to obtain a report covering the time she has been away and to make rounds to see the patients with the nurse who is leaving. She should be thoroughly familiar with the division, its policies, and procedures, and should have a staff member with her who worked on that unit the night before.

When long-range planning of time is not possible, the head nurse will do well to establish a plan for making and receiving requests for special time. This would include a statement of the time when requests must be received in order to be considered. A policy also needs to be established in regard to the method by which decisions shall be made when there are incompatible requests. Staff nurses of course participate in the formulation of such a policy. It is important that the plan be flexible. Some head nurses place a weekly time sheet on the bulletin board permitting the nurses to indicate their preferences for days off duty. Each nurse sees the requests which others have made and makes her own in the light of their choices and the division needs. The nurses themselves usually handle conflicting requests without the head nurse having to make the decision.

In her desire to please the members of her staff, the head nurse should not forget that requests for special time must not interfere with the staffing of the division for good nursing. A sense of fairness and reasonableness are highly important in handling problems related to time. It is a rare occasion when some satisfactory solution to a problem cannot be worked out if it is given thought and is handled in a democratic manner. On the other hand, the planning of time may be a long and difficult task and the head nurse needs to impress upon her staff that changes should only be requested when some very important, unforseen situation has arisen. Planning weekly time from a rotation schedule and handling requests for special time is an activity the head nurse could be relieved of by the unit manager. He would need to be given guidelines relative to strengths and weaknesses of the various staff members.

Time planning for the nursing team. Team nursing is described in Chapter 12, pages 280 to 309, which should be read at this point by those unfamiliar with this method of assignment. When several nursing team leaders function under one head nurse, the customary practice when team nursing is in operation, there is usually some interdependence of teams. However, every effort should be made to provide each one with a consistent staff. Long range rotation schedules are somewhat more difficult to construct as a result of this need. However, it is possible to do so and the values are worth the effort. To permit team leaders to have more than an occasional weekend free, the charge nurse may act in that capacity on Saturday and Sunday. When circumstances do not permit this, it may be possible to reduce the number of teams on the weekend, say from three to two or from two to one to permit one team leader to be off.

Figure 11 shows a weekly time plan for a staff which is organized into teams.[16] The assistant head nurse who is relieving the head nurse on Saturday and Sunday is also the leader of Team I on these days. It will be noted that four persons on the staff in addition to the head nurse—the assistant and three others designated "relief"—are not assigned regularly to a team. These individuals relieve other staff members for days off. For example, the assistant head nurse and the relief staff nurse relieve the head nurse, two daytime team leaders, one evening and one night nurse for a total of ten days during the week. In the same way day and evening nonprofessional personnel are relieved by two relief practical nurses who are not a part of any one team. The night and evening practical nurse and aide relieve one another. Insofar as possible each relief staff member is assigned

---

[16] The plan is suitable for a unit with patients who are not acutely ill. Because the team leader is the only professional nurse on the team, the staff is inadequate for a division in which there are patients requiring close observation and intensive care. Under the latter circumstance, it would be far preferable not to have teams but to assign one or both of the professional nurses to the total care of the acutely ill, to have medications for the rest of the patients given by the second professional nurse, or, if necessary, by the head nurse, and for the head nurse to give the immediate supervision to all nursing personnel.

Weekly Time Sheet — Team Nursing

	Mon.	Tues.	Wed.	Thurs.	Fri.	Sat.	Sun.
Head Nurse							
Ass't Head Nurse	Night Relief	Night Relief			Eve. Relief	H.N. Relief	H.N. Relief
Team Leader I						No relief	No relief
Team Leader II							
Relief Nurse	Prac. T_I	N. Relief T_I			Eve Relief	T.L.II	T.L.II
Evening Nurse							
Night Nurse							
Prac. Nurse-Team I							
" " – " I							
" " – " II							
" " –Relief	Prac. Nurse Eve.	Relief	aide Eve. Relief	T_I			
" " –Relief			T_{II}	aide T_I	relief T_{II}	T_{II}	T_{II}
" " – Eve.							
" " –Night						No relief	No relief
Aide – Team II							
" – Eve.							
" –Night				No relief	No relief		
Total Staff	d e n 7 3 3	d e n 7 3 3	d e n 7 3 3	d e n 7 3 2	d e n 7 3 2	d e n 6 3 2	d e n 6 3 2

Fig. 11. Weekly time for the team is prepared by the head nurse or clerk. If the staff is stable this pattern can be used to plan a long-range rotation schedule like that shown in Figure 10.

to the same team for relief in order that she may identify with its members.

If used consistently the pattern of days off shown in Figure 11 permits the professional staff to have either Saturday and Sunday, Friday and Saturday, or Saturday, Sunday and Monday off on an average of every other week. The practical nurses have these hours approximately every third week. The discrepancy results from the fact that the number of professional nurses needed on the weekends is reduced as a result of the charge nurse acting as team leader. If it were possible to reduce Team II to two members on Saturday and Sunday the nonprofessional staff could have free weekends more frequently. However, the rest of the week would be out of balance as can be seen by the figures giving daily totals.

Forms for recording personnel time. The weekly time sheet with the time planned for each nurse is used by the nursing office to obtain an overall view of the staffing situation. It is used by the department administrator for the same purpose, by the head nurse in planning daily assignments, and by the division staff to learn their hours for the coming week. Even though there may be a master rotation schedule, the names of each staff member are listed. To give a clear picture, days off, leaves of absence, holiday time, evening and night relief are shown. If students comprise part of the regular staff, their class and conference hours are given. Names of student nurses who come for brief periods a few days a week are not always listed on the time sheet. Occasionally they are given in a separate listing, or the time sheet merely states that four junior students will be present from 7:00 to 10:00 AM on Tuesday and Friday.

In large institutions where not all members of the staff are familiar to the entire nursing service personnel, it is customary to designate each individual by her position (head nurse, team leader, night charge nurse, and the like). Unless names of professional nurses, practical nurses, and aides are given in groups, with their category designated, this information is stipulated beside the name of each individual. Students are recorded by class such as "senior" or "preclinical" or by the year the class will graduate. The arrangement of names on the time sheet should be clear and should tell at a glance whether the staff is adequate.

For a division which has a long list of persons on the weekly time sheet, a summary of the number of personnel to be present each day makes daily comparisons easier for the administrator responsible for staffing. At the bottom of the column for each day the number of staff for each period is given. A break down by categories may be desired or only the totals. Thus 6-3-3 means that a total of six staff members are planned for the day period, three for evening and three for night. If another day's total reads 4-3-3, the administrator will check to see whether the day is a less busy one (Sunday, perhaps) or whether it is a heavy weekday. In the latter instance help will be needed for that day unless the head nurse can be assisted in reorganizing her weekly time plan. It is in situations such as this that a key for determining staff needs is of great value.

If one or two staff members have divided time the nursing administrator will gain a better picture of the staffing if summary figures designate the staff planned for morning, early afternoon, and late afternoon. In this instance the numbers 6-2-5 would indicate for a particular day that there were six on duty in the morning, two between 12:00 noon or 1:00 PM and 3:00 or 4:00 PM, five during the late afternoon hours. Since the numbers of evening and night staff are relatively stable they are not included when this form is adopted. When day staff also is stable these figures are unnecessary.

Still another way of summarizing each day's coverage is to state the number of staff hours planned for each day. This involves counting the full-time staff members, multiplying 8 hours by this number and adding the hours each part-time person is to work that day. For example, if the 24-hour staff consists of 11 persons each working 8 hours and a part-time nurse giving 6 hours a total of 94 hours is available. This figure is placed at the bottom of the day's column. By comparing the total for each day, the nursing administrator can tell at a glance whether the hours for the week have been well distributed. If desired, figures may be divided for categories of personnel. Likewise, hours for the day period only may be considered. Consistency in method is, of course, necessary.

When a rotation schedule for personnel time is in use, the weekly time sheet can easily be prepared. Carbon copies are prepared for the nursing office, for the department administrator, and for the bulletin board on the unit. If the division is functioning as an independent unit under a unit director, he, not the nursing administrator, receives a copy.

Time for each day is copied on a daily time sheet by the secretary or clerk. Although there is considerable duplication when a second or third listing must be made (master plan, weekly time plan, and daily time sheet) the daily listing takes into account any changes which have occurred since the weekly plan was prepared. It is possible that in situations where few revisions are necessary the bulletin board copy of the weekly time can be corrected. The department administrator would then be responsible for correcting her copy and the one in the nursing office. When a daily time sheet is used, names of all staff members should appear. As on the weekly time sheet, days off, illness, and absence are so designated. The sheet is easier to use if evening and night personnel are listed separately from the day staff.

SUMMARY

Doctors' orders, reports, and records of various kinds are essential to competent care of the patient. Some of them have legal and scientific value. The doctor's orders are written to protect himself, the patient, the hospital, and especially the nurse. There is probably less likelihood that a nurse would harm a patient by giving a treatment on verbal order than that she would bring the criticism of illegal practice upon herself. The doctor's orders adequately serve their purpose only if they are well written, provide no chance for misinterpretation, and are accompanied by his signature. The order sheet should also indicate the discontinuance of orders. In some hospitals no order for a treatment or medication is valid after 48 hours. This necessitates their review and updating. Standing orders are legal only when ordered by the doctor for the individual patient.

The doctor is limited in his writing of orders by the administrative policy of the hospital. Doctors' orders should be handled promptly and efficiently. The nurse is obligated to understand fully the purpose of the doctor's order, to carry out the order safely and effectively, and to report and record its results. Any inability to comply with the order or difficulty in so doing should be reported promptly to the physician. By the administrative policy of the head nurse or unit director, it is possible to control the doctors' practice of giving telephone and other verbal orders except in an emergency, in which case the order is written and signed by the doctor on his next visit to the division.

Reports are of prime importance to effective patient care, to good administration of the division, and to a well-functioning hospital. The head nurse is responsible for the quality of intradivision nursing reports and for those to the nursing service administrators. Reporting within the division goes on all the time to keep the staff informed. Formal reports occur when responsibility is transferred from one individual to another or to a group. The charge nurse or team leader gives a transfer report to the oncoming staff. The assistant receives a report from the head nurse when she is to be in charge for a few hours or a few days.

Oral reports are given to nurse administrators who come to the division. The department or assistant administrator wishes a general picture of the nursing load as well as information about the sickest patients and any problems which exist. Day, evening, and night reports are customarily prepared on a special form for the nursing office. The content varies with the institution.

Accident and incident reports prepared by the staff members concerned are signed by the doctor and head nurse. They are kept on file in the nursing or hospital administrator's office for legal and study purposes. All reports should be accurate, clear, and complete and should bear the signature of the head nurse. They need to be filed on time.

Records may have historical significance, and they may provide legal evidence or data for research. There should be a specific use, known to the head nurse, for all records kept by the division nursing staff. The patient's clinical chart is by far the most important hospital record. The head nurse has four distinct responsibilities in relation to this document:

First, she, along with the unit director, must see that its content is protected and that it is safeguarded from loss. Second, she is responsible for the content of the nurses' notes. These should give evidence that due care has been taken to safeguard the patient from injury. A complete note on admission of the patient may protect the hospital in accusations of negligence. Well-written daily observations help the physician in diagnosis and in understanding his patient. They are just as important to the nurse in making observations and in diagnosing her patient's needs.

The head nurse's third responsibility in relation to records is to make certain that somewhere in the chart the fact that a doctor's order has been carried out is indicated. This is a protection for the nurse and for the hospital. Each hospital has its own forms for recording these data. The head nurse needs to be fully aware of the importance of the principle. Education of her staff in the writing of valuable nurses' notes and in the use of the doctor's progress record, the physical findings, and laboratory reports to understand their patients and plan their care is the fourth responsibility of the head nurse in this area.

Staffing of nursing care divisions has become a subject of intense research in some institutions and considerable experimentation in many. A key to determine staff requirements based on needs of patients for care and the numbers and categories of personnel which can meet those needs is being sought. Some have developed a formula and index for their own institutions and by means of a computer obtain information which serves as a guide to those who are responsible for staffing. A basic staff for each division is essential plus a float staff which is used to augment the base when necessary. A permanent evening and night staff together with permanent part-time relief for each member reduces staffing problems.

Conventionally the assignment to divisions of both basic and float staff is a function of nursing service administration. In the conceived role of the head nurse, this is her responsibility. The usual nursing care division will have 40 to 60 beds with three to five head nurses functioning with professional autonomy under the administrative direction of a unit director. Sharing of evening and night staff as well as float staff will be likely and will require joint planning by the head nurses. When a workable key for staff assignment has been evolved, the unit director should be able to assume the responsibility for time planning and for placing float staff. Prior to the development of the key a nurse coordinator will probably be needed. This might be a department administrator, or the head nurses may choose one of their members for this responsibility which of necessity involves decision making. The arrangement of working hours for division nursing personnel is a major factor in attracting and retaining staff. Likewise, the ability to care for patients adequately and to provide valuable experience for staff members is influenced markedly by the way in which the head nurse plans the daily and weekly time. She usually has considerable latitude in this area although she is limited by the size of her staff and the general policy of the hospital.

A long-range rotation schedule which indicates days off and relief for evenings and nights makes it possible for staff members to plan their personal lives. A rotation schedule is thus a morale builder and tends to stabilize the staff. On the other hand, it is not possible to make a long-range schedule unless the division staff remains constant, at least in number and category.

QUESTIONS FOR DISCUSSION

1. Were you ever in a position, either as a staff nurse or a student, where you felt impelled to take a verbal medical order? If so, and you took the order, do you now feel circumstances warranted it? Would the same be true for you today? Could the head nurse through her administrative authority or relationships have prevented your being confronted with the need to decide whether or not to take the verbal order? What would she have done?
2. Should the nursing service of your hospital promote the combining of nurses' and doctors' notes? Give reasons for your answer. Philosophically do you consider this a good idea? Explain.
3. Have you ever been called upon to write an accident or incident report? How did you feel about doing it? Did you feel the report was important administratively? educationally? Explain. What was the head nurse's role in the report? What should it have been? Explain in full.
4. As a head nurse how important do you consider your report to the department administrator or director of nursing service to be?
5. If you are a head nurse, how do you feel about the director of nurses making rounds on your floor?

6. How would nurses in the hospital in which you work react to a long range staff rotation plan? Why?

EXERCISES

1. If you are a head nurse or assistant head nurse review the records which are kept on your floor. Which are required by hospital administration? by nursing administration? Which are not required, but are kept because you (or the head nurse) consider them useful? Consider each record you keep in relation to its purpose, its effectiveness in meeting the purpose. If you believe it could be eliminated how would you go about doing so?
2. Review the nurses' notes of a patient whom you do not know who has been hospitalized one to two weeks. Describe the patient as he is pictured. Then read the remainder of the record—medical history, examination, and progress notes. Add to your picture. Then visit the patient and engage him in conversation about himself for about ten minutes. Wherein does the impression gained in the personal interaction vary from that from the chart? How could the nurses' notes have been improved? Should the chart give a picture of the patient as a person?
3. Observe the transfer report between night and day or day and evening staffs on your own division unless you are the person giving, or the primary person receiving the report. If necessary, observe on a floor where you are not working. Is every person who is supposed to be receiving the report hearing it? is she attending? Is everyone involved in some way? What suggestions can you make for improving the report?
4. Analyze the weekly time sheet for the staff on your division in relation to the principles enumerated in this chapter. Relate to the class your findings and your suggestions for improvement with the available staff.
5. Obtain the list of persons who will comprise the staff on your unit for the coming week. Using the formula for planning days off which was presented in this chapter, block in long days and indicate relief. Keep desirable practices in mind. Add nursing hours available each day, according to your plan. Are the hours as equitable as possible? Analyze your plan.
6. Using an actual nursing staff, if you find an adequate one which is also stable, or a realistic hypothetical staff for a familiar situation, plan a long range (six to eight week) rotation plan. Follow the customary pattern in your hospital for evening and night relief. Present the plan for group discussion.

REFERENCES

A British study: Estimation of nurse staffing establishments: Newcastle RHB studies the problem, Nurs. Times, Vol. 61 (August 13, 1965), pp. 1099-1100. Presents a formula for staffing the different nursing care divisions of hospitals in England and Wales.

Banks, Alice W., McKee, Mary E. A., and Moore, David Y. Tape-recorded nurses' notes, Nurs. Outlook, Vol. 14 (October 1966), pp. 42-44. When a nurse completes a patient's care she uses one of four dictaphones placed at strategic locations on the division to dictate her nurse's notes. Notes are transcribed on the patient's chart by a secretary. The nurse signs them. The many advantages of the procedure are listed.

Barclay, Goldia N. From tape to chart, Amer. J. Nurs., Vol. 61 (June 1961), pp. 64-65. Many hours of nursing time are saved by the use of a tape recorder for dictating nurses' notes. Secretaries transcribe the notes to the chart. The nurse reads and signs them.

Barnes, Elizabeth. People in Hospital, London, Macmillan Company, Ltd., 1961, Ch. 5, pp. 55-68. Communication was found to be the big overriding problem in hospitals and is probably due to the natural division of work between medical and nonmedical groups, as well as the isolation of groups and status factors. Actually the patient comes last; illness comes first. The interdependence of groups is clearly portrayed, and ways to improve communication are suggested.

Bellaby, B. Hospital internal communications: Operational research in nursing, Nurs. Times, Vol. 61 (September 10, 1965), pp. 1248-1249. Time, money, and nervous strain have been saved by use of a system for classifying patients according to their nursing requirements: self care, intermediate care, and intensive care. This article is based on a portion of the broader report Problems and Progress in Medical Care (1964) referred to at the end of the article.

Brodt, Dagmar E. Obstacles to individualized patient care, Nurs. Outlook, Vol. 14 (December 1966), pp. 35-36. The writer lists and briefly describes 10 reasons why nurses fail to give individualized care to patients. A good summary.

Committee on Nursing Services, American Nurses' Association. Statement on Nursing staff requirements for in-patient health care services, Amer. J. Nurs., Vol. 67 (May 1967), pp. 1029-1030. This very useful guide for helping nursing service administrators plan staffing will be of interest to the head nurse, especially if she becomes responsible for employing her own staff.

Connor, Robert J. A work sampling study of variations in nursing work load, Hospitals, Vol. 35 (May 1, 1961), pp. 40-41, 111. This study was conducted to investigate causes for variation in the Direct Care Index (see next reference). It is disturbing to learn that the time spent by nurses with patients did not increase or decrease as hours available did.

———— Flagle, Charles D., Hsieh, Richard K. C., Preston, Ruth A., and Singer, Sidney. Effective use of nursing resources: a research report, Hospitals, Vol. 35 (May 1, 1961), pp. 30-39. "A system of patient classification by severity of illness to determine nursing requirements on a day-to-day basis is described by the authors in this report of an extensive research project. How demand for certain supplies, such as linen, can be predicted through this system is explained. The report points out that better utilization of personnel and supplies calls for flexibility in the whole hospital in order to meet the shifting needs." Excellent.

Cuming, M. W. Shift working—an easier way?, Nurs. Times, Vol. 61 (August 13, 1965), p. 1101.
   Rotation of shifts from day to evening to night is proving popular in industry because it permits greater social life. Is this a possible answer for nursing? The writer believes the method of operation should be decided by those involved so long as efficiency of service is not adversely affected.

Deedo, Ann C. The worker you save may be your own, Nurs. Outlook, Vol. 6 (January 1958), pp. 18-19.
   A system for planning division time which stabilizes staff and permits better patient care.

DeMarco, James P., and Snavely, Shirley A. Nurse staffing with a data processing system, Amer. J. Nurs., Vol. 63 (October 1963), pp. 122-125.
   By means of a computer, in ten minutes time per shift, it is possible to show how to distribute the staff to meet the nursing needs of each hospital division.

Ellis, Geraldine L. Communications and interdepartmental relationships, Nurs. Forum, Vol. 5 (No. 4, 1966), pp. 82-89.
   Types of communication between nurses and the importance of quality.

Fagin, I. Donald, and Sister Mary Vita. Who? Where? When? How? An analysis of 868 inpatient accidents, Hospitals, Vol. 39 (August 16, 1965), pp. 60-65.
   A detailed study of hospital accidents to patients reveals the circumstances under which accidents are most likely to occur and the most prevalent types of accidents. The study indicates precautionary measures likely to be effective.

Georgopoulos, Basil S., and Mann, Floyd C. The Community General Hospital, New York, The Macmillan Company, 1962, pp. 500-543; 621-634.
   The findings in relation to nurses' verticle communication and its effect on patient care are highly significant.

Gorlick, Herthe Striker. The working R.N.-mother: her problems and joys, R.N., Vol. 28 (March 1965), pp. 42-49, 104.
   For many reasons nurse-mothers go back to work not the least of which is joy in her profession. This article helps head nurses appreciate the problems of the nurse who has a family.

Haase, Ferdinand, Jr. Shifting to a seven-day week, Hospitals, Vol. 40 (March 1, 1966), pp. 59-66.
   A doctor recommends that for the sake of patients all medical services be available seven days a week. Implications for nursing are obvious.

Hagberg, Earl W. Work analysis cut payroll 14 percent, Mod. Hosp., Vol. 105 (September 1965), pp. 111-113.
   The greatest saving in this work analysis was in the nursing department. Through a qualitative analysis of patient needs (that is, degree to which patient was able to care for himself) daily staffing was determined. As a result fewer nursing staff were needed, and patients received better care.

Hayt, Emanuel, Hayt, Lillian R., Groeschel, August H., and McMullan, Dorothy. Law of Hospital and Nurse, New York, Hospital Textbook Co., 1958.
   Chapter 24 will help the head nurse understand the legal implications of the patient's clinical record.

Healy, Eleanor E., and McGurk, William. Effectiveness and acceptance of nurses' notes, Nurs. Outlook, Vol. 14 (March 1966), pp. 32-34.

A study revealed that nurses' notes, as presently written in one hospital failed to meet the criteria for effective notes. A new procedure and treatment form are being used experimentally. An interesting and useful article.

Hershey, Nathan. Medical records and the nurse, Part I, Amer. J. Nurs., Vol. 63 (February 1963), pp. 110-111; Part II, Amer. J. Nurs. (March 1963), pp. 96-97.
Part I makes it clear that the nurse must know when to disclose and when not to disclose information from a patient's record. A case is cited.
Part II describes instances when the nurse has been held legally liable for failure to record symptoms and for failure to familiarize herself with information on a patient's record. The implications for all nurses are very clear.

——— The apparently erroneous order, Amer. J. Nurs., Vol. 64 (January 1964), pp. 111-112.
A lawyer lays down guidelines for nurses in handling doctors' orders which they believe to be erroneous and suggests that a hospital policy on the procedure under such circumstances is needed.

Hersman, Marybelle R. Staffing a small community hospital, Amer. J. Nurs., Vol. 66 (July 1966), pp. 1588-1589.
A small rural hospital whose census fluctuates widely solves the problem of staffing by a call system for inactive nurses in the community who have been oriented to the hospital and who are happy to help their friends and neighbors.

Hilliker, Floyd. The Flossie Wenger Guild, Nurs. Outlook, Vol. 13 (January 1965), pp. 40-41.
Through their Alumnae Association nurses organized to provide volunteer nursing service to the hospital.

Hopkins, Terence D. Sickness patterns of nursing staff, Nurs. Mirror, Vol. 120 (April 16, 1965), pp. 59-61.
The head nurse who reads this article will find helpful points in preventing and dealing with the "retreat into sickness."

Kriegel, Julia. Tampering with tradition, Nurs. Outlook, Vol. 5 (October 1957), pp. 578-579.
Experimentation with different work hours for nursing service personnel has resulted in a more stable staff.

Livengood, Lindsay. Planned shifts save nurses and dollars, Mod. Hosp., Vol. 104 (February 1965), pp. 101-104, 170.
A detailed description accompanied by illustrations of time schedules show clearly how nursing service can improve staff morale by improving scheduling.

Merrell, Dorothy. Dear Doctor, Nurs. Outlook, Vol. 8 (April 1960), pp. 218-219.
A printed form used for notes to doctors about patients' questions, possible need for changing orders, outdated medications, and similar messages has proved very useful when it is impossible for head nurses to make rounds with all physicians.

Miles, Barbara. Tackling staff problems in hospital, Nurs. Times, Vol. 61 (January 8, 1965), p. 69.
Part time nurses can be used effectively if nursing service uses imagination in determining activities for these people. Rotating shifts can solve the night duty problem.

Morgan, Elizabeth M. New chart forms solve old problems, Amer. J. Nurs., Vol. 65 (March 1965), pp. 93-96.
Following a study by a committee composed of nurses, doctors, and record librarian, the necessary content for a patient's records was defined and new forms devised. Recording of notes is done chronologically with all disciplines writing on the same sheet.

Mott, Paul E. The case against rotating shifts, Nurs. Outlook, Vol. 14 (April 1966), pp. 51-52.
A study of rotating shifts versus a fixed shift schedule in industry is applied to time planning for hospital nurses. Although there are family and health problems involved in both types of schedule, there seem to be more in rotating shifts. Nursing service administrators, including head nurses, would do well to read this article.

Nakagawa, Helen, and Hudziak, Barbara. Effect of increases in numbers of nursing personnel on utilization of time in a psychiatric unit, Nursing Research, Vol. 12 (Spring 1963), pp. 106-108.
Findings of a study in a Veterans Administration hospital showed that the "increases in the proportion of time devoted to direct patient care by each individual was unrelated to the amount of increases of personnel investigated in this study." The researchers believe that personal motivations or work organization are the variables affecting the amount of time spent with patients.

New, Peter Kong-Ming, and Nite, Gladys. Staffing and interaction, Nurs. Outlook, Vol. 8 (July 1960), pp. 396-400.
A study of eight staffing patterns, in which the numbers and composition of the staff varied, showed that the interaction within the group differed when the proportion of professional nurses to practical nurses and aides was changed. Results seem to indicate that looking just at numbers of personnel is not sufficient to determine staffing adequacy.
Report of same study, presented in a different way, will be found in Mod. Hosp., Vol. 93 (October 1959), pp. 104-108.

New York Study charts 10-year change in personnel-patient day ratios, Hospitals, Vol. 40 (March 1, 1966), p. 56.
In this study a marked increase in personnel-patient day ratios was seen. In relation to nursing personnel assigned to inpatient services, which made up 35 percent of all hospital personnel, the study showed that 17.4 percent more persons were employed per 100 patients per day in 1964 than in 1954.

Perillo, Charlotte K. We changed morning report, Amer. J. Nurs., Vol. 66 (December 1966), pp. 2682-2684.
The problem of giving the transfer report created by having one night nurse for two adjoining divisions was solved by having one report taped while the night nurse attended 7 AM surgical rounds giving the report to the head nurse and surgeons jointly.

Plogsted, Helen. Using nursing records to teach, Nurs. Outlook, Vol. 7 (January 1959), pp. 43-45.
Vital, informative nurses' notes serve many purposes one of which is to guide other nurses in their contacts with patients and thus provide smooth continuity. The principles delineated here for recording on patients in a psychosomatic unit are equally applicable in other services.

Preston, Ruth A. Add meaning to your hospital census, Nurs. Outlook, Vol. 10 (July 1962), pp. 466-468.
When the patients who make up the census on a division are classified according to the amount and type of nursing care needed, the census form has value for nursing service administration.

Pullen, Leon C. Modern methods make larger nursing units practical, Hospitals, Vol. 40 (May 1, 1966), pp. 77-80.
This hospital consultant advocates 60 to 80 bed patient care divisions because of the economy in equipping and staffing them. (No mention is made of the quality of patient care.)

Roose, Jeanine A. Interpretation of rest by doctors and nurses, Nurs. Res., Vol. 12 (Spring 1963), pp. 111-113.

For patients with myocardial infarction, there is considerable discrepancy between doctors' and nurses' interpretations of orders. The doctor should be specific or "the nurse must request clarification."

Rosenberg, Mervin, and Carriker, Delores. Automating nurses' notes, Amer. J. Nurs., Vol. 66 (May 1966), pp. 1021-1023.
By means of a carefully devised checklist of patient behaviors and a computer, a private psychiatric hospital has shortened the time required for charting and made nurses' notes more complete and meaningful.

Rutherford, Ruby. What bothers staff nurses, Amer. J. Nurs., Vol. 67 (February 1967), pp. 315-318.
A former staff nurse and head nurse describes the frustrations of the staff nurse and suggests practical ways for alleviating them.

Ryan, Joseph R., and Boydston, Gordon D. This flexible staffing plan puts nurses in right place at right time, Mod. Hosp., Vol. 105 (September 1965), pp. 114-117.
A plan for estimating the staffing needs of a division has been devised. The plan is based on the amount of nursing time of each category of personnel needed by each patient.

Street, Margaret M. Staffing problems in nursing service, Canad. Nurse, Vol. 61 (February 1965), pp. 91-93.
What is meant by "necessary" care has not yet been defined—probably because it is so difficult to do. The writer recommends systematic evaluation of nursing care and analysis of problems related to staffing. "The use to which such information will be put must be predetermined."

Stryker, Ruth P. A staffing secretary releases nursing time, Am. J. Nursing, Vol. 66 (November 1966), pp. 2478-2480.
The transfer of responsibility for time planning to a lay secretary, so clearly described here, is long overdue. Other hospitals would do well at least to consider such a change. No nursing service administrator at any level should fail to read this article—and act upon it!

Testoff, Arthur, Levine, Eugene, and Siegel, Stanley E. The part-time nurse, Amer. J. Nursing, Vol. 64 (January 1964), pp. 88-89.
A study revealed that the number of part-time nurses increased markedly between 1948 and 1962. If there had not been part-time work available the equivalent of 39,000 full-time nurses would not have been in the nursing labor force. The need is to solve the administrative problems which result.

The menace of medicine lists, Nurs. Times, Vol. 61 (March 19, 1965), p. 390.
A study revealed an alarming number (26 percent in one week) of discrepancies between the doctor's prescription and the transcribed order.

Thiessen, Hedwig. A nursing service audit, Canad. Nurse, Vol. 62 (February 1966), pp. 57-58.
Clinical charting improved greatly from the use of a nursing service audit by committees composed of head nurses and staff nurses representing every service.

Walker, Virginia H., McReynolds, Dorothy A., and Patrick, Elsie. A care plan for ailing nurses' notes, Amer. J. Nurs., Vol. 65 (August 1965), pp. 74-76.
A study of nurses' notes revealed that instead of charting being a ritualistic practice as had been thought, notes were practically nonexistent. A committee set up criteria which are being used as a guide in improving the quality of the record.

———— and Selmanoff, Eugene D. A study of the nature and use of nurses' notes, Nurs. Res., Vol. 13 (Spring 1964), pp. 113-121.
A study of nurses' notes in medical-surgical wards of a university hospital showed

that these notes do not serve as an effective means of communication, that though the inaccuracies are few, the number of omissions is high.

Willig, Sidney. Drugs—dispensing/administering, Amer. J. Nurs., Vol. 64 (June 1964), pp. 126-131.
A pharmacist-lawyer discusses the legal implications of a nurse dispensing drugs and administering them without a written order that is clear and understandable.

Wilkinson, Elizabeth. Improving patient care through better communication, Hospitals, Vol. 35 (October 16, 1961), pp. 48-50.
An informative description of the manner in which doctors, nurses, and others concerned with patient welfare work together by services. Examples of committee accomplishment are given.

Williams, D. Joan. Nurse needles plan for flexible staffing. Response by Ryan, J. R. and Boydston, G. D., Mod. Hosp., Vol. 106 (January 1966) pp. 6-10.
A "letter-to-the-editor" re: an article on staffing and the response of the authors point out the problems and values of a scientific system.

Wolfe, Harvey, and Young, John P. Staffing the nursing unit, Part I: Controlled variable staffing, Nurs. Res., Vol. 14 (Summer 1965), pp. 236-243.
One hospital has worked out an index for determining daily staffing needs of the various units. Based on the individual patient's capability for self-care, the index is a guide but judgment of the person allocating staff is still required.

——— Young, John P. Staffing the nursing unit, Part II: The multiple assignment technique, Nurs. Res., Vol. 14 (Fall 1965), pp. 299-303.
Calculations of the number of nursing hours needed and the best mix of professional and nonprofessional staff are made by computer.
Of particular interest to head nurses is the division of nursing activities into task complexes—technical, preparatory, clerical.

part 2 THE HEAD NURSE'S RESPONSIBILITY FOR NURSING CARE ADMINISTRATION

In the preceding chapters a new role for the head nurse has been suggested—a role in which she has professional autonomy and complete responsibility for the nursing care of a small group of patients. A head nurse could play this role only if it were endorsed by hospital administration and if she were well prepared and wholeheartedly accepted as a partner by the chief of the medical service. She would need to be free from responsibility for all unit administration, and it has been suggested that she might function most effectively if a segment of the hospital were decentralized under the administration of a unit director to whom all personnel who worked on the unit, including the doctor and head nurse, would be administratively responsible. Likewise, in the first section, the organization of the hospital and its many services for patients have been discussed, the principles of administration presented, and their application to patient care management made explicit.

In Part Two the kind of nursing care for which the head nurse and her staff should aim will be analyzed. The succeeding chapters will be concerned with the four areas of the head nurse's responsibility for patient care administration: diagnosing the patient's nursing needs, planning his care, assigning or delegating responsibility for his care, and supervising and evaluating nursing care.

chapter 9

THE QUALITY OF CARE THE PATIENT AND HIS FAMILY HAVE A RIGHT TO EXPECT

Who is this person who has left his home and come to the hospital as a patient? The way in which the hospital, the way in which the nursing staff, and the way in which his nurse conceives the patient determines in large measure the care he receives and where its emphasis lies. Every nurse would find it helpful to her development to define her own concept of the "patient."

In this volume he is envisioned as an individual, usually a member of a family from which he cannot be considered apart. In common with every human, he has needs which pertain to the maintenance of life and health and needs which relate to happiness and self-respect. The latter include love, affection, the need to be needed, and other indications that he is respected, that his thoughts and feelings are important, that his well-being is a matter of interest and concern to others. Self-respect grows out of self-dependence, out of a sense of worth or importance and a feeling that he has something of value to contribute to others. Beside these human needs which he shares with all men, the patient has others which result from ill health. The allergic individual or one to whom a respiratory infection might mean exacerbation of a chronic disease needs a controlled environment. A special diet, hormones, medication, an abundance of rest, limited exercise—these and many other special needs may result from less than perfect health. In addition the patient who is confined to the hospital has still other needs—needs which are present *because* he is in the hospital. Each hospitalized person has some degree of fear and most suffer from worry or loneliness resulting from the confinement. For some patients, entering the hospital is a new experience. To others it is an old story. Each one will, as a result of personal experience or that of friends or through hearsay, have certain expectations. He does not know his medical or nursing requirements, but his personal needs are very real to him. His family also has needs, perhaps not clearly defined, but if not met they cause concern, frustration, and sometimes loss of confidence in the hospital.

Thus a situation exists in which the individuals who are most concerned and who have important needs have no clear concept of what they should expect in the hospital. This being the case it is easily recognized that in addition to *needs* the patient and his family have *rights*. Professional persons, in other words, are obligated to meet the needs of patients whether or not the patient or his family knows he has them. This is their right, this they should be able to expect. It is up to the professional personnel to provide the kind of care which will meet the personal as well as the medical and nursing requirements of the patient. The head nurse may, therefore, ask the following questions regarding nursing's responsibility: What do the patient and his family have a right to expect from nursing personnel? This is the same as asking, what *should* patients and families receive in the way of personal consideration, in the way of care?

Primarily people have a right to expect that nurses and doctors are prepared to practice their professions and to anticipate that these individuals will use their full knowledge, judgment, and skill in prescribing and caring for the patient. Second, they have a right to expect that the patient will have freedom to choose, to help make decisions, and plan his care. Third, they have a right to expect that each thing being done to and for the patient will be interpreted to him; that he is free to ask questions and that they will be honestly answered.[1] Fourth, the patient and his family have a right to expect that they will be treated with respect, consideration, and understanding. These expectations will be discussed in terms of the patient's needs and the ways in which nurses can help to meet them. First, however, it is important to review the role of the head nurse in providing the care the patient and his family have the right to expect. Obviously, she cannot personally minister to all the needs of the patients and their families and must have the assistance of her staff, principally her professional staff. The head nurse constantly keeps the needs of the individual patient and his family before the nursing personnel until these needs become for all of them a way of thinking. Not all nurses have the dedication or the skill required to care for the patient as portrayed in this second part of the text. The head nurse who knows the patient from personal contact and is a model for the staff, helps each member become more discerning, more understanding. She helps staff members learn to deal effectively with patients' questions, problems, and needs. One of the head nurse's primary responsibilities to patients is to teach her staff and keep before them the standard of quality care.

As another preliminary to discussing the expectations of patients and families regarding hospital care we need to consider the way individuals feel on admission to the hospital.

[1] That this is not always the case is vividly portrayed in a study by James K. Skipper, Jr., et al. Some barriers to communication between patients and hospital functionaries, *Nurs. Forum,* Vol. 2 (No. 1, 1963), pp. 14-23.

WHAT DOES ADMISSION TO THE HOSPITAL MEAN TO THE PATIENT AND HIS FAMILY?

Admission to the hospital holds high hopes for the young couple who are expecting a new baby. This is true also for the woman who expects to have her hearing restored through stapedectomy or fenestration and for individuals who are to have other types of corrective surgery. These admissions have been planned. On the other hand, the person who comes to the hospital for diagnosis may have postponed coming for some time hoping the symptoms would disappear, fearing what the diagnosis might reveal. He, therefore, enters the hospital with considerable anxiety. Likewise, individuals who are chronically ill may come to the hospital after weeks or months of care at home which can now no longer be managed. Hospitalization is a last resort. Unhappiness on the part of the patient, guilt feelings in the family are often encountered. For the patient who has had an accident, heart attack, cerebral thrombosis, or other sudden illness, the way of life has suddenly changed for him and his family temporarily or permanently. They are stunned, shocked.

It is obvious then that regardless of the circumstance which brings him, entering the hospital is an occasion of great importance to the patient and his family. A sense of excitement and a feeling of uncertainty are always present. Every patient is beset by some anxiety and at times the experience is fraught with fear. What will be the outcome? Will the baby be normal? Will the operation be successful? Will I regain my hearing? Will I survive the anesthetic? Will complications result? What will the diagnosis reveal? Am I going to die? Some of these questions are in the minds of most individuals who are admitted to the hospital. Probably few of them are verbalized even to members of the family. If the patient could express them, his anxiety might be reduced especially if he is fearing needlessly because of misinformation or a misconception. The skillful nurse provides this opportunity should the patient wish to accept it.

Patients and families often have other concerns as well. Expense of hospital and medical care may use funds that have been saved for something else—the education of a child, payment of a debt, a new home. Sometimes the money is not available at all, which necessitates borrowing or calling on parents or children for help. Some persons worry over business affairs or the possible loss of a job. Others, particularly mothers, worry about their children and how the home will run without them. Seldom are readjustments in family life unnecessary and many of them cause great inconvenience in the home. There may have been no time to plan for these changes or to work out a suitable arrangement.

Some people fear pain and discomfort while others are uneasy in a strange environment where they do not know exactly what is expected of them. They hesitate to ask questions and show their ignorance. Some are apprehensive of an impersonal atmosphere where each individual is one of hundreds whom no one knows or about whom no one may care. Many dread being alone, away from loved ones. Children and older women, especially, may never before have been separated from their families. Hospitalization can be a lonely, frightening experience. Families worry too. Their concern is that their loved one will not receive the understanding care he has had at home.

It is individuals with these fears and anxieties whom the nurse greets and "admits" to the division. What care and consideration should she give the new patient? What care, consideration, and attention does he have a right to expect?

MEETING THE NEEDS OF THE PATIENT
ON ADMISSION

Most patients walk into the hospital and go through the admitting office after which they are escorted to the division. A member of his family or a friend usually accompanies the patient. His first need is to be recognized, greeted, and made to feel welcome. This takes but a moment during which the nurse or clerk should give the patient and his family her full attention. This friendly gesture takes priority over everything else at the moment, for the patient at this time is under considerable stress whether or not he shows it. He becomes very uneasy if personnel are too busy to recognize his presence or if they talk about him but not to him. If someone immediately steps up to greet him and learn his name, he feels that he is expected and that preparation has been made for his coming. No time should be wasted in finding the nurse who is to care for the patient and introducing her to him and his family. Patients like to be greeted by name and to have nurses and other personnel introduce themselves.[2]

Every new patient is greeted by the charge nurse as soon as possible. Patients admitted during the absence of the head nurse are welcomed by her when she returns. She should identify herself by name and position to the patient and as soon as possible to members of his family. It is important that they know who is in charge of the division and to feel that she is personally responsible for the patient.

[2] Patients who go to an admitting division for preliminary care need to be shown this interest and consideration there as well as on the unit to which they are permanently assigned.

At no period in a patient's hospitalization is it more important for the nurse and other staff members to show understanding than at the time of his admission. A warm, friendly nurse who appreciates to some extent what the admission means to the patient and his family, by her manner reassures and puts them at ease. The nurse who admits the patient symbolizes to him the hospital. If she is courteous and sympathetic and shows an interest in him, confidence in the hospital will be established. If she is cold and impersonal, the family will dread to leave the patient. There is a feeling of welcome if the patient arrives on the division and finds his room in readiness. Fanning the bed, ventilating the room, and checking to see that all is in order should be routine practice when a new patient is known to be coming.

Both the patient and his family will be more at ease if they are told what to do. It is hard for an unimaginative nurse to realize how little people understand of what they should do in the hospital. Unless they are told, patients do not know whether to undress and go to bed, to unpack their bags or leave them for the nurse. Whether or not he goes to bed may make little difference, but the patient likes to know what is expected of him and if possible, he should be given a choice. It is well to take nothing for granted and to instruct a new patient as one would a guest who is a stranger in one's home. He will appreciate knowing his schedule for the next few hours: the house doctor will be coming to examine him; the orderly to shave him for his operation; blood samples which are collected routinely on all incoming patients will be taken by the laboratory technician; he will have a light supper about 5:30. After the doctor has examined him and he has had his surgical preparation, he may be up and around if he wishes. His family and friends may visit him at any time. If they desire help in controlling visitors, the nurse will be glad to suggest ways in which the situation can be handled.

The new patient will wonder how personal matters are attended to, when and how mail is received, whether it is possible to buy a newspaper, rent a telephone or television set. He will need to know how to summon a nurse and when he will see his own doctor. Most patients can be put at ease in relation to their physical wants by having the nurse foresee their needs. The collection of a specimen helps some individuals to pass a difficult hurdle. The hospital will seem less strange to the patient if he knows his neighbors in the same room and he will be grateful to the nurse who introduces him and opens the way for conversation. From the very beginning of his hospital stay, the patient should be given some choices—to go to bed or to stay up, to keep on street clothes or put on a robe, to stay in his room or go to the solarium.

The nurse's apparent ease and lack of hurry in getting the patient settled help to create an atmosphere in which the patient and his family feel free to ask questions or discuss problems. It may be difficult for the nurse to achieve this relaxed manner when many other important responsibilities await her. The actual time spent with the patient is not necessarily long, however. Much more important than the amount of time spent is the comfort the patient feels in her presence. Mainly, then, she needs to show her interest in him and her concern for his well-being. She needs to give him and his family her undivided attention while she is with them. The patient who is made to feel at ease from the moment he arrives on the division will be less tense and nervous and, therefore, will make fewer demands on nursing time later.

It hardly seems necessary to remind nurses that pain or discomfort should be ascertained early and given immediate attention. Sometimes a patient is too tired or breathless to make the exertion necessary to get into bed. He can be supported in a chair and moved when he feels he is ready unless emergency measures necessitate his being lifted into the bed. When the patient does not feel compelled to move and finds the nurse is in no hurry, he can usually relax sufficiently to gain enough strength and breath to be helped to the bed.

The alert, interested nurse will note when a patient is chilly and add a blanket. A bath blanket around the feet and knees of an elderly or debilitated person brings considerable comfort especially when a short hospital gown is being worn. If a patient has been admitted from the clinic or emergency room in the early afternoon he may have missed his lunch. Fearful of being a bother he may hesitate to say he is hungry. Thoughtful nursing will consider every possible circumstance which may be a cause of discomfort.

In addition to her concern for his comfort, while admitting the patient the nurse observes his general physical condition, his state of consciousness and orientation, and any obvious abnormalities. She may also note the relationships of the family and their social advantages. The latter may be suggested by their hygiene, dress, and speech. Under no circumstances should a patient be caused embarrassment. It takes very little to make an insecure person feel ashamed in a strange environment. Every human being needs to be accepted as he is and treated with respect and kindness. The patient has a right to expect also that his clothing and other personal possessions will be carefully handled and guarded against loss, soil, or wrinkles.

A relatively new and valuable practice is to hold an initial interview with new patients at which time a nursing history is taken. The purpose of the history is to collect data which will help in making a nursing diagnosis and establishing a nursing care plan. The form used for the nursing history is in the experimental stage in most hospitals. Any form is merely a guide and the nurse uses discretion in the questions she asks and in the way she phrases them. Its content includes some or all of the following information:

1) *Patients' perceptions relative to his illness and hospitalization.*
   What brought him to the hospital?
   Has he been hospitalized previously?
   What caused his illness?
   How long has he been ill?
   When did he go to the doctor?
   How long has he known the doctor?
   What changes in his living has the illness brought about?
   What does he expect to be done for *him in the hospital?*
   What does he expect to be done to *him?*
   How does he feel about being in the hospital?
   How long does he expect to stay?

2) *Family, home life*
   With whom does he live? who are family members? their employment?
   Who will be coming to see him?
   Does the family live in a single dwelling? apartment? two-family house?
   On what levels are the bedrooms? bathroom?
   How near do they live to a drug store? food markets? public transportation?
   Where will he go following hospitalization?
   Who in the family will help him when he goes home?
   Has he ever had a nurse come into the home to help care for him or a member of the family? What did she do to help?

3) *Present feelings*
   If he has pain
      Location? severity? is it constant? what brings it on?
      How long has he had the pain?
      How severe is it now compared to previous times?
      What measures are used to relieve pain?
      How much do these measures help?
   If he has discomfort
      Location? severity?
      What brings it on?
      What relieves it? to what extent?
   If he has difficulty in breathing
      When does he have it?
      What brings it on?
      What relieves it and to what degree?
      Over how long a period has he had difficulty in breathing?

Has he been under doctor's care for his breathing problems? Does he have other symptoms which accompany the difficulty in breathing?

4) *Sleep pattern; rest*
   When does he feel tired?
   What does he do to get rested?
   What hours does he spend in bed at night?
   How many hours sleep does he average?
   Does he sleep well?
   Does he have any trouble getting to sleep? What does he do to get to sleep?
   Does he take a sleeping pill? regularly? how often?
   Does he take a day time nap, for how long, and at what time?

5) *Diet and fluids*
   What foods does he eat mostly? Have him describe a usual breakfast, lunch, and dinner.
   What foods does he especially enjoy?
   What foods does he not like?
   What kinds of foods give him distress? What kind of distress?
   What foods does he avoid? Has a doctor ever advised him to avoid certain foods? Which?
   Does he eat between meals? If so, why? what? time?
   What does he like to drink with meals? between meals?
   How much water does he drink in a day? Does he like it iced?
   Have his fluids ever been restricted? restricted now?
   Does he have trouble eating? If yes, what is the cause? What does he do about it?
   Does he consider himself underweight? overweight? about right?
   Is he on a special diet? kind? How long has he been on it?
   Does he have any problems in keeping to his special diet?

6) *Elimination*
   Does he feel his bowels move normally? What makes him think so?
   What is the usual time of day for bowel movement? Is is associated with a meal time?
   Does he take laxatives? If so, what? how often? how effective are they?
   Does he take enemas? If so, what kind? how often? are they effective?
   Does he do anything else to make his bowels move? what?
   Does he frequently have abdominal discomfort? cramping? gas? What brings on the cramping? the gas?
   What does he do to relieve the discomfort?
   How frequently does he get up in the night to go to the bathroom?
   Does he have any trouble with voiding? If so, what kind of trouble?

How does he get relief?
Has he been treated by a doctor for urinary problems? kind of problems?
Is he having any urinary problems now?

7.) *Personal hygiene*
What kind of baths does he take? tub? shower? Frequency?
Time of day preferred? Does he need help?
Is his skin excessively dry? Does he use lotions or ointment on face? body?
Is his skin very oily? What does he do about it?
Does he perspire a great deal? When ? Does he use any measures to control perspiration?
Does he have any sore spots? What has been done about them?
Do his feet require any special kind of care?
How does he take care of his hair? How frequently does he need to wash it?
How good are his teeth?
Is he able to brush his own teeth?
Does he see his dentist regularly? When was his last visit?
Does he wear dentures? All the time? How much of the time?
How does he care for dentures? Is he able to brush them?

8) *Limitation in motion*
Does he need help in walking? getting in and out of bed? What kind of help?
Has anyone told him to stay in bed and not walk? Who? What were the instructions?
How does he feel about staying in bed?
Is there anything he has difficulty doing? Have him give example. In what ways is it difficult?

9) *Vision*
Does he wear glasses? contact lenses? All or part of time? For what purpose?
How well does he say he sees without glasses? with them?
Does he have an artificial eye? How does he care for it? Does he have any instructions he wants to give the nurse?
What difficulties does poor vision cause him?
Does he need any special help because of poor eyesight? If so, what kind?

10) *Hearing*
Is he hard of hearing? How can people help him to hear?
When does he have most difficulty hearing?
In what way does poor hearing handicap him? How does he manage?
Does he wear a hearing aid? When?
How does he care for the hearing aid? instructions for the nurse?

11) Allergies
Does he have any allergies? To what is he sensitive?
How does the allergy affect him? When? any particular time of day, season of year?
To what extent does the allergy handicap him?
What precautions does he take?

12) Interests, hobbies
How does he spend leisure time?
Does he enjoy time thus spent?
Did he bring any means of recreation (reading, games, cards, handwork, radio) with him to the hospital?
Would he be interested in such an activity if his condition and time permit?
Does he enjoy socializing? Would he like to eat or play games with other patients?
What are his special interests?
Does he anticipate a lot of visitors? Does he wish any restrictions on them? If so, in what way?

13) Nurse's observations of condition and appearance:
Activity, orientation, alertness
General build, color, strength or weakness
Condition of mouth, skin, hair, nails, feet
Limitation in range of motion, degree of limitation
Presence of muscular contractures, location, severity, painfulness

14) Nurse's general impressions:
Attitudes
Willingness and ability to communicate, ability to comprehend
Reaction to hospitalization, adjustment to situation
Family relationships

15) Tentative nursing diagnosis

16) Important points to be included in nursing care plan.

The initial interview in addition to giving information for a nursing care plan serves to put the patient at ease by encouraging him to talk about himself. The history taking helps establish a relationship between nurse and patient which gives the patient confidence that he has someone who cares about him to whom he can turn with his problems. If the initial interview is to achieve these purposes, the nurse who takes the history must be skilled in human relationships, capable of freeing the patient to unburden his mind if he wishes, and able to utilize the information so gained to help the patient understand himself and thereby bring about a reduction in tension. The head nurse will wish to conduct these initial interviews whenever possible in order to know the patient, discover his concerns, make a tentative nursing diagnosis, and judge which member or members of the staff are suited to give the care needed. It is very likely the head nurse will wish to care for the patient herself for at least a day to learn more about him and his needs and to verify the preliminary assessment of his needs.

The head nurse makes the acquaintance of the family before they leave the hospital. It is well if she discusses their views on the patient's particular anxieties and needs. If the patient is a very young child or an individual incapable of speaking for himself, the head nurse will obtain the patient's admission history from a family member. However, patients, including children, should speak for themselves in all areas where they are capable of so doing. There may, therefore, on occasion, be two admission histories supplementing one another. Some hospitals which do not take admission nursing histories, collect information from parents on a child's feeding, elimination, and sleeping habits, and words used to express certain meanings. Knowledge in these areas is of great help to nurses in understanding a child and helping him adjust to the hospital. Some institutions use for this purpose a special form with questions to be answered by the mother or father. Needless to say it is far preferable for the nurse to fill out the form in conference with the parents than to request that the latter write the answers. This same type of information is helpful in caring for aged or chronically ill patients. It is incorporated in the plan for the patient's care and made available to all nursing personnel on the unit.

When a patient has been graciously cared for on admission, a forward stride has been made in winning his confidence and his family's trust. However, he continues to have needs which nursing can satisfy. Many of these needs change as the patient's condition changes. Some, on the other hand, remain basically the same.

NEEDS OF THE PATIENT WHICH ARE
EVER PRESENT

When the patient is receiving the care he has a right to expect, he feels that he is an important, respected individual, welcome on *this* unit regardless of his physical or mental condition, his race, color, or creed. He knows that the individuals caring for him are interested in him as a person, not as an example of a disease condition. He is called and referred to by name, not by the number of his room. Even though he may have an unpleasing appearance or odorous discharge he feels accepted. Regardless of his behavior he is treated with understanding. He knows that his religious beliefs are respected by the nursing staff. He is given desired spiritual help through referral to a spiritual advisor and receives strength from nurses who have a deep religious faith.

In addition to having his personal needs met, the patient has a right to expect that his treatments and nursing care will be given in a manner which will produce desired results, safeguard him and cause him a minimum of discomfort. When his treatments are numerous and time consuming, he never feels that his care is a burden. Grouping of his treatments permits him maximum rest.

NURSING NEEDS OF THE ACUTELY ILL

The very ill patient who is well nursed finds it unnecessary to do any thinking for himself. He should of course be free to make a request but should not have to feel it necessary to manage his own care. The confidence of the conscious patient in his nurse should be so great that he has no sense of personal responsibility. His every need is anticipated before he realizes its existence. The nurse senses when he needs to have his position adjusted, his lips moistened, his face bathed, his bed linen tightened. If she is not in constant view she sees him very often to check his condition and reassure him by her presence and her manner.

Good nursing of the critically ill patient insures that every possible precaution is being taken to protect him from injury due to falls, bumps, burns, or pressure and that as far as possible contractures and circulatory complications will be prevented. Adequate nutrition, elimination, fluid and electrolyte balance are the constant concern of the nurse. She is keen in her observations and sound in her judgment, which results in recognition and early reporting of dangerous developments. When the patient receives the care he has a right to expect, nursing ministrations and the technical measures prescribed by the doctor are performed with a minimum of discomfort. The patient's strength is conserved by the nurse's efficient management. A tender, comforting, sympathetic manner on the part of the nurse makes tolerable painful or unpleasant measures. If the patient is conscious or semiconscious, the nurse tells him simply what she plans to do and gains his acquiescence, often through a nonverbal sign.

The members of the acutely ill person's family have rights also. They should be able to take for granted that their concern will be understood and appreciated; that their right to ask questions and to have them honestly answered will be recognized, and their freedom to express their feelings accepted. Because she is more available than the doctor the nurse will receive many of the family's questions. It is frustrating and annoying to the anxious family to be put off by the nurse with vague generalities or the response, "You will have to ask the doctor." There are some things the doctor will wish to explain to the family but the nurse must find out from him to what extent he has informed them of the patient's condition so that she will be able to give them intelligent, meaningful reports. The doctor should expect the nurse to answer direct questions if in her judgment the family is really wanting an answer. She should also be prepared to support the family members in their reaction to a truthful answer. In this type of communication the head nurse is expected to be highly skilled. She in turn helps her staff anticipate and handle such questions. Nonprofessional personnel are taught how to refer matters of this kind to the head nurse.

The family needs to see their loved one frequently. There is no substitute for personal observation. It may be reassuring; it may not. At least the family gains some comfort from seeing for themselves how the patient appears. To deprive members of the immediate family of the right to see the patient, from a distance if that is better for him, does them a very great injustice. If the patient's condition is such that a family member who wishes may help with his care, this need of the family should be satisfied. Likewise, if the presence of parent, husband, wife, son, daughter, or other person calms and reassures the patient, the privilege of sitting quietly at the bedside should be permitted. When the nursing care is of the quality the family should be able to expect, members will not feel it necessary to remain with the patient to assure his safety and comfort. Family members are under dreadful strain and need to take time for rest and to keep the home functioning as well as possible. They can do neither unless they have confidence in the care and attention being given the patient.

GOOD NURSING DURING CONVALESCENCE AND MILD ILLNESS

When the acute phase of illness has passed and the patient starts the uphill climb to health he enters a period of convalescence. He begins to take an interest in his environment. For the first time he may notice the nurse as a person. The convalescent patient needs to know he is improving and to hear from the physician the changes that are recommended in his therapy. He needs to understand that his condition no longer requires the same constant observation, that he is ready to participate in his own care to the degree he feels able to do so. Little by little as he is ready to accept it, the patient should have his improved condition interpreted to him by his doctor and the head nurse and should be encouraged to help decide how much he is able to do for himself. The head nurse will need to assist the convalescent as well as the mildly ill patient to understand that the exercise derived from self care is an aid in regaining strength.

Some patients, who feel better than their pathology warrants, wish to proceed too rapidly to self-dependence. If it is important that the nurse continue to bathe, turn, and feed him, he needs to understand why this is necessary and how long it will be before it will be wise for him to begin to do things for himself. The patient should help make decisions concerning the restrictions to be lifted and those to be retained. He also should expect the staff to be sympathetic and understanding of his feelings about restrictions.

Not all persons are eager to tend to their own needs. Some will expect and even desire to remain dependent. A great deal of interpretation and patience may be needed if these patients are to receive the nursing they really need. Those who desire continuing dependence often look upon mild illness and hospitalization as an adventure which they have no desire to end. In such circumstances, that which the patient feels he has a right to expect is seldom in accord with good practice as seen by doctors and nurses. Good nursing tries to discover the reasons for the patient's attitudes and to make this patient's return to independence attractive. It does not label him "neurotic" or reject him as having "hospitalitis."

Every patient has a right to expect that before any treatment or diagnostic test is begun he will be told what it involves, its purpose, and how he can help to make it effective. Both experience and experimentation[3] have shown that treatments such as the enema are more effective when the patient fully accepts the need for the procedure and understands specifically what he is to do to facilitate it. If he is a conscious adult he is given a chance to refuse a treatment or necessary care if he is not ready or able to accept it. Patients as a rule resent having no choice but to receive the treatment prescribed for them. Accustomed to ordering their own lives and making their own decisions, they dislike being treated as children and expected to accept without question that which the doctor or nurse chooses to do to them. Usually the patient to whom a procedure is properly explained will wish to submit to its performance, for he realizes its value

[3] Phyllis A. Tryon and Robert C. Leonard. The effect of the patient's participation on the outcome of a nursing procedure, *Nurs. Forum,* Vol. 3 (No. 2, 1964), pp. 79-89.

and has confidence in his physician. However, he wishes to feel that he has a choice in the matter, that he may refuse the treatment if he wishes. While the manner of the nurse must be one of confidence, assuming that the patient will understand the value of the treatment and accept it, the door should never be closed to his rejection. If he refuses a treatment there is a reason. The nurse's first obligation is to identify it. Frequently a patient misunderstands something about the measure—something the nurse can clarify and thereby make the procedure acceptable. If she is unable to help the patient see its value to him, he should not be subjected to the treatment. Never should the nurse command or by her manner make the patient feel that he has no alternative but to comply. Neither should the patient feel rejected because he has refused the treatment.

Perhaps after he has had time to think about the matter the patient will decide to accept the procedure. If not, the entire situation should be explained to the physician. He, the nurse, and the patient need to work out an alternative. The success of such a conference—in fact whether it is even held—may very well depend upon the nurse's skill in interpersonal relationships.

Probably no other aspect of hospitalization causes so much comment by patients as the food which is served. The division of responsibility for dietary service varies considerably. Under no circumstances, however, can the head nurse ignore the service even if it is someone else's function. She is responsible for the patient's total welfare and his food is an important item in his well-being. Types of food, methods of preparation, habits of eating vary widely in different national groups, in parts of the country, and in families. Taste is affected by illness. Appetite may be lacking thus making the attractiveness and palatability of food of great importance. Since sufficient calories and proper nutrients are essential to the maintenance of health and regaining of strength, the patient has a right to expect that no effort is too great to make it possible for him to eat well.

In so far as possible, the patients' food preferences should be considered. Leeway in the matter of preferences varies with the institution and unfortunately with the amount the patient is able to pay for his care. Private patients may have more choice in foods than do ward patients and are usually able to select the menu which appeals to them. Within the limits of the menu, consideration should be given to the personal preferences of all patients. With a little thought and effort it is usually possible to give a choice of beverages, the amount of bread can be regulated by the patient's wishes, eggs can be prepared in accordance with the patient's taste, dry cereal can be substituted for cooked. There is a great waste of food if it is served in very large amounts or in a condition unpalatable to the patient, but this fact is less important than the patient's failure to receive the nourishment he needs and the satisfaction derived from an enjoyable meal. A few patients may not care whether the coffee and toast are hot, the milk cold. Enough do care, however, so that these are important considerations for both dietitian and nurse.

If dietary preferences are to be considered, a method of discovering and recording them is essential. The nurse or dietitian should observe the patient's tray when he has finished eating and consult with him regarding any foods not eaten, his special likes and dislikes. These she should record in the proper place. Once recorded, they should be adhered to. There is nothing more discouraging to a patient than to have requested that he receive no tea and stated that he would like an extra slice of bread with each meal and then to have these preferences disregarded.

Psychological as well as physical preparation affects the pleasure with which the patient receives his tray. The meal becomes something of an event when patients have the chance to wash their hands and freshen their appearance, when rooms are tidied, beds straightened, and a place cleared for the tray. Up-patients often enjoy the meal more if they eat with a group in the dining room or in the solarium on the division. This practice should be encouraged.

When diet aides carry trays, the nursing personnel is freed to circulate among the patients, assisting those who need help. Regardless of where the responsibility for carrying trays lies, if the patient is to receive his food in a palatable form, it must reach him within minutes after the food has been placed on the tray. This means prompt transportation and patients ready and waiting for their meals. It is not the purpose of this volume to discuss the various ways of serving diets to facilitate meeting the objectives for tray service. It is important, however, for head nurses to know that in every situation her staff has some responsibility and that the patient has the right to expect that nursing as well as dietary personnel will do their part in providing him food he can eat and enjoy.

Convalescent and mildly ill patients need some form of diversion. The importance to his progress of having some way to occupy time was thoroughly considered in Chapter 3. Patients who do not enjoy reading or who tire of games and handwork sometimes find considerable satisfaction through participation in unit activities such as passing drinking water, wheeling patients, collecting trays, making up charts. There are many such activities which would be therapeutic for patients. Preparing a roster of jobs suitable for patients and classifying them according to degree of energy required would be a useful undertaking for the nursing staff. A compilation of this kind would make possible a planned program of activity graduated in relation to the patient's stage of recovery.

The convalescent and mildly ill patient, when well nursed, not only feels free to ask questions but is encouraged to do so. He is confident that the information given him is accurate. For example, if it is known, the reason for his pain is explained, why it continues, what he can expect in relation to it. Will it ever end or will he have to learn to live with it? What can be done to ease it? Questions of this kind are not evaded. The nurse needs to know the answers, and when there is a team relationship between her and the doctor, she does know. Although she may respond to the patient's queries, at times it is more appropriate for the physician to do so. When this is true the nurse encourages the patient to ask the doctor for answers, helping him formulate the questions should the patient feel this will be useful. By asking his own questions, the patient helps retain his autonomy.

When progress is slow the patient becomes discouraged and often worries about himself. Is everything all right? Am I progressing as I should? He may not verbalize his fears, but an alert nurse notices changes in his behavior which may indicate that something is amiss. He is not ambulating as much as usual. He tells the nurse he is not sleeping well. His appetite has decreased. The attentive nurse listens to the questions he asks and the remarks he makes, and tries to read between the lines to discover discouragement or worry. She verifies her hunches with the patient. "You say you didn't sleep well. You didn't eat your breakfast. You have just told me your daughter isn't coming to see you today." These statements would permit the patient to express any relationship which exists between them if he wishes to do so. If he doesn't respond, the nurse may ask whether there is a connection.

The patient may have misconceptions which she can correct. If he is convalescing normally she can help him to see that recovery seems slow because he is better and hence impatient to get back to normal living. If progress is not being made sometimes it will help if she encourages him to express his concerns, showing that she cares, taking time to be with him. Patients may talk freely if given an opportunity. The nurse needs to listen purposefully, commenting or reflecting as it seems appropriate. If she thinks about what the patient is saying and watches for cues she can often gain a better understanding of his fears and help him verbalize them.

Other patients need real encouragement from the nurse if they are to express the things which are troubling them. The way may be opened by a leading statement such as, "You seem discouraged today, Mr. Burns." If he does not respond she might add, "Would you care to tell me about it?" If the patient's worry is related to his personal or business affairs he may not want to talk about it and should not be made to feel he should do so. On the other hand, if he is concerned about his condition and the nurse shows that his feelings matter to her, a permissive atmosphere may be created in which he feels free to unburden his mind. The nurse knows that there are some problems which she is unable to help him solve. Perhaps there is no solution. It is important to her and the patient that she recognize this and not let him feel that because he has confided in her she will set things straight in his life. A social worker, a clergyman, a psychiatrist may be needed. The nurse's responsibility is to encourage the patient to contact the proper source of help and give him the necessary assistance in doing so. Mainly she must be able to sort out these problems with which, as a nurse, she is prepared to assist him. The patient has a right to expect that his confidence will be respected, that information concerning him, his family, or his illness will be guarded and used in a professional way only.

NEEDS OF THE PATIENT WHO IS WEAK AND DEBILITATED AS A RESULT OF CHRONIC DISEASE

These individuals have special needs which differ both in kind and in degree from the acutely ill and convalescent. Many are old. Since most of their friends are old, too, they are unable to get about easily. Visits from these friends are, therefore, impossible or at best infrequent. An elderly parent may of necessity have been uprooted from his own home to live with a son or daughter in a strange community where no one knows him. He has few if any friends of his own in the new locality, and, therefore, if he is hospitalized for long, his callers are likely to be few. Many younger patients who have been incapacitated for a long time have few visitors. Friends are busy with other things and to find time to get to the hospital is difficult. Sometimes even families cannot come to see the patient daily. Although the patient may understand the situation, still he feels lonely, forgotten, and cut off from the world around him. Life seems to be passing him by.

Since every individual has a need for love and companionship, the patient with long-term illness has the right to expect the nurse to make up in part for its lack. He needs to feel that all members of the nursing staff are interested in him, know his needs, are sympathetic and understanding, and are doing everything in their power to help him regain and maintain his health. The nurse may not have as much opportunity as desired to spend with the patient who is too weak or debilitated to give any of his own care. However, the time she does spend with him should be his exclusively. Regardless of the pressures on the nurse, the periods which she spends in the patient's care should be times for friendliness, for the patient to talk, and for the nurse to contribute a bit of news or a story in which the patient will be interested. The nurse who makes occasion throughout the day for a friendly smile, a few words, or a squeeze of the hand will brighten the day for those who feel they have little for which to live. Most important of all she should, through her approach, encourage the patient to express the thoughts that are in his mind which may be interfering with his improvement or comfort. Their expression often clarifies for him his true feelings. He can then be helped to resolve them.

The night nurse has a special responsibility to see the patient often to learn whether he is sleeping. At night, minutes seem like hours. It is a time of fear if one is wakeful. The imagination often runs wild. If his light isn't answered in a few minutes, the patient worries about what would happen if this were an emergency and the nurse were so slow in coming. Many persons who are inactive sleep poorly at night. Frequent reassurance that the nurse is near and will come when wanted is often satisfying to the wakeful patient. If not, a restful back rub, a clean or tightened draw-sheet, a change in position provide the comfort and diversion which will bring sleep. The patient needs to feel that nothing is too much trouble to make him comfortable.

Good nursing for the person who has been weak and ill for a long time gives him an opportunity to express his wishes and, whenever it is not detrimental to his recovery, to have some choice regarding the way in which his care is given. Little things matter a great deal to these individuals, and they have special ways in which they like their care to be given. The patient is happier and the nurse able to function more easily if some of the major preferences are written in a nursing care plan (see Chapter 11). At all times the patient needs to know on what he can count; that is, that he will receive his bath, medication, and feedings when he is expecting them and that, if circumstances prevent, he will be told. Nothing is more tiring than waiting. The patient also should feel confident that his wishes, his ideas, and his actions are being honestly, accurately, and sympathetically interpreted to the doctor, the hospital personnel, and to his family.

The patient who is always tired and frequently uncomfortable needs special consideration in little things. The thoughtful nurse plans his care so that interruptions to his rest are kept to a minimum. A quiet, peaceful, clean, orderly environment gives him the confidence and security which permits relaxation. He is kept as comfortable as possible by change in position, support, massage, cleanliness, fluids, nourishment, attention to elimination and to his other personal needs. Prone to complications which would add to his suffering, the patient is protected from infection, decubiti, contractures, and other deformities. Supportive care which will prevent impairment of vital functions, such as muscle exercise, joint motion and massage, and the maintenance of a functional position is provided regularly and consistently.

In addition to the care necessitated by his condition and his personality, the patient requires care dictated by his diagnosis and the prescribed medical therapy. It is not the purpose of this text to consider these specific requirements but rather to emphasize that each individual has his own special nursing needs and has the right to expect that they will be recognized and met. The families of patients who are chronically ill also have needs. Often they have guilt feelings for not keeping the patient at home where he preferred to stay. They usually try to make it up to the patient by frequent visits to the hospital. Members of any closely knit family are faithful in visiting the loved one. Nurses who have been through an experience wherein, over a period of months, daily visits were made to a parent, husband, or child appreciate the way in which home life is affected and the drain on human energy. Such family members need understanding. If they wish to participate in the patient's care, this should be encouraged. However, if they are tired, they may prefer to have the patient fixed up and looking his best when they come to call. Nurses need to discover family preferences just as they do the patient's and not to assume that a daughter *wants* to comb her mother's hair everytime she comes to visit. It often helps the staff to have the family assume part of the patient's care, but the family's and the patient's wishes in the matter should be determined. If the patient is returning to his home and will be unable to care for himself the family must, of course, learn to perform technical procedures in which they are not skilled. (See pp. 229-230.)

NEEDS OF THE PATIENT WHO HAS PERMANENT DYSFUNCTION OF HIS MUSCLES OR JOINTS

A major objective for the patient with motor incapacity is to prepare him to be as self-sufficient as his condition will permit. Many of his limitations can be partially overcome. The patient and his family have the right to expect that the patient will be helped to gain the will and the ability to perform all the activities of daily living of which he is capable. Rehabilitation starts in the hospital although it must be completed elsewhere.

No time should be lost. Maintenance of joint motion and prevention of muscle atrophy have high priority in the care of one whose power of movement is impaired.

For many of these persons disablement has come suddenly. After the first shock has passed, the realization comes to the patient that he no longer has a hand or that his leg is permanently paralyzed. He has a right to expect the nurse to understand his despair and to know that it is a stage necessary to his acceptance of his disability. Only when he has really accepted his loss can he think about his future. One of the hardest tasks for the nurse and one of her greatest challenges is to help this patient through his depression to the point where he can accept his loss. He needs time. He must not be hurried. The empathetic nurse will use every means at her disposal to gain understanding of the way to help him. She encourages him to express his feelings and listens carefully while he does so. She observes him closely for signs of hope. She seeks information and help from his family, his doctor, the physical therapist, other nurses. When he is ready she helps him think through his personal resources—his interests and skills, mental capacity and education, and the individuals he may know who can help him. His clergyman is often a source of strength and may know persons who can serve as contacts in finding a new type of work. The patient may feel his family, his employer, a club, or lodge to be potential sources of help. Although the patient may appear to have accepted permanent disability and the need to change his way of living, he will have discouraging days ahead during which he will need a great deal of support. Until he has become adjusted and feels he is once again living a useful life and making a contribution to his family and to society, he will need someone with whose help he can obtain renewed courage. That someone may very well be the head nurse who maintains continuity throughout his stay in the hospital.

For some persons disablement comes gradually. Arthritis creeps from joint to joint. The patient who needs an amputation usually has time to make up his mind, to get used to the idea, and to accept it. Although the shock may not be as great as when the patient is faced with the accomplished fact of a severed spinal cord or hemiplegia, nevertheless he has to adjust to the disability. The nurse's responsibility is to help him accept his limitations, build on his strengths, and develop new resources.

Good nursing helps the family of the patient to understand him and to assist him in accepting and living with his limitations. They need to understand the extent of the patient's disability and its emotional effect upon him, the precautionary measures which should be taken to prevent accidents and injury, and follow-up medical care. They need help in learning the skills necessary for the patient's continuing care at home. It is important also that the patient's family understands that he needs to *want* to do things for himself and that they have an important responsibility to let him do them. They should be able to expect that definite plans will be made with them for the patient's discharge from the hospital so that he and they know how and where he is going. To provide continuity in care he is referred to a community agency if this is indicated.

If the nurse meets her obligation to the family, she recognizes that they have needs of their own. The family and the patient are intricately bound to one another. That which affects one affects all. If father loses his leg, mother develops multiple sclerosis, or Johnny gets poliomyelitis, the disabilities which follow affect the way of life of all who live in the same household. Members of the family as well as the patient need empathy. They may need to express their feelings and to release their tensions. Here again the understanding nurse realizes their need to speak and makes herself psychologically available to them. She may also suggest others who might be of assistance if the family wishes help. The family members may try to hide their emotions for the sake of the patient. They feel their problems are minor in comparison to his and feel guilty if they mention concern about themselves. As is true in every situation when good nursing is given, the needs of the family are recognized and the personnel show that they care.

NEEDS OF THE PATIENT WHO HAS LOST HIS SIGHT

The newly blinded individual and his family are likely to have many of the same problems in acceptance and adjustment that are suffered by the patient with motor impairment. In addition the patient is deprived of the pleasures that have heretofore come to him through sight. He cannot read; he cannot see the things that go on about him in this strange place, the hospital. If the sightless patient is to be protected from harm, articles which could cause injury are kept out of his way. Keeping the things he needs within easy reach and helping him know how to locate them are essential for his peace of mind. Although he may learn to do most things, the learning takes time and for some skills special training is required. The patient and his family have a right to expect that hospital personnel will instigate and participate in long range planning to help the patient become self-dependent.

NEEDS OF THE PATIENT WHO HAS A PROBLEM
IN COMMUNICATION

The ability to communicate may be impaired by many means. Inability to make his wishes known and to gain answers to his questions isolates a patient, frustrates him, and can easily produce anxiety. Add this problem to another, such as impaired sight or locomotion, discomfort, and lack of visitors, and the patient may indeed suffer. A language barrier can usually be overcome to some extent. Seldom is there no one in the hospital who speaks a language in common with the patient. Since this person cannot be ever present, a sign language needs to be established with the help of the interpreter. The person interpreting to the patient may be a maid or a porter who has neither the information nor the experience of the nurse in dealing with the ill. The nurse, therefore, has the important responsibility of explaining to the interpreter a little about the patient and the consideration he should be shown. Some type of diversion is almost essential for the patient who cannot understand the language of those about him.

The patient with aphasia also has difficulty in communicating. Here the family may be the best help since they know the things to which the patient is accustomed. However, the nurse must use her powers of observation to the fullest in an effort to determine what he is trying to say. To ease the situation for the patient she asks questions which can be answered with a nod or shake of the head. Later when the patient is being re-trained to speak, she learns from the speech therapist the ways in which she can be of help. At all times infinite patience and full attention are needed when an aphasic patient is trying to make his wishes known.

It is less difficult to communicate with the individual who is hard of hearing and the tracheotomized patient unless they have handicaps which prevent them from reading or writing. The patient who has difficulty in hearing may be able to hear a well-modulated voice and to understand if the nurse enunciates clearly and does not speak too rapidly. He may be embarrassed to be shouted at and unable to understand if the nurse speaks too loudly. Many can at least partially read lips. The patient who has a laryngectomy should know that he can learn to speak and where he can get the necessary training. In the hospital he is supplied with a slate and chalk or a pad and pencil on which to write the messages he cannot convey by sign language. He is not asked questions which require long answers. The nurse who knows her patient's interests should learn to carry on a conversation in which the patient is a silent but active participant.

NEEDS OF THE PATIENT WHO IS CONFUSED
OR DISORIENTED

Confusion and disorientation result from a number of causes, including vascular changes, brain damage, infection, and functional disorders. If the patient realizes he is confused, he may find the confusion perplexing and disturbing. The good nurse tries her best to reorient him. If he seems to have illusions, she attempts to determine whether anything in the environment is contributing to them. The writer knows of a very ill patient who was frequently disturbed because she saw red and green balls being thrown about. It was not until the nurse, in leaning over the bed to turn the patient, happened to notice from that position the traffic lights on the street corner turning from green to red. The "balls" were explained to the patient, who, for the moment at least, understood and felt more comfortable. In another instance, an elderly patient, sexton of a nearby church, kept insisting he had to get up to unlock the church. He pounded on the wall, rattled the side bars on his bed, pulled at his ankle restraints. The nurses tried to reassure him that everything was all right, he was in the hospital now, he shouldn't worry. Finally someone suggested calling the parish priest. The nurse was told that the sexton did have the keys and always opened the church for early mass. The priest sent word to the patient that he had a second set of keys and would unlock the doors. The patient immediately relaxed and was no longer "disoriented."

The patient has a right to expect that the basis for his apparent irrational behavior will be sought, and, if necessary, patient reiteration will be used to help him think more clearly. If he is confused but not disturbed, all he may need is someone to whom to talk and loving care which will help him feel secure. Special protection is necessary for the confused individual who tries to get out of the bed or chair to attend to his personal needs or to perform some task for which he thinks he is responsible.

NEEDS OF THE PATIENT WHO IS GOING
HOME FROM THE HOSPITAL

Patients and their families often do not realize the problems they will face when the patient comes home from the hospital even after a short illness. Suddenly he is home and all kinds of questions come to mind. In the hospital he has been up and about, has taken his own bath, seemed so well. Sometimes he has even administered his own treatments; often he has not. He has taken no real responsibility for his care. The proper diet has been served him. Medications and treatments have been given or supervised by the nurse. If he had discomfort or couldn't sleep, the nurse was there to reassure him and help him relax. Now, at home, he may have a loving family eager to help him. At least there is usually someone to oversee his care. But they don't know as much about his care as the patient, so the responsibility is his. He must make the decisions. This is a step necessary to progress toward health and for some it creates no problems. For others, however, return home can be accomplished with less anxiety and less risk of mistakes which might undo some of the good that has been done in the hospital if the nurse recognizes the rights which are the patient's due. She needs to realize that his care does not end when he leaves the hospital and that his convalescence may be shortened if he has help in his adjustment to home life.

The head nurse is responsible for seeing that necessary steps are taken to insure the patient having proper care at home. His questions are answered and he is given the general information needed for home care and for good health. If tests or treatments are to be administered at home he is taught to perform them and helped to obtain the necessary equipment. The assistance of a community agency is provided through referral if this is indicated and desired. All patients do not need assistance in all areas, but the head nurse must know the kinds of help which each patient needs and, therefore, has a right to expect.

General Information Needed by the Patient Who Is Going Home

Nurse, doctor, patient, and family should collaborate in seeing that the patient has the information he will need to carry on at home. One effective method is for the nurse to suggest to the patient as soon as discharge is anticipated, that he should begin thinking about information he will wish to have at home. To assist him the nurse may suggest that he start by writing down his questions. Since for most operative and postpartal patients hospitalization is only a matter of a few days, there should be no delay in his starting the list. Family members may wish to include their questions with those of the patient or they may make separate notations. Assurance should be given that the questions will be answered. Many, the head nurse will answer. Some she may suggest the patient discuss with the physician. One gynecologist, when shown a list of questions his patient had prepared, was so impressed that he wrote out the answers and asked that the list be typed and given to all his patients who have had hysterectomies.

Some patients will not be able to think of questions or may not be able to list them. For others they may cause worry. The nurse through her scientific knowledge and her knowledge of the patient and his home situation will be able to provide much of the information he needs. Any patient who is sent home with directions for taking medications needs to know their purpose and importance, the expected effects, dosage, methods and frequency of administration, length of time the drug is to be taken, where it may be procured, possible undesirable effects if the medication is to be taken over a long period, and the need for reporting symptoms. He needs to be instructed in the hazards of self-medication and of resuming medications prescribed for another illness.

Almost every patient needs specific instruction in the care he will require when he reaches home. Unless told, he does not know how much activity he should permit himself. To leave the judgment to the patient by telling him not to get too tired will result in far too much exercise for some and not enough for others. He needs to be given some idea of the number of times a day he may go up and down stairs, approximately how much time he should spend up and about and how much reclining, the circumstances under which to rest, the advisability of taking a tub bath, the types of activity and work which are to be avoided such as lifting, stooping, reaching, sweeping, ways to return gradually to normal activity, how soon he may travel or drive the car.

Private physicians tell their patients when to report for a check-up and the conditions they should report prior to the visit should they occur. Instructions relative to the care and precautions specific to his diagnosis or condition are usually given by the doctor but may be left to the head nurse if she has participated in long-range planning. The clinic patient also needs information about home care. The head nurse makes sure the intern or resident has a chance to instruct the patient before he is discharged. Included in the instructions are the types and amounts of food the patient should eat and items to be avoided. The patient and his family need to understand the reasons for any dietary restrictions. The importance of elimination and methods for its control are also made clear to the patient. The head nurse is competent to give this information but in a teaching hospital it is usually considered a necessary experience for the young doctor.

It is especially important that some patients be taught the dangers of infection and the methods of avoiding it. Patients with nephritis and cardiac disease need to be warned against contracting respiratory infections and instructed to avoid crowded, congested rooms, contact with people known to have colds, drafts which may cause chilling, wet feet, and insufficient clothing in winter. The relationship between fatigue and respiratory infection is pointed out. The postpartal patient is taught how to prevent mastitis by handling breasts with clean hands, using clean wash cloths and towels and clean clothes.

The head nurse should assume the responsibility for seeing that the new mother is instructed in her baby's needs for affection and security and in methods of handling, holding, bathing, clothing, and feeding him. The mother also welcomes information on the care of diapers and other clothing, normal elimination and its control, ways to avoid infection, sleep and feeding schedules, indications of normal development, and the need for medical supervision.

The patient's family often needs help in assisting him to make a readjustment to home life and in enabling him to progress as rapidly as possible through convalescence to health. If they recognize the patient's need to regain his independence and to feel useful, the members of his family need not prolong the period of invalidism unnecessarily. If they understand that a degree of stimulation is restorative, they will encourage visitors and bring in news of the outside world. However, they will need to be on the alert for signs of overfatigue. Both the patient and his family should understand that there will be periods of discouragement. The patient who tends to become restless during a long convalescence can often be persuaded that it is a time in which to do many of the things for which he has never found time. Some will find it an opportunity to develop hobbies. Others may need the convalescence made less attractive in order that it will not be needlessly prolonged.

Instruction in Treatments and Dressings

Another need of the patient before discharge is for instruction in the performance of treatments which he is to receive at home and to insure his learning through return demonstrations. The patient's learning is likely to be more successful if he practices with equipment similar to that which he will use at home. He may need to be prepared for insulin administration, urinalysis, diet calculation, colostomy dressings and irrigation, eye compresses and drops. He needs help in selection of home equipment, its care and handling, necessary precautionary measures to prevent infection or injury. If it is necessary for him to be taught to dress a wound, he should know to use clean hands and avoid touching the lesion. He needs to be told where to procure and shown how to handle sterile dressings as well as ways to dispose of soiled ones. Often it is insufficient to teach the patient alone. There will be times when he will be incapable of caring for himself and it is wise for a member of the family to be prepared to assist him. If the patient will need bed care, his wife, mother, or daughter or the practical nurse who will care for him at home should come into the hospital, if possible, to work with the nurse. It will help greatly if this person knows how to get the patient in and out of bed with ease, give him a bed bath and back rub, exercise a paralyzed limb, and prevent contractures.

Referral to a Community Agency

The third need of the patient who is being discharged is to have arrangements made for his continued care after he leaves the hospital if this is necessary. A system of interagency referral between the hospital and the health and social agencies of the community has been established in some localities with excellent results. Following a report from the hospital, a public health nurse or social worker visits the patient in his home to observe his condition and give him any help that he may need. The patient may or may not have been known to the community agency before his hospitalization. If the head nurse, the social worker, or the doctor feels that the patient needs care, assistance, or observation after leaving the hospital, any one of these workers may take the initiative in referring the patient to the proper agency. In some hospitals this is done by telephone, but those which have used the written report have found this method more satisfactory (Figs. 12 and 13). The written form, which may be made out by the head nurse or the patient's nurse, usually contains information about the treatment which the patient has received in the hospital and that which is to be carried on at home. If the patient has been taught to perform his own treatments, this should be indicated and a brief description given of the method. The public health nurse also needs to know how well the patient has mastered the technique and the kind of help he will need in the home. If members of the family have been taught also, the public health nurse should have this information. There is space on the referral form for the doctor's orders and his signature. He may also indicate the need for follow-up medical attention and state when the patient is to return to the clinic or his office. The head nurse usually writes a note explaining how

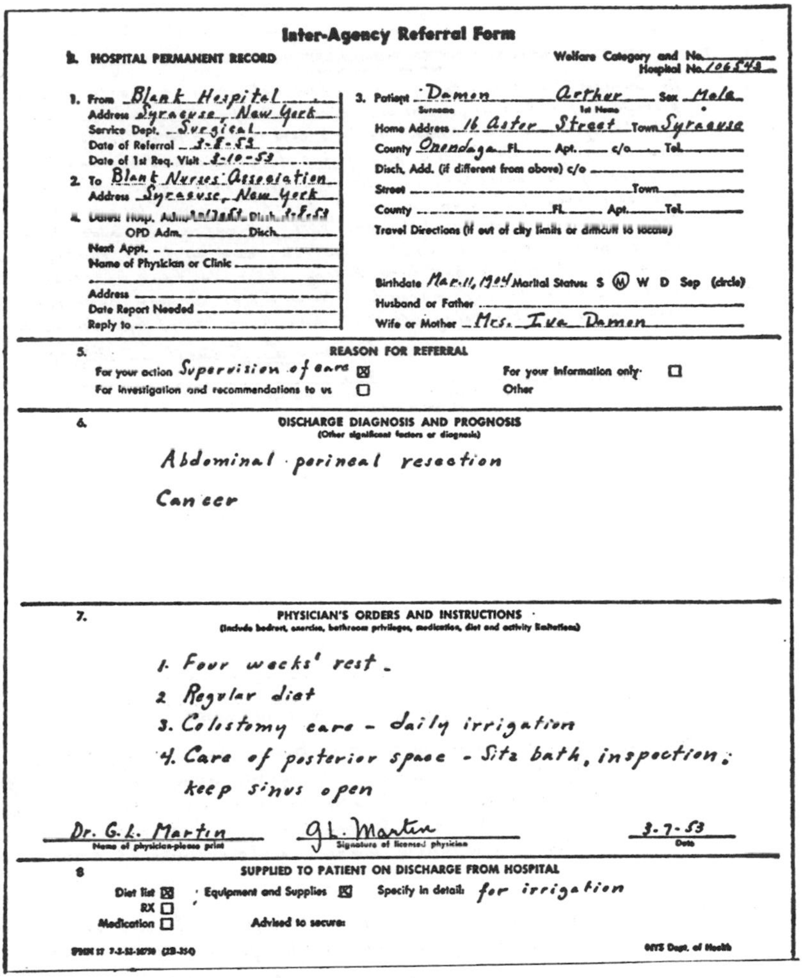

Fig. 12. Interagency referral form (front). Referral may be initiated by any member of the health team in a hospital and community. Form is completed in triplicate (or quadruplicate if copy is required for private physician). One copy is retained by the receiving agency; two are returned to the sending agency. One copy is attached to the patient's permanent hospital record. Each sheet is a different color. (Courtesy of the New York State Department of Health.)

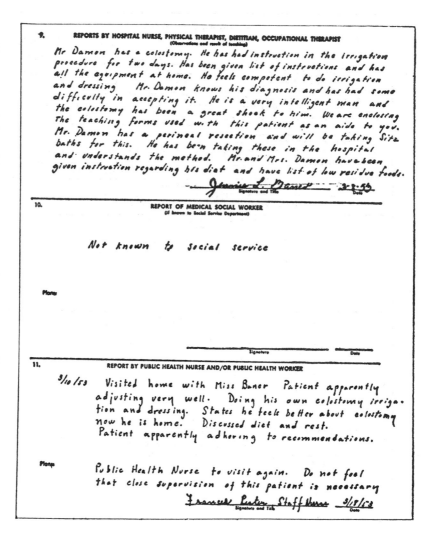

Fig. 13. Interagency referral form (back). A continuation sheet may be used if necessary. (Courtesy of the New York State Department of Health.)

much the patient knows and understands about his condition and tells the attitude of the patient and the family toward his illness. The social worker includes a brief explanation of any existing social problem. Other individuals such as the dietitian or physical therapist may make notations if the patient is known to them.

If possible the report should reach the community agency the day the patient leaves the hospital. When this cannot be managed a telephone call from the head nurse may precede the written report. If the public health nurse is notified of the patient's discharge several days in advance, she may visit the home and assist the family in making necessary preparations. After the patient has been seen in his home, the public health nurse or social worker sends a report to the hospital describing the home situation, the patient's adjustment and his ability to carry out instructions given in the hospital (Fig. 13) The report is read by the head nurse and others who cared for the patient. Both reports are filed with the patient's clinical record.

Without an adequate referral system there is too little coordination between hospital care and home care. Agencies often work in the dark in regard to the patient's past treatment which results in duplication of effort and loss of time. The patient may be the loser. For continuity of care there needs to be a close working relationship between the hospital and other community agencies. If the head nurse were to receive a report from the public health nurse or social worker who knew the patient in his home prior to his admission to the hospital, she would have a better understanding of his reactions and would be greatly helped in adapting the health teaching to his particular needs. Likewise, the hospital nurses should be interested in what happens to the patient after his departure and how effectively he has been prepared to take up life in his home surroundings. If the patient is admitted to the hospital in the future the insights provided by the follow-up report of the public health nurse are invaluable to the hospital nurses in planning for home care the next time. This is continuity of care of a high order.

Immediate Preparation for Discharge

It is important that the head nurse help decide when the patient is ready to go home. She knows the progress of his instructional program. She is in the best position to judge his state of psychological readiness. The time of discharge, then, is one of the most important occasions for a group decision by patient, doctor, nurse, and family. There is no excuse for a unilateral spontaneous decision by the physician to send the patient home. Instruction for home care given in the excitement of home going will not likely be remembered. The family, too, needs time to prepare the home to receive the returning member. Transportation must be provided; work schedules often have to be adjusted. Tentative plans for discharge can be made several days in advance with all who are concerned concurring, each understanding that the schedule is tentative and knowing the circumstances upon which discharge is contingent.

When a patient is to be discharged the head nurse must know that he has proper clothing to wear home and if he does not, to see that it is provided through his family or social service. The patient needs suitable transportation and a member of his family or a friend to accompany him to his home. The head nurse should assure herself that these facilities are available and that he has the necessary medications and equipment to take with him. She should see that there is someone to assist the patient to dress, if necessary, to help collect and pack his personal effects, and if he is unable to walk, to transport him to the business office and assist him to his conveyance. It is important that the patient be able to reach his car or taxi easily and that he not be expected to walk down stairs if his condition does not favor that amount or type of exertion.

The head nurse will wish to talk personally with the patient and his family as they are leaving. As hostess on her division she bids them farewell. To the great majority of patients, going home is an occasion for rejoicing. They wish the nurses to share their happiness. The patient cannot but feel slighted if the nurses sit at the desk when he is leaving and bid him a perfunctory good-bye. The patient and his family should be able to expect that friendliness and courtesy will be shown as long as they are within the hospital.

SUMMARY

The patient is an individual who has needs and rights. He and his family are not familiar with all the needs which they should expect to be met by the nursing personnel of the division. They have a right to expect, however, that the nurse knows most of the things the patient should have for his happiness and well-being and that she will find out those others which he feels are important to him. Since many nurses do not meet these expectations of the patient, one of the head nurse's chief responsibilities is to motivate and help her professional staff develop ability to determine patient's needs and become increasingly effective in meeting them.

Admission to the hospital means something different to each individual based on his experience and the immediate circumstances which brought him to the hospital. All are excited and anxious even when their condition is not serious. They are never quite sure what hospitalization will bring, and what its outcome will be. An understanding nurse helps put the patient and his family at ease in the hospital setting. Everything possible is done for the patient's comfort, from letting him know he was expected to explaining the schedule for the day. Pain and discomfort are given immediate attention. The patient is observed for signs of abnormality and body lesions. Family relationships are noted as an aid to understanding the patient's behavior. An admission history taken by the head nurse helps her in making a tentative diagnosis and setting up a nursing care plan. Families can often be of help by describing the patient's preferences, habits, and special anxieties. The patient has the right to expect that he is accepted regardless of his economic status, his color, or condition. He also should be able to anticipate that his treatments and nursing care will be effectively and safely performed without unnecessary discomfort to him.

The well-nursed, acutely ill patient knows he can put his entire trust in the nurse. His every need is anticipated and promptly met in a skillful, comforting manner. He is guarded from harm and observed closely for signs of complications. The needs of the convalescent or mildly ill differ in many respects from those of the patient who requires intensive care. His needs tend to relate more specifically to the kind of person he is. The good nurse endeavors to discover and to satisfy the individual's personal needs and at the same time to see that he receives the rehabilitative care his condition requires.

Because the patient who has been ill a long time often feels lonely and unneeded, the nursing personnel try to fill some of the gaps in his life. A period when he feels the nurse's attention is his alone helps make the day brighter as do little attentions which show that she cares. A consistent pattern of care is usually welcome to the weak, debilitated patient who gets used to a system and is not comfortable when it is changed.

The individual who has just suffered a permanent disability needs physical rehabilitation and special protective measures. More difficult to deal with is his depression. His problems in adjustment are frequently extreme. He needs understanding and acceptance by all personnel. The nurse, members of the other healing professions, and his family must help the patient mobilize his resources and find his way back to happiness.

Any interference with the patient's ability to communicate places a burden of responsibility on the nurse to find ways for the patient to make his wishes known, to prevent frustration, and to keep him occupied with appropriate diversion. Confused and disoriented individuals are often troubled by their inability to think clearly. A considerate nurse tries to remove sources of psychological discomfort and explains repeatedly if necessary where the patient is and how he happens to be here. Special protective measures are instituted.

The family, regardless of the patient's condition, has many needs and a right to expect that they will be met so far as it is in the power of the hospital to do so. Their need for understanding, for accurate information, for support, for complete trust in the personnel is recognized by the nurse who has the ability to empathize. She never fails to be considerate nor to do everything possible to be of help.

The patient's discharge should be planned days in advance with the patient, his family, and the nurse participating with the doctor in the decision. Patients and their families many times do not realize that they should expect any help from the hospital in relation to home care. However, they should be helped to make careful plans for the patient's homecoming and to think through the questions which will likely arise once they are away from immediate sources of information. The nurse makes sure the family has the general information and skills necessary for comfortable, safe home care. If indicated, she refers the patient to a community agency for further assistance. At the time of discharge the patient receives final instructions and is given a gracious farewell by all staff members who are at hand. Thus he leaves the hospital feeling that the importance of the day is recognized.

QUESTIONS FOR DISCUSSION

1. If your community has no system for referral, what could the head nurse do to arouse a feeling of need for this service?
2. How do you react when a patient tries to tell you how to give his care? Do you think your feelings are "normal"? "healthy"? If you were a patient would you care how your treatments were given? whether you were screened for personal care? whether the bedside equipment was arranged in a particular way if you were unable to do this yourself? Would you express these wishes if you knew it bothered the nurse to be asked or told? How can a nurse who dislikes having a patient make requests for things she has already anticipated avoid such feelings?
3. What are the barriers to patients asking questions of doctors? If you, a

member of your family, or a friend has been hospitalized recently were there any barriers felt in asking questions of nurses? If so, what were they?

4. How would you feel if you were a patient on a stretcher in a hot elevator, crowded with hospital staff? with visitors?

EXERCISES

1. Define your concept of a patient. Concepts of each class member could be presented to the group, common elements isolated, key points agreed upon, dissenting ideas noted. Discuss ways the different concepts could influence the patient's care.

2. Develop criteria for a good admission procedure. Then, accompany a relative or friend or, is this is not possible, observe any patient being admitted to a hospital. Preferably your identity should be unknown to hospital personnel. Every effort should be made not to let your presence color the situation. Identify with the patient. Evaluate the admission procedure from the patient's point of view, that is, as though you had been the patient. Compare the actual situation with the criteria previously established. What implications do your findings have for the head nurse?

3. Observe visitors on your division for an hour or more, identifying as far as possible, with each one in turn. Describe your feelings.

4. With the help of the division staff make a list of activities which patients on your floor might undertake. At what stage of the patient's recovery would each be advisable? What values do you see in the activities? What, if anything, is there to prevent the encouragement of patients to undertake such activities?

5. Establish criteria for good tray service from the patient's point of view. Observe tray service on another floor than your own. Evaluate it. How could the service be improved from the point of view of the dietary department? nursing care?

6. Using the descriptions of patients according to their needs as presented in this chapter, select a patient on your division who appears to fit one of the descriptions. Compare the nursing care pictured in the text with the care that the patient is receiving. Is there a difference? Wherein? How should the description be augmented? Should the patient's care be altered in any way? Is there a problem in communicating (in its broad sense) with the patient? Can the class make suggestions for getting at the problem?

7. If sending referrals is not a regular procedure in your hospital, select two patients on your division who could profit from follow-up nursing care after discharge. What facilities are there in your community for home care? Even if there is no accepted procedure for referral, determine what the head nurse can and should do to provide continuity in care for these two patients.

8. Select one patient on your division who will be going home in about a week to convalesce for a week or more. Preferably the patient should have little or no need for technical skill. Ask the patient to list the questions that he would like to have answered. The family might be asked to make a list also. Before looking at these lists make your own notations of information you think the patient should have. It will be helpful to think of yourself as the patient and to consider his home situation, occupation, and other pertinent information. Compare all three lists. To how many of the questions do you *not* have answers? Obtain the answers and transmit them to the patient or ask the physician to answer them if it seems inappropriate for you to do so. In the latter case, consider why it is inappropriate. Of what value is this exercise to a head nurse?

REFERENCES

Aasterud, Margaret. Defenses against anxiety in the nurse-patient relationship, Nurs. Forum, Vol. 1 (Summer 1962), pp. 34-59.
Certain nursing areas are charged with feeling for both patients and nurses—intrusive procedures, pre-danger anxiety, death. Only with some understanding of situations can nurses function intelligently to relieve tension. Helpful illustrations are given.

Abdellah, Faye G., Martin, Almeda, Beland, Irene L., and Matheney, Ruth V. Patient-Centered Approaches to Nursing, New York, Macmillan Co., 1960.
This little book was written to assist in the development of ways to bring about patient-centered nursing which is a generally recognized goal. A list of 21 so-called nursing problems is presented as an aid in providing this type care.

Adamek, Mary Elaine. Some observations on death and a family, Nurs. Science, Vol. 3 (August 1965), pp. 258-267.
An interesting presentation of the needs of the dying child for his family and of the family for support.

Baker, Joan M., and Sorensen, Karen C. A patient's concern with death, Amer. J. Nurs., Vol. 63 (July 1963), pp. 90-92.
The way in which one nurse answered a patient's direct question about the imminency of death. "The difficult part of death is not the act of dying itself—but in preparing for coming death." In this the nurse can play a significant part.

Barnes, Elizabeth. People in hospital, London, Macmillan and Co., Ltd., 1961, Ch. 1, 2, 3, pp. 1-36.
This little book resulted from an international study of general hospitals by many small study groups.
The first three chapters describe the person who becomes a patient and his relationship to the doctor. The nurse gains a better understanding of both from reading Chapter 3.

Bender, Ruth E. Communicating with the deaf, Amer. J. Nurs., Vol. 66 (April 1966), pp. 757-760.
A speech expert describes the responsibility of hearing persons to take time and to be thoughtful enough to talk with the deaf. Suggestions for facilitating understanding by the hard of hearing are presented.

Bettelheim, Bruno. To nurse and to nurture, Nurs. Forum, Vol. 1 (Summer 1962), pp. 60-76.
Interesting and challenging, this article describes what nurses can do for the emotional health of children.

Bozian, Marguerite W. Nursing in a geriatric day center, Amer. J. Nurs., Vol. 64 (April 1964), pp. 93-95.
The writer's philosophy is that health is "a state of complete physical, mental, and social well-being within the framework of one's limitations and capacities, irrespective of the presence or absence of disease or infirmity."

Brauer, Paul H. Should the patient be told the truth?, Nurs. Outlook, Vol. 8 (December 1960), pp. 672-676.
A psychiatrist suggests that in deciding whether the patient and his family should be told the truth about terminal illness the doctor or nurse should ask himself, "which patient? what truth?" A very helpful discussion of a question which troubles many nurses.

Brooks, Helen Louise. The Golden Rule for the unconscious patient, Nurs. Forum, Vol. 4 (No. 3, 1965), pp. 12-18.
The rights and needs of the unconscious patient are vividly portrayed in this interestingly written article.

Brown, Esther Lucile. Newer Dimensions of Patient Care, Part 3: Patients as People, New York, Russell Sage Foundation, 1964.
This third volume discusses "patient care as seen in the social science perspective." "Patient care cannot be individualized . . . unless staff have some appreciable knowledge about the persons to whom care is given, as well as their medical conditions." A data sheet for collecting information about the patient is suggested.

Brown, J. P. Faith and nursing, Nurs. Times, Vol. 61 (October 15, 1965), p. 1428.
". . . one's faith is of paramount importance and the ability to communicate it to patients is vital." The writer believes this should be done through action rather than words.

Brueggen, Stella L. Nurses' opportunities to conserve sight, Nurs. Outlook, Vol. 10 (October 1962), pp. 658-660.
Opportunities of the nurse for detecting eye disease and teaching eye health.

Dennis, Robert J. Ways of caring, Amer. J. Nurs., Vol. 64 (February 1964), pp. 107-108.
The writer's personal experience with nursing during nine months of hospitalization following a serious accident. His descriptions may help each nurse to see herself and the possible effect of her behavior on patients.

Dudgeon, M. Y., and Davidson, T. W. Patients' reactions to their stay in hospital, Nurs. Mirror, Vol. 120 (May 28, 1965), pp. 203-206.

Report of a very interesting study in Royal Victoria Hospital, Belfast brings an important message, especially to head nurses. Of special interest are the quotations from patients relative to the information and reassurance the patient received or failed to receive on admission to and on discharge from the hospital.

Durocher, Mary Ann. Parent educator in the outpatient department, Amer. J. Nurs., Vol. 65 (June 1965), pp. 99-101.
A nurse employed as parent educator in an outpatient department is "someone with whom parents can identify in time of crisis . . . someone to whom they can turn when they are confused, overwhelmed, or bewildered."

Eckelberry, Grace. The nurse as a patient, Nurs. Outlook, Vol. 12 (December 1964), pp. 20-23.
A beautifully written, revealing account of a nurse-patient's hospital experiences, the way she feels about nursing and empathizes with both patients and nurses.

Engel, George L. Grief and grieving, Amer. J. Nurs., Vol. 64 (September 1964), pp. 93-98.
Some positive suggestions to help the nurse understand the process of grieving and to support families and patients through the period of grief.

Errera, Paul, and Dye, Mary C. Emotional steam clouds emergency care, Mod. Hosp., Vol. 104 (February 1965), pp. 87-92.
A study of 20 patients who visited the emergency room in a large urban hospital indicated many lacks in care, especially in meeting emotional needs. Lack of concerned medical leadership is blamed for the situation by the researchers—a psychiatrist and a nurse.

Fulton, Robert, and Langton, Phyllis A. Attitudes toward death: an emerging mental health problem, Nurs. Forum, Vol. 3 (No. 1, 1964), pp. 104-112.
A reorientation to death and dying is needed by nursing and medical personnel as well as by the laity. The process of dying and the dead body must be accepted. Present practices are hypocritical.

Gardner, E. Grief in our hospitals and homes, Int. J. Nurs. Studies, Vol. 2 (February 1966), pp. 293-296.
To help health workers deal with grief of patients and families the writer suggests that future doctors, nurses, ministers, social workers should be concerned with care of patients in the home as well as in the hospital, that they have opportunity to study together.

Georgopoulos, Basil S., and Mann, Floyd C. The Community General Hospital, New York, The Macmillan Company, 1962.
This intensely interesting report of extensive research carried out in ten community hospitals describes in detail factors which influence the quality of patient care.

Gleason, Doris. Tightening the loopholes in newborn identification, Hospitals, Vol. 40, Part I (August 1, 1966), pp. 60-63.
A detailed account of precautionary measures that need to be taken if the hospital is to be legally protected against a mixup of newborn babies.

Goodland, Norman L. Putting the patient in the picture, Nurs. Mirror, Vol. 121 (December 31, 1965), pp. VII, X.
Patients should have their questions answered truthfully if their minds are to be at ease. If doctors fail to satisfy the patient's need for knowledge, the nurse must assume this responsibility regardless of future consequences. Possible reasons for the nurse's reluctance to answer questions are given.

Gordon, Beulah M. A feeding plan for geriatric patients, Hospitals, Vol. 39 (April 16, 1965), pp. 92-98.

An unusual mealtime plan for older patients in a rehabilitation hospital has proved successful. It is based on the needs and preferences of patients.

Gregg, Dorothy. Reassurance. Reprinted from Amer. J. Nurs., Vol. 55 (February 1955) In Social Interaction and Patient Care, Skipper, J. K., Jr., and Leonard, R. C., eds. Philadelphia, J. B. Lippincott Company, 1965, pp. 127-136.
Communication between a distressed patient and two nurses in turn—one non-reassuring, the other reassuring—are analyzed.

Hands spread more infection than air, physicians report in California, Mod. Hosp., Vol. 104 (March 1965), p. 174.
A well-controlled study in one hospital nursery indicated "that physical contact between nurse-carrier and the infant was necessary for effective transmission." Similar studies are recommended for surgical divisions and operating rooms.

Hanson, Daniel J. Intramuscular injection injuries and complications, Amer. J. Nurs., Vol. 63 (April 1963), pp. 99-103.
Many important technical points in the administration of intramuscular injections which are enumerated here should be studied by nurses.

Hay, Stella I., and Anderson, Helen C. Are nurses meeting patient's needs?, Amer. J. Nurs., Vol. 63 (December 1963), pp. 96-99.
These nurses turned to the literature and determined patient needs and patient expectations by analyzing the writings of ex-patients about their illness experiences.

Hays, Joyce Samhammer. Analyses of nurse-patient communications, Nurs. Outlook, Vol. 14 (September 1966), pp. 32-35.
Many examples of patient questions and ways—poor and good—in which student nurses responded to them.

Hershey, Nathan. Informed consent, Amer. J. Nurs., Vol. 65 (July 1965), pp. 101-102.
The patient has a right to accept or reject treatment. The doctor who leaves explanation of procedures to others runs a real risk. The nurse who fails to refer to the physician patient's questions which she cannot satisfy is increasing the risk.

Horner, Ada L. and Jennings, Muriel. Before patients go home, Amer. J. Nurs., Vol. 61 (June 1961), pp. 62-63.
An active program of instruction for patients, families, and attendants who will help with nursing care is essential when severely disabled individuals are sent home.

Horty, John F. How to avoid emergency room lawsuits, Mod. Hosp., Vol. 106 (January 1966), pp. 44, 46.
Every person presenting himself in the emergency room must be examined immediately. "The nurse has a continuing duty to see to it that he [the doctor who has been summoned] is coming and to check this at reasonable intervals."

Jackson, George D. How blind are nurses to the needs of the visually handicapped?, Nurs. Outlook, Vol. 13 (September 1965), pp. 34-37.
A blind psychologist tells the thoughtless way in which persons in general treat the visually handicapped and suggests that nurses should be educated to understand the problems and relate more effectively than do others.

Jaco, E. Gartly, ed. Patients, Physicians, and Illness, Glencoe, Illinois, The Free Press, 1958. Ch. 25.
"Illness, therapy, and the modern urban American family" by Talcott Parsons and Renee Fox indicates that the tendency to hospitalize the ill person has values other than the technical care opportunities thus made available—values to the

family and values to the patient in the form of deprivation and loneliness which hopefully help him recover more quickly.

Jourard, Sidney M. To whom can a nurse give personalized care?, Amer J. Nurs., Vol. 61 (March 1961), pp. 86-88.
Every nurse should aim to become a "general practitioner," able "to get into empathetic contact with anybody who is sick," not just patients who have certain personal characteristics or diagnoses. A stimulating, thought-provoking article by a clinical psychologist.

Kottke, Frederic J., and Blanchard, Russell S. Bedrest begets bedrest, Nurs. Forum, Vol. 3 (No. 3, 1964), pp. 56-72.
Two doctors describe the skeletal, neuromuscular, and cardiovascular deterioration which occurs as a result of bed rest and inactivity. The article is full of suggestions for maintenance of normal body function in those who are incapacitated. No nurse should miss reading this article.

Lewis, Wilma R. A time to die, Nurs. Forum, Vol. 4 (No. 1, 1965), pp. 6-27.
Although the entire article with its two case studies is interesting, of special value are the conclusions (pp. 22-26).

Litwack, Janice, and Litwack, Lawrence. Four stages of nursing care, Amer. J. Nurs., Vol. 62 (January 1962), pp. 95-96.
Four of the eight stages of human growth can be applied to the aims of nursing care in nurse-patient relationships.

Macgregor, Frances C. Uncooperative patients: some cultural interpretations, Amer. J. Nurs., Vol. 67 (January 1967), pp. 88-91.
The writer, a medical social scientist, illustrates the way in which a patient's cultural heritage may influence his behavior. She suggests that nurses recognize that there are cultural differences and make allowances for them.

Mahaffy, Perry R., Jr. Admission interviews with parents, Amer. J. Nurs., Vol. 66 (March 1966), pp. 506-508.
Based on a research study this interesting report illustrates by specific examples the ways nurses can relieve tension in parents of the newly admitted child.

May, Karen H. What nursing means to me, Amer. J. Nurs., Vol. 64 (January 1964), p. 87.
Excerpts from a prize wining Nurses Writing Contest manuscript. In six succinct statements the writer conveys a depth of feeling.

May, Philip R. A., and Wilkinson, Mary. Admitting a patient is therapy, Nurs. Outlook, Vol. 11 (June 1963), pp. 447-449.
Radical changes in admitting procedure were made in a psychiatric hospital when it was realized that the admission had therapeutic potential. General hospitals could learn from this study.

Moyer, Lawrence N., Collette, John P., and Ludke, Richard L. Family-centered care helps new parents, Mod. Hosp., Vol. 106 (March 1966), pp. 130-134, 174.
It has been assumed that rooming-in, father privileges during labor and delivery, and visiting and handling the baby make for easier postpartal adjustment in the home. A study reveals the assumption to be correct but suggests further research to determine the effects of each facet.

Newton, Marjorie E., and Folta, Jeannette. Hospital food can help or hinder care, Amer. J. Nurs, Vol. 67 (January 1967), pp. 112-113.
A dietitian and a nurse-sociologist discuss the meaning and importance of food to the patient.

Neylan, Margaret Prowse. Anxiety, Amer. J. Nurs., Vol. 62 (May 1962), pp. 110-111.
A certain amount of anxiety is normal and desirable in unfamiliar or trying situations, but it needs to be understood and controlled. Thinking about causes

of anxiety may help the nurse, who should be skilled in recognizing it, in reducing that which is unnecessary and in helping patients tolerate it and use it constructively.

Novick, Louis J. Understanding makes the difference, Canad. Nurse, Vol. 62 (January 1966), pp. 21-25.
An article showing great understanding of the aged patient. All nurses should read it.

O'Neill, Paul C. Understanding your blind patient, Canad. Nurse, Vol. 61 (September 1965), pp. 728-730.
A most interesting account of the ways in which nurses can help the blind to be comfortable and to enjoy their hospitalization.

Owens, Evelyn J. From one O.R. nurse to another, Amer. J. Nurs., Vol. 63 (February 1963), pp. 106-109.
An operating room nurse thinks safety is taken for granted to some extent and reviews for her colleagues their many responsibilities to the patient as operating room nurses.

Powers, Maryann E., and Storlie, Frances. The apprehensive patient, Amer. J. Nurs., Vol. 67 (January 1967), pp. 58-63.
A beautifully written presentation of the fears and the rights of the patient having open heart surgery and the qualities needed by nurses if the patients are to be cared for effectively. Every nurse should profit from this article. It has special value for those who nurse the critically ill.

Prentice, W. E. What the patient wants, Nurs. Times, Vol. 61 (June 11, 1965), p. 808.
In this summary of a paper given by Miss Prentice, seven needs of the patient are stressed. Especially emphasized is the lack of privacy of patients in the out-patient department.

Privacy for dying patients, Nurs. Mirror, Vol. 122 (May 6, 1966), p. III.
A nurse-patient tells her experience of being in a ward near a dying patient and the suffering this caused. She suggests a means of attaining privacy for the dying.

Quint, Jeanne C. Awareness of death and the nurse's composure, Nurs. Res., Vol. 15 (Winter 1966), pp. 49-55.
Influence of ward social structure on nurses' ability to maintain composure when a patient is dying. A comparison of nurses' behavior in two units where death is common—the intensive care unit and the cancer floor. ". . . there are important consequences for patients when physicians and nurses are unable to cope with the interactional aspects of dying, and the dying patients are prevented from making decisions about their final days.

———— Obstacles to helping the dying, Amer. J. Nurs., Vol. 66 (July 1966), pp. 1568-1571.
Nurses are hindered in their care when patients are not told they are dying and when the patient's dying behavior does not conform to staff expectations. Staff reacts by withdrawal which may have serious consequences for the patient because dying is a social as well as a biological experience.

Reeves, Robert B., Jr. Emotional stress and healing, Hosp. Manage., Vol. 88 (December 1959), pp. 38-39.
A hospital chaplain in a very meaningful way points out the necessity for a "staff member to match the patient's feelings with appropriate feelings of his own." Failure to do so becomes an obstacle to healing. Excellent.

Roberts, Gordon, Jr. Brief encounter in a hospital waiting room, R.N., Vol. 28 (April 1965), pp. 78-79.
An example of *good* nursing.

Rusk, Howard A. Rehabilitation belongs in the general hospital, Amer. J. Nurs., Vol. 62 (September 1962), pp. 62-63.
It is only in the general hospital that rehabilitation services can be brought to the patient in time to avoid costly damage.

Saunders, Cicely. The last stages of life, Amer. J. Nurs., Vol. 65 (March 1965), pp. 70-75.
An English doctor, who is also a nurse and social worker, describes a philosophy of life and death which creates a peaceful serene atmosphere for patients terminally ill with cancer.

―――― Watch with me, Nurs. Times, Vol. 61 (November 26, 1965), pp. 1615-1617.
Beautifully written by a devout Christian woman—a doctor, nurse, and social worker—the article portrays the atmosphere which surrounds the patient terminally ill with cancer at St. Christopher's Hospice in London.

Schade, Julia Ann. Comprehensive nursing in an outpatient clinic, Amer. J. Nurs., Vol. 60 (September 1960), pp. 1259-1262.
The changed role of the nurse in the outpatient clinic from clerk to observer, interviewer, and teacher has greatly improved patient care.

Schreiber, Frederick C. Dental care for long-term patients, Amer. J. Nurs., Vol. 64 (February 1964), pp. 84-86.
A dentist emphasizes the need of the elderly for clean mouths and dangers which result from lack of care.

Singeisen, Fred. Hospitals need more patience with patients, Mod. Hosp., Vol. 95 (December 1960), pp. 79-81.
This splendid article writen by a psychiatrist emphasizes the needs of patients for understanding, friendliness, and consideration and suggests that these result from a good spirit or atmosphere and do not involve losing or wasting time.

Sister M. Timothy. Spreading the gospel of rehabilitation, Nurs. Outlook, Vol. 10 (September 1962), p. 586.
This article which is one in a series on rehabilitation describes the collaboration between nurses in the rehabilitation hospital and those in the general hospital and the aid given to hospitals in other communities.

Sister St. Augustin. Safeguarding human personality, Canad. Nurse, Vol. 61 (September 1965), p. 740.
The responsibility of the head nurse for safeguarding respect for the patient as a human being. The writer suggests the head nurse put herself in the patient's position and look at all things from his angle.

Skipper, James K., Jr., Mauksch, Hans O., and Tagliacozzo, Daisy. Some barriers to communication between patients and hospital functionaries, Nurs. Forum, Vol. 2 (No. 1, 1963), pp. 14-23.
Although communication with hospital personnel affords patients a way to secure information and desired interpersonnel contact, patients hesitate to ask questions or make requests of doctors and nurses. A study revealed some of the reasons.

―――― Mauksch, Hans O., and Tagliacozzo, Daisy. What communication means to patients, Amer. J. Nurs., Vol. 64 (April 1964), pp. 101-103.
Three sociologists in a research project designed to explore the patient's perception of the patient role, conducted interviews with hospitalized patients to determine the meaning of communication to these patients. Results are revealing.

Spitzer, Stephan P., and Sobel, Raymond. Preferences for patients and patient behavior, Nurs. Res., Vol. 11 (Fall 1962), pp. 233-235.
A study in a pediatric division showed that nurses, physicians, and aides liked those patients best who did not interfere with the individual's execution of hospital duties. It is suggested that liking or disliking plays a decisive role in the type of hospital care that children receive.

Stevens, Leonard F. What makes a ward climate therapeutic?, Amer. J. Nurs., Vol. 61 (March 1961), pp. 95-96.
A clear description of the needs of patients, the practices conducive to a happy, healthful environment for patients and personnel, and the forces which produce tensions and anxiety.

Stillar, Edith M. Continuity of care, Nurs. Outlook, Vol. 10 (September 1962), pp. 584-585.
The value of an initial interview as a means of planning care in the hospital and after discharge is made very clear in this article.

Thomas, Victoria. Your patient is no moron, R.N., Vol. 29 (January 1966), pp. 58-64, 94.
This article is based on an interview with Dr. Bernard Kutner, Ph.D., social psychologist. Patients need three basic kinds of information: what is happening to him, what is expected of him, and whether he is accepted socially. Each of these points is discussed in a clear, interesting way.

Thompson, LaVerne R. Thermometer disinfection, Amer. J. Nurs., Vol. 63 (February 1963), pp. 113-114.
Scientific studies show that cleansing thermometers before disinfection is essential to effectiveness. Ineffective disinfectants are still being used by some hospitals. This is an interesting and enlightening article.

Travelbee, Joyce. What do we mean by rapport?, Amer. J. Nurs., Vol. 63 (February 1963), pp. 70-72.
The meaning of the term is described and illustrated by the writer who also suggests ways in which to establish it with patients.

———— What's wrong with sympathy?, Amer. J. Nurs., Vol. 64 (January, 1964), pp. 68-71.
Contrasts empathy and pity with sympathy which has warmth, "feels another's distress," and "wants to do something to alleviate it." Unless we (nurses) are able to "relate as one human being to another, and unless we deem it important to give of ourselves personally, then we shall interact but not establish relationships. . . ." A beautifully written article.

Tryon, Phyllis A., and Leonard, Robert C. The effect of the patient's participation on the outcome of a nursing procedure, Nurs. Forum, Vol. 3 (No. 2, 1964), pp. 79-89.
A controlled experiment on the effectiveness of the pre-delivery enema in which patients in the experimental group were encouraged to participate in the procedure. The findings have meaningful implications for the carrying out of any procedure.

Vander Bergh, Richard L. Let's talk about death, Amer. J. Nurs., Vol. 66 (January 1966), pp. 71-73.
Since little is known about death, research in this area is greatly needed. To study death it is necessary to look at it objectively. Time must be spent with the dying rather than abandoning them which is so often done.

Vander Zanden, James W., and Vander Zanden, Marion V. The interview: what questions should the nurse ask and how should she ask them?, Nurs. Outlook, Vol. 11 (October 1963), pp. 743-745.
Direct suggestions for talking with and responding to patients are given and discussed. Many nurses will find this a helpful presentation.

Wygant, W. E., Jr. Dying, but not alone, Amer. J. Nurs., Vol. 67 (March 1967), pp. 574-577.
A hospital chaplain tells how he helped a young woman and her husband face death. Implications for the nurse are stressed throughout.

chapter 10

DIAGNOSING NURSING NEEDS
OF THE PATIENT

The last chapter considered some of the physical and emotional needs of the patient as related to his condition, his diagnosis, any disabilities he might have, and the newness of the experiences he was undergoing in the hospital. These needs encompass curative, preventive, and comforting measures. The knowledge and skill required to perform the techniques involved in these measures are a part of every nurse's preparation. Most nurses are able to diagnose the patient's physical nursing needs, but the preparation of many nurses for determining and meeting the emotional and social needs of the patient is limited because those who teach and supervise them often are not themselves equipped in this area. While many good nurses have intuitive understanding of the patient's feelings and behavior, they frequently do not have the scientific knowledge to understand the reasons for his behavior nor the ways to deal with it.

The term "diagnosis," when referred to as a nursing responsibility, is one that has been criticized by nurses brought up to believe that diagnosis is the prerogative of the doctor alone. Medical diagnosis is his responsibility but the intelligent nurse cannot carry out many of his orders without making a decision about the patient's condition. That to some is nursing diagnosis. Carrying out any p.r.n. order calls for such a decision as does calling the obstetrician in time to deliver the baby.

Webster defines diagnosis as a "conclusion arrived at through critical perception or scrutiny." Nursing diagnosis, then, involves 1) systematic collection of medical and personal information about the patient through observation, discussion, study of records, and the like; 2) analysis of the data so gathered; and 3) drawing a conclusion in terms of the patient's nursing needs and problems. The nurse looks for and carefully appraises symptoms relative to the patient's condition, disorder, age, and disabilities. She observes his behavior, facial expression, his body movements, his conversation, responses to questions and actions of nurses, his relationships to his family. On the basis of all these observations, her scientific knowledge and her knowledge of human behavior, the nurse draws conclusions relative to the patient's nursing needs. It is important that the nurse make the same careful study that the doctor uses in making a medical diagnosis.

COLLECTION OF DATA

The first step in making a nursing diagnosis is data collection. To what sources of information does the nurse have access? The best source, of course, is the patient himself. The nurse picks up clues by giving him opportunity to talk about himself, his illness, hospitalization, and personal problems thereby created and what he thinks the nurse might do to help. His family also may have a great deal to contribute through the information they volunteer and the answers to questions. A source of information immediately available in most instances is the admission slip, which, if read thoughtfully, gives a great many hints or clues about the patient. It tells where his home is, whether he has a telephone; his age, marital status, nearest relative; his occupation, race, religion, citizenship, where he and his parents were born; whether he has previously been a patient in this hospital, his diagnosis or the purpose of his admission, his doctor. Each of these bits of information suggests something about the patient's socio-economic status, his family relationships; his education, mores, beliefs; his familiarity with the hospital routine, his probable symptoms, his medical regimen.

Shortly after the patient is admitted, other data become available for the head nurse to use in determining the patient's needs. The purpose of the nursing history is to provide information on which to make a diagnosis and to build a plan for nursing care. The patient's clinical record is a resource with which the nurse will wish to remain up-to-date. It tells a story which helps the nurse to understand the patient's symptoms and sometimes his behavior. The nurse who is not entirely abreast clinically will find real value in reading up on the diagnoses represented by the patients for whom she is caring. Up-to-date medical and nursing texts and journals give research findings on the subject and report the experience of others in the field. In addition nursing periodicals publish excellent articles dealing with human behavior which can help the thoughtful nurse in understanding the patient. With information from these sources the nurse is better prepared to make meaningful observations. She knows what to look for in the way of physical and emotional needs relative to the patient's medical diagnosis or general condition. The amount and quality of reading undertaken by the staff will in many instances depend upon stimulus from the head nurse who will also need to help in the application of knowledge so gained.

Sharing observations with others who know the patient usually results in a more accurate assessment of the patient's needs. When special needs exist, many individuals may participate. The physical therapist and occupational therapist recognize physical problems the nurse is not prepared to diagnose but with which she can be of help. The head nurse, doctor, social worker, public health nurse, and other members of the division staff may have made observations and be in a position to assist in determining the patient's needs, the reasons for his behavior.

The physician has information which, if shared, will help the nursing staff understand the patient. He may have known the family and the patient for many years, in which case he should understand something of their immediate concerns and worries: what *this* operation means to *this* patient, the adjustment that has had to be made to make hospitalization possible. The patient's clergyman may also assist the nurse to understand the kind of person the patient is, the meaning of hospitalization to him and his family. Regular conferences provide opportunity for this exchange. Where they are nonexistent, if the nurse is to gain this information from doctor or clergy, the chances are she must seek it.

New information is added to the nurse's storehouse of knowledge every day. Likewise, the patient's needs change as his condition changes. Some needs are met and no longer create problems for the patient. When he feels fully accepted he is no longer demanding. Because new needs of the patient are frequently discovered, diagnosis should be under constant scrutiny.

ANALYSIS OF THE PATIENT'S NEEDS AND DRAWING A CONCLUSION

The patient's physical needs are not difficult to analyze when the nurse considers carefully the medical data which she has collected. Thus she knows that the dyspneic patient is more comfortable sitting up. The nurse also recognizes potential needs and prepares to handle them should they occur. It is better to have the oxygen tank and mask in the patient's room if he is having difficulty in breathing, even though they may never be needed. If Mr. Andrews has a history of convulsions, a mouth gag is placed on his stand, padded side rails on his bed, and a member of the nursing staff is given the responsibility of observing him at stated intervals. An analysis of the patient's personal needs is difficult for most nurses because they often do not have the fund of knowledge to help them understand human behavior. If the patient moans and wails with pain which seems to the nurse to be out of all reason, she should try to find out what the pain symbolizes to the patient. He may not have been prepared for its severity and believe that he is much worse off than is the case. He may think he is dying. When he understands and when he recognizes that pain under the circumstances is to be expected, it becomes more bearable because it no longer frightens him. However, there may also be other reasons for the patient's seemingly exaggerated discomfort or his refusal to receive certain examinations or kinds of care. The nurse needs an understanding that acceptable and fitting behavior varies with one's cultural and family background. The data she has collected tell her the patient's nationality, where he lives, where he was born, how long he and his family have lived in this country. Consideration of this information may at least cause her to question whether his behavior is cultural rather than individual.[1] The nurse has her own culture, Margaret Mead points out, which influences her attitudes and actions. How has she been brought up to behave when in pain? Awareness of her own cultural behavior helps the nurse to understand that individuals with other cultural backgrounds have different attitudes and values. For them, they are acting in a perfectly "normal" way. Although the nurse may not be familiar with the cultural patterns of many peoples, she can observe and compare behavior of individuals from ethnic groups frequently cared for in the hospital with which she is associated. Likewise, she can read the literature in this area.[2] Just an awareness that cultural differences exist and should be taken into account helps the nurse to be nonjudgmental and to look for combinations of circumstance which please or displease the patient.

If the patient asks an unusual number of questions, the nurse, instead of being annoyed, should seek the reason. Perhaps he has had a good deal of experience with illness and hospitals and is rather sophisticated in his knowledge. He, therefore, has many questions which he needs to have answered. A highly educated individual or a patient with intellectual curiosity will need a different kind of explanation of hospital policy and therapy than do others. His questions are often probing. He has a need to understand the purpose of the laboratory work, what the gall bladder test is like, how the diagnosis is made. To be told to ask the doctor indicates to the patient that the nurse does not know the answer. If put off with a superficial reply, he may doubt her scientific knowledge and question her ability to care for him properly. As has been repeatedly said in these pages, the nurse must be

[1] Margaret Mead. Understanding cultural patterns, *Nurs. Outlook,* Vol. 4 (May 1956), p. 261.
[2] One very helpful reference for nurses is the interesting book written for nurses by an anthropologist. The material is based on a study made over a period of years at the New York Hospital. See: Frances Cooke MacGreagor, *Social Science in Nursing,* New York, Russell Sage Foundation, 1960.

aware of what the patient knows about his condition. Direct questions should be answered honestly and the nurse prepared to support the patient if need be. On admission she can ask the questioning patient what the doctor has already told him about the plan for his care and clarify the information. There are certain things the doctor will wish to explain himself, but, if he trusts the nurse's knowledge and judgment, he will expect her to answer questions completely and truthfully. Why should a patient not know the purpose and effect of the drug he is taking? Why should a nurse not explain the rationale of the gall bladder test? All patients have a right to have their questions about themselves answered if the answer is known. If it is not, they should know this, too. The fullness of the explanation, the words used, the timing depend upon the individual patient. It is obvious that if the patient is a nurse or doctor explanations given will be couched in different terms from those used if he is a plumber. A teacher of physics or an engineer will have some understanding of x-ray but in all probability will need an explanation of the reasons for fasting and enemas in preparation for a gastrointestinal x-ray series. The college president who has lost a baby at birth because of defective embryonic development may know enough about genetics to ask questions about the part the genes play in such development.

In analyzing the needs which pertain to the purely personal side of the patient it is necessary to hypothesize about his behavior until the nurse knows him well enough to understand him. In addition to the information about the patient which the nurse has assembled, her hypothesis is based on experience with others—patients, family, friends—under similar circumstances or on the way the nurse herself would feel were she the patient. Her hypothesis will also be influenced by the concepts other nurses have of him.[3] It is good to have a working hypothesis, provided the nurse recognizes it as a guess, the best guess possible for the moment, and provided she tests its validity and revises it. In testing hypotheses the nurse will discover that patients do not always feel as she expects them to nor do they behave as she anticipates. The patient whose biopsy showed malignant cells and who, when wakened from the anesthetic, finds she has had a radical mastectomy may have the utmost confidence that surgery was performed early enough. Secure also in the love of her husband and family she goes through none of the tortures which are expected when one learns she has cancer.

When a person is 80 years old he is expected to be forgetful, to like special little attentions, to need to be needed. Some, however, are mentally alert, very self-sufficient, and physically quite vigorous. It is anticipated that indi-

[3] Sidney M. Jourard. How well do you know your patient? *Amer. J. Nurs.,* Vol. 59 (November 1959), p. 1569.

viduals, on learning they have a permanent disability and will not be able to do many of the things they have always enjoyed, will go through a period of depression. Most do. The nurse is watchful and ready to help. But some patients respond, "Well, if I have to spend the rest of my life in a wheel chair, I'm certainly going to enjoy myself!" And they do, not because they would choose invalidism, but because they have a source of strength which helps them to accept adversity with good grace and make of it something rich and meaningful. These patients have needs, but they are not the anticipated ones. The nurse, however, must be mindful in such circumstances that the patient may be masking his true feelings, preferring not to talk about them but to weep alone. His wishes should be respected. More than ever the nurse needs to listen for possible indications that the patient *would* like to talk about his personal tragedy and to make it possible for him to do so. It takes a very perceptive nurse to discover what the patient really wants.

How does the nurse learn to know the patient's real feelings and needs? First, she must have opportunity for frequent direct contact with him. Then, while caring for and conversing with him she creates an atmosphere in which the patient is free to express himself. She is unhurried, relaxed. She gives him a chance to talk, showing interest and encouraging him through carefully chosen words. Comforting, soothing physical care often makes the patient feel very close to the nurse and tells him that she cares and wants to help. The nurse is ever mindful that he may be trying to communicate with her. She knows that words are not the only means of expressing feelings, desires, and needs. The voice, its feeling, tone, and inflection, body tension and movement, all convey meaning to the nurse who is astute and caring enough to read it. Through the expression in his eyes and his clutching of the nurse's hand, the patient may be fairly crying out, "Love me! Give me some indication that you care whether I get over this pain and get to sleep." "Tell me that you understand what this operation means to me, that my whole world has collapsed as I face the future without my arm." "Tell me that *you* don't think I will die if I submit to the operation on my heart." The nurse should constantly ask herself what the patient is trying to say, what is it that he needs. Observing, listening, thinking, reasoning are essential. Jourard [4] suggests that most important, of all, is the nurse's ability to empathize; that is, "to imagine the inner experience of another person at a given moment." Without this it is impossible for the nurse to make a diagnosis of the patient's emotional needs.

Mr. Bastow, a salesman by occupation, had all the courtesy and charm

[4] Jourard, *Ibid.*, p. 1570.

expected of one in this type of work. One day, while recovering from an abdominal perineal resection, he suddenly threw a cup of coffee at the nurse who had been caring for him and with whom he had apparently established an excellent relationship. Why? The nurse needed help to understand that his outburst was not directed at her personally but resulted from the fact he had just been told by the doctor that he had cancer. With this understanding the nurse could be accepting and helpful instead of hurt or angry.

Dolores, a 20-year-old girl with diabetes, would not adhere to her diet in the hospital or at home. Following discharge she returned several times in acidosis. Unable to hold a job because of her health she was on welfare. In the home provided by the welfare agency several old men and Dolores were housed and fed. Because she cheated on her diet every time she had been pulled through her acidosis, the nurses gave up in despair, the interns and dietitians rejected her. When nurses who had an understanding of human behavior gave Dolores the love, respect, and trust she needed so badly, she began conforming to her diet. Through vocational rehabilitation she was trained for a job. The welfare department made other living arrangements for her. A girl was salvaged because her needs were diagnosed and met.

A middle-aged, chronically ill woman was very untidy in her habits, throwing paper on the floor, expectorating on the wall, wetting the bed. No organic basis for her incontinence could be found. She complained the nurses never came in time. Her signal light was on frequently. When answered she usually wanted the shade adjusted, the screen moved, or some apparently trivial request satisfied. Scolding, disapproval, threats were ineffective in changing her behavior. The nursing staff decided to try showering her with attention. She was moved to the cubicle near the office. Everyone who went by either stopped to see if the patient needed anything or waved in passing. Pains were taken to fix her hair attractively. She was asked how she wanted her care organized. The diagnosis—a need for acceptance and attention—proved to be correct. The patient responded by being friendly and cooperative. Her bad habits and incontinence disappeared. The plan for this patient's nursing care was based on assumptions. Could a more scientific approach have been used? If so, would outcomes have been more sure? Could the patient have been helped earlier before she had to resort to attention-getting mechanisms? Research in nursing practice and experimentation with various approaches to the patient indicate that answers to these questions may be affirmative.[5]

[5] See references at end of chapter by Anderson and Mertz, Elder, Elms and Leonard, Hall, Orlando, Peplau, Wiedenbach.

THE HEAD NURSE'S RESPONSIBILITY IN DIAGNOSING THE PATIENT'S NEEDS

Since a correct diagnosis of the patient's needs is of such importance to his well-being, the head nurse must assume immediate responsibility for it. She gets acquainted with the patient and his family, gathers information, and analyzes it. Her experienced eye may see things which other nurses miss. Her knowledge of behavior and the factors which influence it make it possible for her to interpret the patient's actions and attitudes to others. The patient may not wish to discuss his real feelings with more than one nurse. The head nurse in many instances will become the patient's confidante. However, she is responsible for helping members of her professional staff develop this relationship and increase their skill in diagnosing patients' nursing needs. The head nurse promotes this learning by assuring continuity in patient-nurse relationships through keeping the same nurse with the patient during his entire stay in the hospital (see Chapter 12). The head nurse also encourages group participation in diagnosing the patient's needs when problems exist. One of her greatest responsibilities is that of leadership through which she stimulates desire to find causes of behavior and to experiment with methods of satisfying needs.

RESPONSIBILITY OF THE NURSING PROFESSION

To have practicing nurses skilled in nursing diagnosis should be a goal of the nursing profession. Essential for its achievement is continual research to develop nursing diagnostic methods and test their effectiveness. For the latter, measures must be evolved. To achieve the goal, nurses now practicing must be helped to study and criticize their communication skills and to find more effective ways to detect patient needs which are not readily observable, namely those of a psychosocial nature. Most important to achievement of the goal is its inclusion in the objectives of basic nursing education, but before this can be accomplished, nurse teachers and head nurses must know what makes an approach to the patient effective, what helps to liberate the patient so he can and, if he so desires, will express his needs. The teacher and the head nurse who sets the standards for nursing care in the field where the student practices must be skilled in nursing diagnosis. They themselves may need help in learning the art. In addition they must have ability to guide students as they strive to learn to determine patients' needs and analyze reasons for their success or failure in particular instances. Teachers, head nurses, department administrators have opportunity and responsibility to add to the body of knowledge in this area through controlled experimentation, testing and retesting, then making their findings available to others.

SUMMARY

"Diagnosis" is a term just as applicable to nursing as to medicine, and nurses should not hesitate to use it. Most nurses are able to diagnose the patient's physical needs. Meeting those which pertain to him as a person is more difficult because frequently nurses have had little preparation in the behavioral sciences. Many who are successful in diagnosing the reasons for behavior and meeting emotional needs rely on intuitive rather than scientific understanding.

Sources of information available in making a nursing diagnosis are the patient's admission slip, his nursing history, his chart, clinical nursing texts, references on the behavioral sciences, as well as the patient himself, his family, his doctor, his clergyman, and the members of the hospital staff. From the assembled data an analysis is made of the patient's physical and personal needs. In analyzing reasons for his behavior and the needs this behavior expresses, the nurse must know the influence on his beliefs and attitudes of the patient's cultural, educational, and socio-economic background and his family relationships.

Until the nurse really knows the patient, she formulates a hypothesis about the reasons he behaves as he does, and the way in which the nurse should respond. It is important that she accept the hypothesis as the guess, which it is, and as quickly as possible prove or disprove it through personal knowledge of the patient. Knowing him is possible only if she has direct contact with him. The nurse creates an atmosphere in which the patient is free to express himself. By observing, listening, thinking, reasoning, and above all by empathizing with him the nurse comes to know and understand him. She can then diagnose and meet his needs. The head nurse in most instances will carry major responsibility for gathering the data and drawing the conclusions relative to the patient's needs. However, she makes use of the observations and suggestions of all staff members. She assumes the obligation to help professional nurses who work with her, increase their powers of perception and their ability to make a nursing diagnosis. Goals for the nursing profession should be the addition to knowledge in this area through experimentation and analysis, and teaching future generations of nurses skill in observation and determination of patients' psychosocial needs.

This chapter has dealt primarily with the sources of information for making a nursing diagnosis and the factors affecting patients' needs. Only in a very general way has it considered methods of assessing these needs. Methods will be considered in detail in Chapter 13, Supervision and Evaluation of Nursing Care.

QUESTIONS FOR DISCUSSION

1. Are *judgment* and *diagnosis* synonymous when used in relation to patient's needs? Substantiate with illustrations.
2. To justify the use of the term "nursing diagnosis" what specifications are necessary?
3. How do you react to a patient who asks you questions about his condition and therapy? Do you believe he is justified in asking them? Are you, the nurse, justified in answering every question to which you know the answer? If yes, why? If no, under what circumstances? How, at these times, should the nurse answer the questions? How would you answer a patient who asked you, "Do I have cancer?" when you know the doctor and his family have felt it better for him not to know? Would the patient ask if he did not want an answer? Why might he want to know?

EXERCISES

1. Study references at the end of the chapter analyzing the approach various writers have described. Wherein does each differ from your own approach in trying to determine whether a patient has psychosocial needs and whether you can be of help? Do you feel your approach is usually successful? To what do you attribute your success or lack of it? What ideas have the readings given you? Plan an approach to the patient to help you in making a nursing diagnosis. It should be a *guide* not a *formula*. Try it out. Evaluate it. Class discussion prior to use should be helpful.
2. If you have friends of another culture or ethnic group who have been hospitalized try to find out their reaction to things which happened to them—the physical examination, bed bath, and treatments such as suctioning and injections. What were their feelings? fears? What if anything helped? What *could* have helped? What could the nurse have done to

lessen problems? What did the patient do? Did he refuse the examination or treatment? As a nurse, would you have been aware of the patient's feelings? Could you have helped him express them?

3. At the end of a morning or midafternoon go around the unit to see what patients are doing. Are they reading, talking with one another, just sitting, walking around? Are any patients talking with personnel? If so, with whom? about what? Does the patient seem to be enjoying the talk or is he dissatisfied with the situation? Select two patients who appear aimless, and open the way for them to talk to you. Encourage this by reflecting what he says or by asking a leading question such as, "Life in the hospital is pretty dull sometimes, isn't it?" Then listen for clues of the patient's satisfaction or dissatisfaction with the situation, following up with an appropriate comment meant to encourage his continuance. As a result of this conversation, judge whether you believe the patient has a need. Then, or later after you have thought about it, ask the patient for verification of your judgment. Is he bored? Would he like to have some type of diversion? If so, what? Or is he restless? worried? What can the nurse do to help? This exercise will be of greater value if you reconstruct your conversation with the patient including remarks about the patient's and your own nonverbal actions. Reconstructions shared with classmates help the individual to see wherein she helped the patient, wherein she missed an opportunity.

REFERENCES

Allen, Shelly. Nurse attendance during labor, Amer. J. Nurs., Vol. 64 (July 1964), pp. 70-74.
An experiment in which uterine contractions and fetal heart beat were measured indicated that the presence of the nurse had a marked physiological effect on strength and frequency of contractions.

Anderson, Barbara J., Mertz, Hilda, and Leonard, Robert C. Two experimental tests of a patient-centered admission process, Nurs. Res., Vol. 14 (Spring 1965), pp. 151-156.
Results of this study support the contention that the admission procedure is of crucial importance to the patient's well-being. Two studies indicated that an experimental approach concentrating on the patient and his needs resulted in less tense behavior, lower blood pressure and pulse than were presented by patients who received a "task oriented" admission procedure.

Blake, Florence. In quest of hope and autonomy, Nurs. Forum, Vol. 1 (Winter 1961-62), pp. 8-32.
Miss Blake describes the third stage (second postoperative period) of her study

of a four year old child who underwent open heart surgery. Miss Blake's deep understanding of children and her clear description of the child's behavior, its meaning, and her way of helping Suzie regain autonomy make this essential reading for pediatric nurses and is highly valuable for all who care for patients.

Burrill Marjorie. Helping students identify and solve patients' problems, Nurs. Outlook, Vol. 14 (February 1966), pp. 46-48.
The student, at the end of each day, analyzes the care she has given her patient in terms of 1) the patient's problems; 2) nursing care given to meet the problem; 3) diet; 4) drugs given; 5) reasons for nursing care, diet, and drugs. The mental processes involved would be valuable for all nurses giving nursing care.

Carnevali, Doris L. Preoperative anxiety, Amer. J. Nurs., Vol. 66 (July 1966), pp. 1536-1538.
A study of variation in perceptions of patients and the nurses caring for them regarding causes of preoperative anxiety, and the measures which brought relief. Includes a thought-provoking summary.

Chambers, Wilda. Nursing diagnosis, Amer. J. Nurs., Vol. 62 (November 1962), pp. 102-104.
The process of evaluation involves assembling data from many sources and applying it in the identification of problems.

Davidson, Ramona Powell. To give care in terminal illness, Amer. J. Nurs., Vol. 66 (January 1966), pp. 74-75.
A helpful description of ways in which nurses in one hospital studied inevitable death and learned that the two most important needs of the dying patient are physical comfort and communication.

Durand, Mary, and Prince, Rosemary. Nursing diagnosis: process and decision, Nurs. Forum, Vol. 5 (No. 4, 1966), pp. 50-64.
Nursing diagnosis has two aspects: 1) the process of diagnosing through collecting information, observation, thinking, recognizing a pattern, and 2) the decision or actual diagnosis.

Elder, Ruth G. What is the patient saying,? Nurs. Forum, Vol. 2 (No. 1, 1963), pp. 25-37.
Patients need encouragement to express their *real* needs and require help in doing so. The nurse should learn this and how to do it. Time is a factor, but, later, time is often saved by an initial encouragement of the patient to express himself.

Elms, Roslyn R., and Diers, Donna K. The patient comes to the hospital, Nurs. Forum, Vol. 2 (No. 3, 1963), pp. 88-97.
Although the patient usually needs little technical care on admission, his psychological needs are great and can best be met by a professional nurse. This study indicates that the patient's adaptation to the hospital can be accomplished when the nurse concerns herself with the patient's reactions to hospitalization, focuses on his feelings, and explores his fears.

——— and Leonard, Robert C. Effects of nursing approaches during admission, Nurs. Res., Vol. 15 (Winter 1966), pp. 39-47.
An experimental nursing approach was found to be effective in relieving distress experienced by patients during elective admission to a general hospital.

Field, William E., Jr., Patterson, E. Gene, and Dayton, Mildred. The senses taker, Amer. J. Nurs., Vol. 66 (December 1966), pp. 2654-2656.
When placeboes are effective in relieving pain it is probably because the patient has faith in medical treatment and what is being done to heal him. A thought-provoking article.

Geis, Dorothy P. Mothers' perceptions of care given their dying children, Amer. J. Nurs., Vol. 65 (February 1965), pp. 105-107.
The writer interviewed mothers of 26 children who had died in the hospital 6 weeks to one year previously. The mothers were most concerned with areas dealing with relationships. There is much for nurses to learn from this study.

Hall, Lydia E. A center for nursing, Nurs. Outlook, Vol. 11 (November 1963), pp. 805-806.
One of a kind, The Loeb Center offers professional nursing service "in an institutional setting midway between the hospital and the home." One unique feature is that "medicine and allied fields offer ancillary therapy." Mrs. Hall tells in this brief article the way nurses help patients learn to face problems and find ways to solve them.

Henderson, Ian W. D., and Henderson, Jane E. Psychological care of patients with catastrophic illness, Canad. Nurse, Vol. 61 (November 1965), pp. 899-902.
This husband-wife, doctor-nurse team has shown exceptional insight in this presentation. No nurse should fail to read the article. Reactions of patients and their families at various stages of catastrophic illness plus suggestions for the medical and nursing staff in dealing with these reactions are very helpful.

Hewitt, Helon E., and Pesznecker, Betty L. Blocks to communicating with patients, Amer. J. Nurs., Vol. 64 (July 1964), pp. 101-103.
Five major verbal blocks to communication between nurse and patient have been identified and illustrated. These could be very useful to a nurse who wished to increase her ability to talk with patients.

Hilliard, Mary E. One dimension of nursing, Amer. J. Nurs., Vol. 67 (April 1967), pp. 756-759.
This nurse tells how she discovered the true meaning of nursing. No nurse should fail to read the article.

Jaco, E. Gartly, ed. Patients, Physicians, and Illness, Glencoe, Illinois, The Free Press, 1958, Ch. 26, 27, 55.
Chapter 26, How the Sick View Their World, by Henry D. Lederer, describes three phases of illness—transition period from health to illness, period of "accepted" illness, and convalescence. The reactions of patients during these periods, and the ways in which the physician can be of greatest help are very pertinent to the nurse.
Chapter 27, Cultural Components in Response to Pain, by Mark Zborowski, should help the nurse in her understanding of patients' behavior in response to pain.
Chapter 55, Culture and Nursing Care, by Lyle Saunders, stresses the nurse's need "to recognize and adjust to many aspects of cultural and sub-cultural differences." He points out that "the most difficult thing about culture difference is the recognition that 'difference' is a two-way word. In other words, not only are others 'different'— we are 'different' too."

Johnson, Betty Sue. The meaning of touch in nursing, Nurs. Outlook, Vol. 13 (February 1965), pp. 59-60.
Touch has different meaning with different individuals and in different cultures. The nurse's own attitude toward touch influences her interpretation of its meaning and her behavior. She needs to be aware of the varying effects of touch in communication.

Jourard, Sidney M. How well do you know your patients,? Amer. J. Nurs., Vol. 59 (November 1959), pp. 1568-1571.
A clinical psychologist defines terms which nurses use loosely and frequently—interpersonal relationships, insight, empathy—and explains their importance in the effective practice of nursing. The importance of extra-professional activities is stressed.

Kelly, Katharine. Clinical inference in nursing, 1: a nurse's viewpoint, Nurs. Res., Vol. 15 (Winter 1966), pp. 23-26.
Clinical inference or making a judgment about the state of the patient and his needs is now a legally recognized function of the nurse. The writer differentiates between the responsibilities of the physician as a diagnostician and the nurse as a diagnostician.

Komorita, Nori I. Nursing diagnosis, Amer. J. Nurs., Vol. 63 (December 1963), pp. 83-86.
"Nursing diagnosis involves discriminative judgment, is based on a body of scientific knowledge, and is a process which provides nursing with a systematic way of assessing patients' problems and needs."

Lambertsen, Eleanor C. Education for Nursing Leadership, Philadelphia, J. B. Lippincott Co., 1958, Ch. 6.
Chapter 6 is an excellent discussion of the process of diagnosing patient's needs and problems. Ways in which such factors as age, sex, culture, and intellectual capacity influence needs.

——— Professional Education for Leadership in Nursing Practice, Doctoral dissertation, Teachers College, Columbia University, 1957, pp. 144-159.
The necessity for diagnosing patients' needs and problems indicates that "the admission and orientation of any patient to a hospital requires competencies of a professional nature."

Loder, Eileen R. A gift for the nurse, Nurs. Outlook, Vol. 13 (December 1965), p. 21.
An editorial describing a patient's need to *give* to the nurse and the importance of the nurse accepting the gift.

MacGregor, Frances Cooke. Social Science in Nursing, New York, Russell Sage Foundation, 1960.
Written by a medical social scientist this book expresses the need for incorporating in nursing education instruction in the social sciences. It is rich in illustrations which will be very helpful to nurses in understanding patient behavior.

McCain, R. Faye. Nursing by assessment—not intuition, Amer. J. Nurs., Vol. 65 (April 1965), pp. 82-84.
Nursing is primarily intuitive. However, some attempts have been made to develop guides for assessing a patient's condition and situation, and determining his nursing needs. The assessment here described is of patients' functional abilities and disabilities. The assessment is used as a guide in diagnosing needs and planning care.

Mead, Margaret. Understanding cultural patterns, Nurs. Outlook, Vol. 4 (May 1956) pp. 260-262.
"Understanding differences among the patterns of behavior in peoples of different cultural backgrounds has obvious relevance to nursing." A helpful article by a renowned anthropologist which will be of interest to all nurses.

Mercadante, Lucille T. Leadership development seminars, Nurs. Outlook, Vol. 13 (September 1965), pp. 59-61.
In a series of seminars held with the same group of nurses over a three-year period, team leaders, and the director of nursing services studied ways to carry out the nurse's independent function, ie, determining a patient's needs, developing a plan for care, and appropriate delegation of responsibility for the patient's care.

Murray, Jeanne B. Self-knowledge and the nursing interview, Nurs. Forum, Vol. 2 (No. 1, 1963), pp. 69-78.
The nurse listens and observes in order to help the patient understand himself. To do this she must understand herself.

Newman, Margaret A. Identifying and meeting patients' needs in short span nurse-patient relationship, Nurs. Forum, Vol. 5 (No. 1, 1966), pp. 76-88.
Can the nurse be equipped to diagnose and meet the patient's needs and will there be enough time available for each patient? These are questions raised. "The key to the answers . . . seems to be in the nurse's ability to utilize whatever time she has available, whether it be five minutes or an hour, to provide an atmosphere of receptivity to patient needs."

Norris, Catherine M. Toward a science of nursing—a method for developing unique content in nursing, Nurs. Forum, Vol. 3 (No. 3, 1964), pp. 10-45.
A study which attempts to identify the unique content in nursing through concentration on determining and meeting the nursing care needs of the hospitalized psychiatric patient at bedtime and during the night. Has meaning for all nurses.

Orlando, Ida Jean. The Dynamic Nurse-Patient Relationship, New York, G. P. Putnam's Sons, 1961.
This small book is filled with illustrations of nurse-patient interaction, together with clear analysis of each situation. Should be in the library of every nurse, read and reread.

Owens, Charlotte, Parents' reactions to defective babies, Amer. J. Nurs., Vol. 64 (November 1964), pp. 83-86.
A psychiatric nurse tells nurses how to help families adjust in a positive way to a crisis such as the birth of a handicapped baby.

Peplau, Hildegard E. Psychiatric nursing skills and the general hospital patient, Nurs. Forum, Vol. 3 (No. 2, 1964), pp. 28-37.
"The unfortunate aspect of intuitive functioning is that it requires an 'every man for himself' approach and ignores the possibility of generally applicable principles."

Prange, Arthur J., Jr. and Martin, Harry W. Aids to understanding patients, Amer. J. Nurs., Vol. 62 (July 1962), pp. 98-100.
Two psychiatrists suggest that in making a nursing diagnosis the nurse can use certain guideposts to help her select information which is important.

Rhodes, Martha. Nursing the acutely ill psychiatric patient, Nurs. Outlook, Vol. 14 (February 1966), pp. 25-26.
Expected behavior of the acutely ill psychiatric patient should be interpreted to him on admission and consistently demanded by the entire staff.

Rothberg, June S. Why nursing diagnosis?, Amer. J. Nurs., Vol. 67 (May 1967), pp. 1040-1042.
The writer makes a strong case for the nursing diagnosis as essential to a nursing care plan. Three elements of diagnosis are identified: 1) identification of individual need, 2) establishment of goals, 3) selection of appropriate methods.

Schwartz, Doris. Uncooperative patients?, Amer. J. Nurs., Vol. 58 (January 1958), pp. 75-77.
Study of 50 clinic patients considered "uncooperative" by members of at least three professional groups and the behavior changes which resulted from an attempt on the part of the staff to determine the cause of the behavior and from a careful plan to help each patient with his problems.

Sister Irene Pepin, and Howe, Del. Nursing the patient in pain, Canad. Nurs., Vol. 61 (June 1965), pp. 446-448.
Ways of diagnosing and methods for relieving pain. Prevention through preparation for pain experience and through early alleviation.

Talking about patient care, Amer. J. Nurs., Vol. 61 (May 1961), pp. 56-59.
"At four A.N.A. conferences across the country, nurses raised questions and sought ways to improve their practice."

Katherine R. Nelson stresses that assessing the patient's needs and designing a plan for his care are the prime responsibilities of the professional nurse. The plan may be carried out by herself, or others may do so under her direction as team leader. Only the professional nurse has the intellectual competence to design the plan for care (p. 58).

Tarnower, William. Psychological needs of the hospitalized patient, Nurs. Outlook, Vol. 13 (July 1965), pp. 28-30.
A psychiatrist graphically describes the feelings experienced by many patients in the hospital—feelings unrecognized and, therefore, unrelieved by nurses and other staff members.

Thomas, Betty J. Clues to patients' behavior, Amer. J. Nurs., Vol. 63 (July 1963), pp. 100-102.
"Psychiatric nursing principles can be applied in medical-surgical nursing." Three patient situations and the way they were handled by nurses are described.

Wastage of nursing staff: Report of S. E. Metropolitan Regional Hospital Board conference, Nurs. Mirror, Vol. 120 (May 14, 1965), p. 169.
Report of Mr. John Simmonds is of interest to head nurses in that 1) he was impressed by the Platt Report's criticism of the failure of the hospital to provide a therapeutic environment due in part to inflexibility of ward routine and authoritarian approach, and 2) he sees "nursing diagnosis" a responsibility of the nurse alone though it must "enmesh with the doctor's diagnosis."

What man shall live and not see death,? Nurs. Outlook, Vol. 12 (January 1964), p. 23.
The nurse has grave responsibilities in caring for the dying. She needs to understand that the "attitude of the individual toward death is tempered by many factors."

Wiedenbach, Ernestine. Clinical Nursing: a Helping Art, New York, Springer Publishing Company, Inc., 1964.
In this small volume Mrs. Wiedenbach has described a philosophy and way of nursing which involves knowledge, judgment, and communicative and procedural skills. Filled with illustrations and anecdotes this thoughtful book should be helpful to all practicing nurses.

chapter 11

PLANNING THE CARE OF THE PATIENT

To be effective the patient's care must be carefully planned on the basis of his personal requirements and be consistently followed by all nursing personnel. Assessment of the patient's needs begins immediately upon his admission to the unit, if not prior to it. If the head nurse knows his diagnosis and condition and has the responsibility for assigning rooms, she decides, before his arrival, in which room he shall be placed. A patient with a bleeding peptic ulcer or one in diabetic coma is placed near the office even if other patients must be moved to make this possible. Consideration is given to age and nationality as well as to diagnosis in deciding with which patients a newcomer will be placed. When the patient arrives on the division his condition is immediately observed and steps taken to guard him from possible injury. From this time on, continuously throughout his hospitalization, the patient's care is planned, the plan is evaluated and revised as necessary.

In some hospitals planning is done entirely by the head nurse. In others, plans are formulated by the individual nurse who is assigned to care for the patient over a period of several days or weeks. In still others, plans for patient care are made by the members of the nursing team which is responsible for the patient. The last method has the advantage of group participation. The several individuals who have contact with the patient, including the head nurse, pool their information and together think through a plan for nursing care which will meet the patient's needs. Definite arrangements are made for the patient himself to play a part in making the plan for his care. The degree to which he actively participates depends upon his physical condition. When he is able, he should help to decide how frequently he shall be bathed, how he shall dress, how much fluid he shall drink in an hour to attain his quota. Although this may sound like an impossibility on a busy unit, patients who get used to taking responsibility for their care are better adjusted. It should follow that they will recover more quickly and the demands on nursing time will be fewer. Why should a nursing division staff not be able to adjust to the needs of a business man, confined in the hospital with a fractured femur, to carry on his business from his room? Is there any reason why his nursing care should not be given and his room cleaned in time for him to work with his secretary at 9 AM and have his day planned so that he will be free from interruption until noon?

OBJECTIVES OF PATIENT CARE

Planning the patient's care involves more than organization of the activities which concern him on any one day. Daily care should be fitted into a long-range plan. This plan is revised as the patient's condition changes and as further needs are discovered, but not with each change in staff. Nursing must always be planned within the limits of the medical regimen. The plan for care is based on objectives, whether or not they are clearly defined. It is well to spell them out. For example, two objectives for a patient in congestive heart failure might be: 1) to maintain adequate oxygen supply to the body cells and 2) to minimize the strain on the patient's heart. Objectives are the specific *outcomes* to be achieved for the patient's welfare. They are *not* the *process* by which the nurse achieves them. Thus to keep the oxygen flowing at a specific rate is not an objective but one of the means by which the nurse hopes to maintain an adequate oxygen supply. Objectives should be simply stated and clear to all who have responsibility for the patient's care. Likewise, nurses should know the signs which indicate that the objectives are being met.

The two objectives stated above are objectives of medical as well as of nursing care. Part of the doctor's obligation in meeting the first one is to prescribe the oxygen and to observe its effects on the patient. The nurse assumes her responsibility when she maintains the proper concentration of oxygen by periodically checking gauges, regulating the flow, testing the concentration in the tent, and seeing that the tent does not leak. Even if an inhalation therapist takes much of this responsibility the nurse must be aware that the system is functioning effectively. Her responsibility also includes observing the patient's color and respiration. The fact that the patient has dyspnea and is in an oxygen tent imposes two additional objectives on the nurse. The first is to keep the patient comfortable; the second, to protect him from harm. Responsibilities related to these objectives for the dyspneic patient include maintaining optimum position for breathing, keeping him warm, using blocks and foot boards to prevent tightening of heel cords, protecting him from fire by use of "No Smoking" signs and instruction of the patient and family in the danger of fire from use of matches or cigarettes. Responsibility also includes making sure he understands the reason for the oxygen tent, has a chance to express how he feels about it, and has any misconceptions and fears dispelled. These activities must be properly performed if the objectives are to be met. The activities and the manner of doing them make up the nursing care plan to be used by the nursing staff for the particular patient.

Objectives for other patients might include some of the following:

To have the patient accept his salt free diet.
To have the patient drink 1000 ml of fluid a day.
To have the patient learn to get out of bed unassisted.
To prevent decubiti.
To prevent contractures.
To protect the patient from self destruction.
To keep the infection from spreading.
To have the patient overcome his discouragement.
To have the patient accept his limitations and look with hope to the future.
To have the patient learn to administer his insulin.
To have the patient feel accepted and wanted.

AREAS OF NURSING RESPONSIBILITY

Each objective listed above falls in one of the areas of patient care for which the nurse has a major concern—comfort measures, therapeutic or rehabilitative measures, protective and preventive measures, support, teaching. Specific nursing care in these areas is planned to meet the diagnosed nursing needs of the individual patient. There are many ways to carry out therapeutic measures but one may be more effective than another with this patient. He should be consulted. Even though the method used may not be of great concern to some patients, others care a great deal that their baths and treatments be given in the same way by each person. Especially is this true if the patient has been brought into the planning. It is annoying, to say the least, when he has helped to decide that he will be given his irrigation at 10:00 so that he may go back to sleep after breakfast, to have the nurse waken him at 8:30 to administer it.

When a nurse has come to know the patient, has determined the desired outcomes of his care, the nursing measures which keep him comfortable and safe, the personal approach which makes him happy and brings favorable responses, the *next* step is to make an over-all plan for his care. This plan requires a great deal of thought and often some experimentation. When it has been formulated, it serves as a guide to those who know the patient less well. It is never static but is changed as the patient's condition and the situation change.

Comfort Measures

Many nursing measures contribute to the comfort of patients. The nurse figures out the least painful way to turn a patient who has extensive areas denuded of skin, the most successful way to keep him from sliding down in bed. She determines not to show offense at unpleasant odors, appearance, and habits. In her planning she arranges to see the nervous, apprehensive patient frequently. She remembers to take a glass of hot water before breakfast to Mrs. Saunders who always had this at home. In giving a colostomy irrigation she takes time to protect the bed the way the patient wants it. The nurse arranges for the patient who likes to know in advance about new procedures to be told 20 to 30 minutes before a treatment is due, then checks to be sure he is ready before she sets up for it. The nurse with a research attitude continually analyzes results of her ministrations. Why did this happen? What measures might have proved more effective? The head nurse encourages this questioning and promotes experimentation.

Therapeutic and Rehabilitative Measures

The nurse thinks through and plans these measures so they will meet the needs of the individual patient. Included are such things as the procedure for bowel and bladder training, the specific solution which will keep the patient's mouth clean and moist, effective ways to get him to take fluids orally.

Prevention

Prevention is one of the nurse's most important responsibilities. When hazards for a patient have been determined, a plan is immediately made for his protection. Complications are foreseen when possible and preventive measures instituted. The nursing care plan for a patient with hepatitis includes isolation precautions. The nurse's plan in caring for Mr. Black, who has hemiplegia, includes frequent massaging of his back with a body lotion, observing for signs of pressure, putting joints through the range of motion, keeping a roll in his paralyzed hand.

Support

Measures to support the patient in discouragement, loneliness, fear, and decision-making are planned for patients who have these problems. "To reassure" and "to cheer" him are not specific enough to guide the nurse in her approach. Methods for achieving reassurance need to be planned by the nurse. What approach will be effective in helping Mr. Quinn, who is thoroughly discouraged? Being cheery is not the way to reassure him.[1] To show sympathy may make him think there is good cause for his discouragement. In planning his care in this area, the fact that all nursing personnel who enter his room will contribute to his feelings must be taken into account. It is, therefore, the responsibility of the head nurse to suggest that staff members assume a quiet, friendly, encouraging manner, that they make no attempt to engage him in conversation in order to "take his mind off his troubles." She recommends that not everyone attempt to get him to express his worry but that all observe him for contradictions in what he does and says which might suggest the nature of his concern. She suggests also that attention be paid to his physical comfort as a means of encouraging relaxation. In addition, planning provides for the day, evening, and night nurses assigned to the patient's care to have enough time for ministration of general nursing, for the patient to feel free to talk about his feelings should he desire to do so.

TEACHING

As the patient becomes better known to the nurse and his need for health instruction becomes evident, plans are made whereby he may receive the necessary information in a way that he will be likely to accept it. Sometimes instruction is merely a matter of giving information about home care which the patient has requested or helped to decide that he needs. All that may be required under these circumstances may be to use terms which have meaning for the patient and to space the telling so that he can grasp and remember the information. Sometimes, however, there is resistance to instruction which is necessary to the patient's regaining his health. In this case, it is necessary to discover and deal with the reason for the patient's unfavorable reaction. The nurse also should be aware that for those who are forgetful, old, or do not fully comprehend, instructions may need to be

[1] Lucile Petry Leone. Wanted: good nursing, *Nurs. Outlook,* Vol. 5 (October 1957), pp. 576-578.

repeated and understanding tested. In such situations, the responsibility for teaching an individual patient should be assumed by one person making sure that the rest of the staff knows the plan and progress of her instruction. If all are kept informed, questions which are asked by the patient can be answered in a way that will reinforce the instruction given. The staff also needs to know the nurse responsible for the instruction so that several persons will not "teach" the patient with nephritis that he should avoid contact with individuals who have colds for fear of reactivating his disease.

Hospitalization provides opportunity for the patient to gain information on a wide variety of health matters which are not necessarily associated with his present illness or condition. Much of the information pertains to preventing disease and injury. Every nurse has an obligation to stimulate interest in health and to create opportunities for teaching it to her patients. For example, women patients who are not already informed should be taught the importance of breast self-examination and Papanicolaou ("Pap") smears in early detection of cancer. Every middle-aged adult should know the danger of glaucoma, the simple test which will reveal beginning symptoms, the treatment required to prevent blindness. Awareness of the new measles vaccine is important for parents of young children.

The nurse needs to have and be able to pass on the latest *scientific* information on smoking; the effect of car seat belts and shoulder harness in saving lives and reducing injuries; the danger of burns and fire from frayed, worn electric cords and other defective household equipment; causes of poisoning in young children and preventive measures. In all probability none of this information will be related to the patient's reason for being in the hospital, yet it all has a bearing on his health and well-being and that of his family. The hospital's purpose is not only to cure but to prevent disease and promote health. The nurse has a better opportunity to teach than does any other health professional. What is the head nurse doing to encourage the teaching of patients by her staff?

METHODS OF TRANSMITTING THE PLAN FOR CARE OF THE PATIENT

From the foregoing discussion the value of planning in providing good nursing should be obvious. The nurse responsible for the patient's care cannot be present 24 hours a day, yet care needs to be consistent. A question to be answered, then, is how shall a plan for care be transmitted in order to serve as a guide for all members of the nursing staff? A beautiful plan can be made and followed without being written, provided one or two persons are responsible for its execution. Private duty nurses, if they confer and agree on a plan, are able to give their patient consistent care. Staff nurses who are responsible for many patients and who are absent from the division at least two days a week cannot be expected to remember details of the plans for those with whom they have had little or no close contact. Writing the plan is, therefore, essential if the patient is to profit from the experience of nurses who know him best. Depending on oral reports is to lose valuable information. The information which is written about the patient in a plan for his care need not, as a rule, be detailed. Indeed, for two reasons, the amount of written material should be kept to a minimum compatible with effectiveness. *First,* there is usually not much time to write and keep up the outlines, and the content may vary frequently as the patient's condition changes. *Second,* the nurse who especially needs the information and finds it most helpful is the one who is new to the floor or for some reason does not know the patient. Helpful as long, detailed descriptions might be to a new nurse, there would seldom be time for her to read many of them before starting the day's work. Brief statements, however, prove exceedingly helpful to a nurse who does not know the patient.

Each hospital has its own form for transmitting the nursing care plan. Most frequently it is a part of or an addendum to the cardex containing current medical orders and identifying data such as date of admission, patient's age, the doctor's name, and so forth. By placing the nursing care plan with the cardex, duplication of information is avoided and the plan can be easily checked against the medical orders within which it must operate.

Some nursing care plans include the aim or objective for the patient's care, information about him personally, the methods for meeting the objective, and the patient's specific needs. Since there are many objectives and all cannot be listed, it is well to omit the obvious ones and state the one which is not being fulfilled. For example, there are many objectives in the case of 85-year-old Mrs. Newcomb, admitted with a fractured femur. These include: to prevent decubiti, to keep her from falling out of bed, and to keep her oriented to her surroundings. The objective which is not being met, however, is to get her to eat and drink. This, then, is the objective to be stated on her nursing care plan. Directions for attempting to meet this objective are given. So also are those for meeting the unstated objectives.

Many nursing care cards or forms have two columns. One gives personal data about the patient. This may be in the form of a portrait or word picture, or it may list only his needs and problems. Preferably it includes both. The second column tells the actual plan for care, including the approach to the patient when this is needed. The following is an example of the kind of information which is of value:

Portrait	Approach
Mr. Jones is an elderly, lonely man who needs all the consideration possible in the course of his fatal disease. He has no family; his only friends are his landlady and her husband. He may be disoriented at times but is generally much interested in his surroundings.	*Explain everything you plan to do for him. Encourage suggestions. Question him to be sure he understands and approves the plan. Stimulate self-help where possible. Commend achievement.*

Needs and Problems	Plan for Care
Likes to smoke. Must not be left alone.	*Permit four cigarettes spaced throughout the day in accord with his wishes. Have someone with him.*
Incontinent.	*Check bed linen frequently.*
Will not move by himself.	*Change position every hour. Lift, do not drag, when moving. Suggest ways he can help.*
Uncomfortable on paralyzed side.	*Encourage to lie for short periods on right (paralyzed) side. Place in semi-side position with pillow tucked firmly against back. Use small pillow to elevate left arm.*
Fearful of getting into chair.	*Have two people help.*
Will not wear dentures which do not fit. Cannot eat solids.	*Encourage to eat. Explain why he must take food and fluids. Takes eggnogs readily and they supply needed protein. Vary flavor.*

Specific instructions for physical nursing care should be a part of the nursing care plan but are all too frequently omitted. One way to include such measures as special back or mouth care, instructions for turning, positioning, observing, protecting, and so forth is to write them as nursing orders in the treatment column of the cardex. They are less likely to be overlooked there because the nurse who has once familiarized herself with the patient does not read the entire nursing care plan each day.

Another important part of patient care is related to the way treatments and medications are given. Methods of administration are a nursing responsibility for which directives are often necessary. Clarification of the doctor's orders, a responsibility of the head nurse or team leader, gives greater assurance that they will be performed in a consistent manner. A description of the method or the clarification may accompany, in parentheses, the transcribed order. For example, the nurse supplements the doctor's order for periodic intramuscular injections with instructions about rotating the site. For another patient the doctor's order reads:

"Hot wet 10% magnesium sulphate dressing to right foot and ankle for 12 hours."

The plan for patient care states:

"Hot wet 10% magnesium sulphate dressing (sterile) to right foot and ankle for 12 hours. (Moisten with solution at $105°$ F. q 4 hours.)"

The parenthetical instructions are the method used by the head nurse, or the patient's nurse, to transmit this part of the plan for the patient's care.

The plan for instruction of the patient and his family, if brief, is included in the second column of the nursing care card. However, if a detailed plan is necessary, it is prepared by the patient's nurse and placed in the back of the patient's chart. Either on this sheet or in the nurses' notes, the teaching done and evidence of the patient's learning should be recorded so someone in addition to the patient's nurse knows to what extent the plan has been fulfilled. A notation is made on the nursing care plan that an instruction guide is in the patient's record.

As the patient's needs change his nursing care plan must be changed. The habit of reading plans for care is soon lost unless they are kept up-to-date.

THE HEAD NURSE'S RESPONSIBILITY IN PLANNING PATIENT CARE

The quality of nursing care plans for patients on the unit, indeed their very existence, depends upon the head nurse's conviction that written plans improve patient care and, in the end, save nursing time. If she believes in their value and has leadership ability she will convince her staff of their worth and together they will find a way to get the essentials written. Responsibility for the writing of nursing care plans must be clearly established and the individual so designated held accountable. The failure to prepare nursing care plans, which is all too prevalent, results from a lack of conviction of their worth, and failure to delegate responsibility for their preparation. The head nurse or team leader who takes the nursing history makes the first plan or guide and may be the person who will continue to be responsible. Usually, however, the professional nurse who knows the patient best, that is, the one assigned to his care over a period of time, will make changes in the plan as necessary. She should be the person held accountable for keeping the guide up-to-date. Preparing nursing care plans for her patients can easily become an accepted regular practice for the nurse in the same way that she has come to accept responsibility for charting.

Many nurses in the beginning will need considerable assistance with the content of the plans and also in writing them. To help with the former the head nurse provides for group planning through nursing care conferences on individual patients. Then, since the head nurse has herself prepared many of the first nursing care plans for patients the staff will have models which should assist them in knowing what to include and how to write it simply and clearly. The head nurse will also need to give individual help to nurses in the preparation of plans. Perhaps she will find it useful to work with a group of staff nurses who express a need for assistance. The head nurse sets standards for content and quality of expression against which she assists staff members to evaluate their work. Since the head nurse knows all patients and reads each plan she knows when changes are indicated.

Only a few nursing care plans will, as a rule, be long and detailed. For many patients, all that is needed in a portrait are a few brief statements. For example:

This is the first hospitalization of Mr. Carleton, a prominent local businessman. He is active in the Chamber of Commerce and a leader in his church (Congregational). May be more concerned about his forthcoming surgery than it appears.

When personal problems are known, a brief description of them together with the approach that the patient's nurse has found effective will help others.

Mrs. Clancy's husband died suddenly last Friday. Having finally started to cry, she has not been able to stop. Let her know it is all right to do so. Do not try to cheer her. Show interest in what she tells you. Reflective technique appears to relieve her tension.

For the portrait to be of value, the nurse who prepares it must have had enough contact with the patient to possess accurate information about him and to know how he thinks and feels. If this is to be achieved the head nurse must establish a policy whereby patients, consistently, have the same nurse or the same team assigned to their care. Where this is impossible the head nurse herself writes the portrait and plan.

NURSING CARE PLAN

PHYSICAL - PHYSIOLOGICAL NEEDS	PSYCHO - SOCIAL PLANS
1. Foot board @ all times	1. Provide for company while eating
2. Use ace bandages on both legs from	2. Needs to reduce smoking
toes to knee	Try week of 12/3 - 3cig./da. p.c.
Remove and elevate legs 3x/da. in	Week of 12/10 - 2cig./da. p.c.
a.m., after lunch, @ bedtime	3. Encourage family to visit one @
3. Complete bed rest except:	time for short, frequent intervals
a. May use commode @ bedside	4. Rests well with T.V. Likes latest
b. " bathe own face, arms, chest.	editions of all newspapers
c. " feed self	5. Encourage his discussion of fears
4. Provide for an hour of sleep after	of heart disease when he indicates
bath and during afternoon	readiness
5. Save dessert from evening meal for	
bedtime snack	TEACHING AND DISCHARGE PLANS
6. Check elimination carefully	Will probably convalesce @ home for
Use milk of magnesia freely	2 months. Company expects him to
7. Watch for signs of bleeding from	return
mucous membranes	Will be referred to cardiac evalua-
	tion clinic after 2 months.
	Discuss this with him when he
	seems interested

DATE	MEDICATIONS	TIME	DATE	TREATMENTS	TIME
11/26	Morphine sulphate 10mg. (H) q̄ 3h.	P.R.N.	11/26	B/P. Pulse and Resp. B.I.D	9-9
	Nembutal 0.1gm. H.S.	P.R.N.			
	Milk of magnesia 30cc H.S.	P.R.N.			
	Daily Coumadin ordered to be				
	written after prothrombin				
	level is reported.				
11/30	Digitoxin 0.1 mg. q̄d.	9A.M.			

RESTRICTIONS Bed Rest
Limit Smoking

ADM. DATE Nov. 26, 1960 SURG DATE	PRIVILEGES Commode at bedside
DIAGNOSIS AND SURGERY	May feed self

Posterior myocardial infarction

DIET 1400 cal. 800 mg. sodium	BATH Self with help
FLUID ad. lib.	✓

| ROOM 52 | LAST NAME Cohen | FIRST NAME Jacob | DOCTOR Peters | SERVICE Med. | HOSP. NO 41698 | RELIGION Heb. | AGE 52 | SPEC. NUR. | I-O | FEED | SPEC. DIET |

Fig. 14. Double cardex. Nursing care plan, prepared by team or in staff conference. Thoroughly reviewed by same group at least once a week and rewritten as necessary. See Figure 15 for back of nursing care plan.

PATIENT PORTRAIT

Mr. Cohen is president of manufacturing company. Worked up from laborer in company. Will need to make occupational adjustments. Married. Two college age sons. Responds to many verbal stimuli with laughter. Brother-in-law died two weeks after "heart attack".

Fig. 15. Back of nursing care plan (Fig. 14) gives a word picture of the patient.

Nursing care plans for some patients need to include all the sections illustrated: objective, portrait, needs and problems, approach, plan for care including teaching, nursing orders, and clarification of doctor's orders. For many, only a portion of this information is applicable. A brief portrait, as suggested above, is important for all patients to aid the individuals who have not had the chance to know them. Likewise, the inclusion of orders for nursing measures and clarification of medical orders, if any are indicated, are essential if the care of the patient is to be efficient and consistent in method (Figs. 14 and 15).

Joint planning by members of the health services involved in the patient's care is often customary in teaching hospitals. The chief of the medical service, the house medical officers, the head nurse, department administrator, social worker, and, if they are concerned with the patient's care, the physical and occupational therapists confer at regular intervals. They discuss patients on the service and plan their care. Problems are brought out by members of the group. Together they decide on an approach for the solution. This sharing of many minds and varying points of view results in a broad program for care. Provision is made for staff nurses to attend the sessions in which plans for their patients are considered. As a result of discussion in this conference, doctors and nurses confer with the patient and confirm the plan suggested by the group. Nursing care plans are revised accordingly.

SUMMARY

Following the assessment of the patient's needs, a plan is made for his care. The plan is started on the patient's admission and is continuously revised as his condition changes. The patient shares in the planning. As soon as he is able, he should be encouraged to participate in his own care as a step toward self dependence.

The plan for the patient's care is based on objectives which should be formulated in simple, clear terms. Objectives are related to comfort, therapeutic and rehabilitative measures, protection and preventive measures, support, and teaching, in all of which the nurse carries important responsibility. If the patient is to benefit from the planning for his care and if one member of the nursing staff is to profit from the experience of another, the plan for patient care must be transmitted accurately. Accuracy and thoroughness can be assured only if the plan is written.

There are many forms for nursing care plans. Usually a card is provided as part of the cardex for doctor's orders. The content, in general, includes one important objective, a portrait of the patient, his needs and problems, the plan for his care including approach, a teaching plan, nursing orders and clarification of medical orders. For many patients much of this detail is unnecessary. A brief portrait, together with nursing orders and clarification of doctor's orders, is often sufficient when the patient is hospitalized for a short period and is well-adjusted.

The head nurse's responsibility for nursing care plans is primarily one of leadership in helping the staff to see their value, making it possible for nurses to know patients through long term assignments, arranging for joint planning when it is thought this will benefit the patient, specifically delegating responsibility for the preparation of nursing care plans and giving the necessary instruction and supervision.

QUESTIONS FOR DISCUSSION

1. If you were a new staff nurse what help would you like to have the head nurse give you in preparing nursing care plans?
2. How high on your priority list would you put the writing of nursing care plans? Give reasons for your answer.

EXERCISES

1. Using the content of the form in Figures 14 and 15 prepare a nursing care plan for a patient for whom you are caring. Ask others who are sharing in the patient's care—the evening nurse, night nurse, and others—to use your plan. With their assistance, evaluate the form and your plan. Is there any information in the portrait which is valueless to the nurse? Any other which would be of help?
2. Devise a form for a nursing care plan which you believe will be most useful to you. Use and evaluate it as in 1, above.
3. Prepare a short portrait and effective approach to a patient you know well which you think would give helpful information to other nurses and result in better or more satisfying care to the patient. Portraits should be presented in class with an opportunity for members to decide whether they would find the content and form useful.

REFERENCES

Amend, Edith L. A parent education program in a children's hospital, Nurs. Outlook, Vol. 14 (April 1966), pp. 53-56.
Parents are partners in the health team which is furthering the recovery of their hospitalized child. An active program of education for parents which has for its aim the provision of physical and emotional security for the patient, the parent, and the nurse should stimulate other hospitals to examine their own procedures for the care of children.

Among other things, prescribing nursing care, Nurs. Outlook, Vol. 15 (February 1967), pp. 64-65.
Description of the organization of the nursing service in a private mental hospital. Registered nurses prescribe nursing care and work closely with the doctor. Practical nurses are responsible for nursing service, unit administration, supervision of aides, and implementation of nursing care prescribed by the registered nurses.

Bailey, June Teig. The critical incident technique in identifying behavior criteria of professional nursing effectiveness, Nurs. Res., Vol. 5 (October 1956), pp. 52-64.
Annotation with Chapter 13 reference.

Bardsley, Christine, Fowler, Helen, Moody, Edith, Teigen, Elizabeth, and Sommer, Joan. Pressure sores—a regimen for preventing and treating them, Amer. J. Nurs., Vol. 64 (May 1964), pp. 82-84.
The unique feature of this article is the expectation that all lucid patients can help to prevent pressure sores.

Barnes Elizabeth. Patients in Hospital, London, Macmillan and Company, Ltd., 1961, Chapter 10, pp. 116-124.

Visitors although often thought of as a hindrance to the unit staff can be a help and visiting hours may be used for family instruction.

Berkowitz, Norman H., Malone, Mary F., Klein, Malcolm W., and Eaton, Ann. Patient follow-through in the outpatient department, Nurs. Res., Vol. 12 (Winter 1963), pp. 16-22.
This study has implications for the teaching of hospitalized patients as well as for outpatients. It was found that patients comply with instruction related to return appointments, referrals and tests better than to instruction related to medication, treatments, and restrictions which are the patient's exclusive responsibility for his own care at home.

Blumberg, Mark S., and Drew, Jacqueline. Methods for assessing nursing care quality, Hospitals, Vol. 37 (November 1, 1963), pp. 72-80.
Annotation with Chapter 13 reference.

Campbell, Lucy. Clinical nursing conferences, Nurs. Outlook, Vol. 14 (March 1966), pp. 63-64.
Chronically ill patients, in one city, may be referred to a Health Department clinical nursing conference, held near their homes, where a public health nurse counsels them on health and personal matters.

Donny, Ethel. Imagination in maternity care, Amer. J. Nurs., Vol. 60 (January 1960), pp. 46-49.
An inspiring article stressing the tremendous opportunity of the nurse in helping mothers with adjustments needed in the home as a result of the arrival of a new baby, whether it be her first or her fourth.

Drummond, Eleanor E. Impact of a father's role, Amer. J. Nurs., Vol. 64 (August 1964), pp. 89-91.
"Basic disturbances to the family occur when the father has a disability. The nurse's knowledge of the common disturbances will help her care for the patient, help him adjust to his altered role, and guide her plan of family teaching." Excellent!

Glaser, Barney G., and Strauss, Anselm L. The social loss of dying patients, Amer. J. Nurs., Vol. 64 (June 1964), pp. 119-121.
Social values are placed on patients based on their age, social class, education, accomplishments, etc. Awareness of this fact should help nurses avoid letting their responses to social loss interfere with their nursing care.

Goode, Margaret A. The patient with a cerebral vascular accident, Nurs. Outlook, Vol. 14 (March 1966), pp. 60-62.
A thorough and interesting description of the nursing needed during both acute and chronic phases of the illness.

Hagen, Elizabeth, and Wolff, Luverne. Nursing Leadership Behavior in a General Hospital, New York, Institute of Research and Service in Nursing Education, Teachers College, Columbia University, 1961, p. 137.
In this study the researchers noted the absence of any long-range planning by the head nurse and "the tendency to take action related to the immediate problem and to treat symptoms rather than causes . . ."

Henderson, Lilian M. Nursing care in acute cholecystitis, Amer. J. Nurs., Vol. 64 (May 1964), pp. 93-96.
The observations the nurse must make, the medical dianostic procedures used, together with physical nursing care needed are clearly described.

Hulicka, Irene M. Fostering self-respect in aged patients, Amer. J. Nurs., Vol. 64 (March 1964), pp. 84-88.
A research psychologist graphically describes the behavior of elderly hospitalized

patients and the reasons for it. Very helpful are her descriptions and illustrations of what nurses can do to make the lives of these individuals happier, their behavior more acceptable to staff. Every nurse should read this article.

Hungler, Bernadette P. What every patient needs, Amer. J. Nurs., Vol. 64 (October 1964), pp. 112-115.
A nurse tells the story of her mother's heart surgery and stresses the importance of T.L.C. (tender, loving care) in recovery.

Kelly, Mary M. Exercises for bedfast patients, Amer. J. Nurs., Vol. 66 (October 1966), pp. 2209-2213.
The great need for the patient to exercise is made clear. Diagrams of range of motion for joints are very helpful.

Kelly, Nancy Cardinal. Nursing care plans, Nurs. Outlook, Vol. 14 (May 1966), pp. 61-64.
Report of a study of nursing care plans and excellent suggestions for a guide to be used in formulating plans for patient care.

Kempf, Florence C. This I believe about nursing's responsibility to society, Nurs. Outlook, Vol. 13 (January 1965), pp. 63-64.
". . . nursing in its broadest interpretation is doing for the patient what he cannot do for himself then assessing his potentials for self-care and teaching him to do for himself are the nurse's foremost activities." Are we educating for this responsibility?

Leavitt, Helen B., A statewide patient referral system, Amer. J. Nurs., Vol. 64 (March 1964), p. 101.
The Washington State Nurses Association with the help and support of other health agencies in the state has developed a form which is being used to refer patients from one agency to another. Other benefits besides the standardized form have resulted.

Leone, Lucile Petry. Wanted: good nursing, Nurs. Outlook, Vol. 5 (October 1957), pp. 576-578.
Written in an interesting, challenging manner, this article describes nursing at its best.

Leventhal, Bette. An intern's experience, Nurs. Outlook, Vol. 14 (February 1966), pp. 44-45.
This is the fourth part of an article entitled, *An Internship for Leadership*. This nurse intern describes her experiences and makes very clear the value of the nursing care plan and the circumstances under which it is useful.

Lewis, Garland K. Communication: a factor in meeting emotional crises, Nurs. Outlook, Vol. 13 (August 1965), pp. 36-39.
"We must evaluate our communication and whether it has been effective for the other person, and then be willing to assume the responsibility for correcting the error if we have not been effective."

Linehan, Dorothy T. What does the patient want to know?, Amer. J. Nurs., Vol. 66 (May 1966), pp. 1066-1070.
A study in one hospital showed that patients have many unanswered questions. As a result of the study an interdisciplinary committee made recommendations regarding what patients should be taught, who should teach, and the methods for patient education. Resulting changes are presented.

Little, Dolores, and Carnevali, Doris. Nursing care plans: let's be practical about them, Nurs. Forum, Vol. 6 (No. 1, 1967), pp. 61-76.
Full of helpful suggestions for initiation and use of nursing care plans. Of particular interest is the groups of nurses who would find nursing care plans helpful.

Mansfield, Elaine. Use of patient care plans by aides, Nurs. Outlook, Vol. 15 (April 1967), pp. 72-74.
In several wards of a state hospital aides were taught and made responsible for preparing nursing care plans for a group of 4-5 patients. Questions about patient behavior were used as a guide. As a result interest in patients increased, their care improved, and staff morale was enhanced.

Melody, Mary, and Clark, Genevieve. Walking-Planning Rounds, Amer. J. Nurs., Vol. 67 (April 1967), pp. 771-773.
At the completion of the transfer report, the nursing team makes rounds to see patients and together they plan the patient's care. Since instituting walking-talking rounds, team nursing has functioned more effectively in this institution.

Monteiro, Lois A. Notes on patient teaching—a neglected area, Nurs. Forum, Vol. 3 (No. 1, 1964), pp. 27-33.
Teaching, an integral part of nursing, is done individually or in groups, informally; it may be planned or spontaneous. If teaching is considered important, time must be allowed for it and nurses helped to learn ways to be effective.

Muhs, Eleanor J. and Nebesky, Marjorie T. A psychiatric nursing care plan, Amer. J. Nurs., Vol. 64 (April 1964), pp. 120-122.
A nursing staff devised a nursing plan to meet the needs in their own situation. The plans serve to promote good nursing and one means to this end is their use in inservice education.

Nelson, Katherine R. How will individualized care, based on the patient's nursing needs, be provided? Pamphlet: Improvement of Nursing Practice, New York, American Nurses' Association, 1961, pp. 19-26.
This experienced public health nurse describes, by means of a specific patient situation, a method for assessing a patient's needs and planning her care. This, she says, is *professional* nursing. Excellent reading.

Otto, Herbert A. The human potentialities of nurses and patients, Nurs. Outlook, Vol. 13 (August 1965), pp. 32-35.
Taking inventory of personal assets and potentialities increases self-esteem, instills hope, and encourages the development of health processes. The nurse can utilize this process with patients, students and herself and receive rich rewards.

Park, Wilford E., and Hughes, Anne. Minneapolis forges a new communication tool, Hospitals, Vol. 39 (May 16, 1965), pp. 62-65.
A committee of nurses and doctors developed a simple but comprehensive referral form which can be used in any nursing referral situation. Objectives are listed as are the services from and to which patients are referred.

Reiter, Frances. Choosing the better part, Amer. J. Nurs., Vol. 64 (December 1964), pp. 65-68.
Miss Reiter believes "that the long-term care setting is the place in which some of the problems of independence in nursing practice may be resolved." Nursing in a chronic disease hospital has implications for practice, for education, and for research.

Robinson, Geraldine, and Filkins, Marilyn. Group teaching with outpatients, Amer. J. Nurs., Vol. 64 (November, 1964), pp. 110-112.
Clinic patients waiting to be seen by the doctor meet in classes with a nurse. Each clinic has developed content around specific needs of its patients.

Rosencrans, Emily. This committee gives more than advice, Nurs. Outlook, Vol. 14 (February 1966), pp. 38-39.
Story of the way in which one Visiting Nurse Service developed a referral plan for discharged hospital patients.

Schwartz, Doris R. Toward more precise evaluation of patients' needs, Nurs. Outlook, Vol. 13 (May 1965), pp. 42-44.
Needed in nursing is a systematic means for collecting data and making a nursing assessment. In the study here reported, Miss Schwartz is using a progress record based on an initial assessment and a prediction of the outcome. A nursing care plan is prepared and is revised as indicated by 6 week evaluation reports based on the original assessment and nursing prognosis.

Smith, Dorothy M., Myth and method in nursing practice, Amer. J. Nurs., Vol. 64 (February 1964), pp. 68-72.
Miss Smith makes a plea for a system in nursing which will indicate clearly what is to be done for the patient and what we must do to accomplish it.
Realistically we cannot meet all the needs of the patient but we can, systematically according to a plan, determine what these needs are and what we will do in dealing with them.

Stephens, Gwen Jones. The time factor—should it control the patient's care?, Amer. J. Nurs., Vol. 65 (May 1965), pp. 77-82.
A fascinating description of the differing effects drugs have when given to mice at different periods of the day. Has implications for nursing if research shows similar variations in effect on humans of activities performed at different times of day.

Sullins, Della D. The "G" plan works, Nurs. Outlook, Vol. 12 (July 1964), pp. 31-32.
The G plan—ie, giving of material things, time, opportunity, and responsibility—is often an effective way to nurse the "demanding" patient.

Sykes, Eleanor M. No time for silence, Amer. J. Nurs., Vol. 66 (May 1966), pp. 1040-1041.
Through preoperative planning for postoperative communication, the patient who is to have a laryngectomy can be greatly reassured.

Turner, Charlotte, and Mahoney, Robert F. After hospitalization, Amer. J. Nurs., Vol. 64 (September 1964), pp. 137-139.
As a result of a pilot project in a Veterans Administration Hospital more and better referrals are being sent out. On admission and periodically during his stay the patient's likely need for follow-up care is evaluated. "Staff is obtaining much more pertinent information about patients than was previously the case."

Wahlstrom, E. Dorothy, and Weston, Jerry L. Initiating referrals: a hospital-based system; a health department approach, Amer. J. Nurs., Vol. 67 (February 1967), pp. 332-335.
Referral systems of two institutions are described together with the values which occur.

Wang, Mamie Kwoh. The intramural nursing referral, Nurs. Outlook, Vol. 7 (June 1959), pp. 346-347.
A means by which continuity of care can be maintained when a patient is transferred to another unit within the hospital. The procedure was developed over a period of time by a committee of the nursing service. The referral is now an accepted part of nursing's responsibility to patients.

chapter 12

DELEGATING RESPONSIBILITY FOR NURSING CARE OF THE PATIENT

Nursing service personnel who give direct care to patients on a hospital division are made up of professional nurses, practical nurses, and many times nurses' aides. Registered as professional nurses are graduates of two-year associate degree programs, three-year diploma programs, and four- to five-year degree programs.[1] Their capabilities vary, but nurses from all three types of programs meet the minimum requirements for state registration in most states. State laws regulating the practice of practical nurses vary considerably. In some, licensure is mandatory; in others it is not. Graduation from an approved school of practical nursing is generally recognized as necessary except for some older, experienced women who have been licensed by waiver. Head nurses need to know which practical nurses have had formal preparation.

Nurses' aides are prepared on the job. Usually they are given a six to eight week training period with classes and demonstrations by the professional nurse responsible for inservice education. It is now being recommended that their preparation be received in vocational education institutions with other health occupation workers.[2] The aide group sometimes includes middle-aged women who have had no more than a grade school education but who have good personal habits and a liking for people. Young married women who need to help support their families may choose to become nurses' aides because no preparation is needed except that gained while working. Some hospitals, as part of a nursing recruitment program, employ as aides high school students between their junior and senior years. This not only helps the student decide whether she wishes to enter nursing, but it assists the hospital during the summer vacation period.

These, then, are the members of the nursing staff who participate in

[1] Some attempt is presently being made by national nursing organizations to differentiate "professional" and "technical" nurses. See: American Nurses Association's first position on education for nursing, *Amer. J. Nurs.*, Vol. 65 (December 1965), pp. 106-111. Since at this writing no such designations have been generally accepted or recognized, the term "professional" nurse as used in this text refers to all who have state licensure to practice as a professional nurse.
[2] *Ibid.*, p. 108.

nursing care. The condition of some patients demands that their entire care be given by a professional nurse. No day goes by but that all patients need some ministration from the professional nurse. The majority of patients can be well nursed if, during part of their hospital stay, they are cared for in part by a practical nurse or possibly an aide. The person who is responsible for the patient's general care, including his bath and simple nursing measures, is the individual to whom he is "assigned." Other parts of his care may or may not be carried out by this staff member. The professional nurse gives medications and treatments, observes, and teaches any patients assigned to the aide and usually also the patients for whom the practical nurse is caring. The head nurse or team leader decides which members shall participate in the care of each patient and in what ways they shall do so.

On what basis shall this decision be made? This is a question the head nurse must answer and, to do so wisely, necessitates a great deal of thought. It is necessary that she know the needs of each patient and the qualifications of each staff member. Unless she has this information and takes it into account, good judgment in selection of a person competent to handle the responsibilities entailed in the patient's care is impossible.

KNOWLEDGE OF THE PATIENT'S NEEDS

The new patient whose nursing needs have not yet been determined should be cared for by the head nurse or team leader to provide opportunity for making a nursing diagnosis. When this is not possible the patient is assigned on the basis of the best knowledge available. The head nurse or team leader makes this initial assessment. When the patient's needs are more fully known a change in assignment may be indicated. Because worries and fears are not readily disclosed by some patients, the head nurse needs to have enough contact with each person to detect the seriousness of his concerns and to learn whether the patient desires to talk about them. All individuals have some uneasiness resulting from hospitalization. This is to be expected and many patients will have no need or wish to share their feelings. The individuals who may be helped by talking should be recognized by the head nurse who will be guided in her assignment by this knowledge. All too frequently, if the patient is ambulatory, takes his own bath, has no special treatments, he is automatically assigned to the aide. This assignment takes into account the patient's physical needs only.

When a practical nurse or aide gives the patient his care she may be the one to hear about his worries. It is a sad commentary on professional nursing when a doctor reports that, while a patient in the hospital, his greatest support came from the nurses' aide. Not that it is undesirable for an aide to be supportive, but professional nurses should have more scientific understanding, insight, and ability to help a patient through pain or discouragement or fear than has an aide. Some patients who are assigned to the care of an aide have the opposite reaction. These patients cannot talk with the aide and feel quite disassociated from the nurses. There is cause for concern, too, when studies of staffing patterns[3] show that baths and bedmaking are considered to be "aide work" and that professional nurses suffer considerable frustration if they are called upon to give this care to any but the sickest patients.

QUALIFICATIONS OF THE PERSONNEL

Staff members, on the basis of their education, their experience, and their personal characteristics, vary in their qualifications for meeting the nursing needs of patients.

Professional Nurses

It is usually expected that graduate professional nurses have the ability to give intelligent care to any patient. Head nurses need to realize, however, that a graduate nurse may have been a student yesterday or last week or that she may not have practiced her profession for a number of years. In her previous experience, perhaps she failed to care for patients following some of the more intricate operations which are performed today in large hospitals. Therapeutic and diagnostic methods change frequently and vary in different institutions. It is important, therefore, that the head nurse, in making assignments, know the graduate nurse's past experience in caring for patients suffering from the various disorders found on the service. A conference with the nurse will give the head nurse the information which she needs. If the nurse has been employed by the central office, the department administrator can usually assist by furnishing data on the nurse's previous experience. Although the graduate nurse may be deficient in certain areas of preparation, she usually has the basic technical knowledge

[3] Peter Kong-Ming New and Gladys Nite. Staffing and interaction, *Nurs. Outlook,* Vol. 8 (July 1960), pp. 396-400.

on which to build greater understanding and skill through a program of staff development (see Part 3). Her need for experience must be taken into account in planning assignments. If she has not cared for a patient with thoracic surgery she should be assigned to the care of an individual having this therapy and given the instruction and supervision needed.

Professional Student Nurses

In most instances the school of nursing instructor, not the head nurse, assigns patients to students. The head nurse under all circumstances should assist. In situations where the head nurse does carry the responsibility for making student assignments, she should have guides to determine the ability of the student to give the care needed. The *first* guide is the stage of the student's development. Is she a first, second, third, or fourth year student? On what services has she had previous experience? Has she been assigned to the present unit or to another unit on the same service at an earlier date? Has she had her obstetric experience before coming to the pediatric floor? medicine before surgery? the operating room before obstetrics? pediatrics before her public health experience? Have her classes relating to the clinical subject been completed or will they correlate with her division experience? Has the student's experience been interrupted by a long illness or leave of absence? If so, how long has she been back in the school? Answers to these questions the head nurse should be able to obtain from the department administrator or the school of nursing office. This information helps the head nurse plan assignments which safeguard the patient.

A *second* guide to the head nurse in determining the student's ability is the knowledge and skill which can be expected of students at various levels of experience. To what extent can the head nurse expect a first year or a third year professional nurse student to handle skillfully a patient with emotional strains? to recognize symptoms and interpret their significance? to be able to turn and move a critically ill patient with skill and conservation of the patient's energy? Can the student be expected to assume responsibility for general activities if they are not assigned to her? How well should she be able to recognize the patient's need for health teaching and to make good use of her opportunities? How much technical skill and knowledge of procedure principles and methods should she have at her stage of development? Without information of this nature the head nurse might well place a student in situations for which she is not ready, to the detriment of both the patient and the student.

Information pertaining to the competence which can be expected of student nurses at different levels of experience is difficult to acquire. There are a great many variables particularly if students are not assigned to a service at a specific stage in their educational program. With the help of the clinical instructor the head nurse needs to analyze the abilities which can be expected of students who come to her floor.

If this division receives students who have had no previous clinical experience, the head nurse knows the student has very few nursing capabilities but that even these will vary with the type and length of her preclinical education. Usually, in the preclinical period, the student learns procedure principles and methods. She probably has little, if any, instruction in clinical nursing. In her first hospital assignment following the preclinical period she can be expected to know procedures but to have limited skill in their performance. She is unable to organize a large assignment. She may have little ability to win the patient's confidence and cooperation. She has no real understanding of the emotional and social factors which enter into the picture of illness. She knows very little about the organization of the division.

Having decided the things which the young student is and is not able to do, the next step is to list the types of activities which she should be capable of undertaking safely in the early stages of her first experience. She should be able to care for convalescent or mildly ill patients who have no unusual physical or emotional problems. It is expected that the student will be able to perform simple treatments and to participate in general activities such as preparing patients for rest hour or for visitors. She should be allowed the time and opportunity to practice nursing procedures without having to make many adaptations until she is thoroughly familiar with technique and fairly skillful in performance. The patient whose condition requires wide variations in method should not be assigned to the young student early in her experience. However, as the student becomes adjusted to the situation and gains in ability, she is assigned to patients whose care requires increased knowledge, skill, and understanding.

Perhaps the students who are assigned to this division have had part of their clinical experience. How much ability can be expected of a student at the various stages of her educational career? As with the beginning student her previous experience is analyzed. For example, if the student who is assigned to the obstetric service has already had experience in pediatrics it is anticipated that she will possess skill in handling babies. If she has not had experience in caring for infants, less can be expected of her at the beginning of her period in the nursery.

If the head nurse knows in what year of their course the students are assigned to the service and if she determines the experiences which customarily precede the assignment, she will be able to judge to some extent the students' ability at the beginning of their assignment. It is possible to establish standards of ability, knowledge, and appreciations by which students can be judged.

The capabilities which are not present when the student starts the service she must acquire with the assistance of teaching and supervision. Students who have not had experience in handling infants before their nursery assignment, for example, are taught ways to do so and are closely supervised until proficiency is developed. Students learn by doing but the doing needs to be closely observed for the protection of the patient and to insure the student's correct learning. The head nurse must have assurance that students are competent to meet patients' needs or that they will have enough supervision from a clinically prepared instructor to be able to do so.

A *third* guide in determining whether the student is able to meet the patient's needs is the ability of the individual student. How well does she measure up to the expectations for her group? Students differ widely in ability to adjust, in manual and organizing skills, in personality, and in many other ways. Records of her past experience in the school are very helpful in knowing how well a student will be able to care for certain patients and how much help she will need.

The clinical instructor should provide the head nurse with information about the student before she comes to the division. Possession of such information will influence the student's assignment to patients. This is not to say that a student cannot and should not learn to care for all patients but for her sake and that of the patient, no activities should be assigned until the student is ready to deal with them with at least minimal skill.

Practical Nurses

The role of the practical nurse has changed rapidly and markedly over the last few years. There seem to be two points of view regarding practical nurse education. *One* takes the position that in addition to nursing patients in situations relatively free from scientific complexity, under the supervision of a professional nurse or doctor, the one-year practical nurse program prepares its graduates to assist the professional nurse in more complex situations. She is considered equipped to teach patients self-care and to participate in medical therapy.[4]

[4] Neva M. Stevenson. Prospective on developments in practical nursing, *Nurs. Outlook,* Vol. 8 (January 1960), pp. 36-37.

In most hospitals today the practical nurse is deeply involved in caring for patients who have all types of needs. In fact there seems to be little differentiation made between nursing care activities delegated to the professional nurse and those assigned to the practical nurse. For this reason a *second* point of view toward education of the practical nurse has been expressed recently.[5] Because the job demands on the practical nurse approach those for which the registered nurse has been educated, and because practical nurse schools are endeavoring to prepare their graduates to handle assignments which require this higher level of ability, some think it advisable to take steps to replace these schools with associate degree programs in community colleges. Be that as it may, at the present time most hospitals include practical nurses on their staff and to the professional nurse falls the responsibility for analyzing the particular patient's present needs and deciding which patients can be assigned to a practical nurse. In general, patients who require highly technical observations or the exercise of professional judgment should not be assigned to a practical nurse. On the other hand, she is able to perform most nursing procedures and is capable of developing a high degree of technical skill in their performance. She needs close direction and supervision.

Individual hospitals reserve the right to decide that certain treatments may not be performed by practical nurses. Thus some institutions will permit them to catheterize, give eye treatments, administer medications. Other hospitals will not. Since far more drugs are given in the hospital than in the home, there is more possibility of error in dosage and greater need for recognition of contraindications. Many hospitals, therefore, are not willing to take the responsibility for the administration of medications by a practical nurse. There are pharmacists who consider the practice dangerous.

Some hospitals are utilizing the services of practical nurses in intensive care units and postoperative recovery rooms *where a professional nurse has the patient in constant view*. Skilled in the use of their hands, gentle in manner, many practical nurses give beautiful care to the very ill. They should be told what to look for, what to report, precautions to take, with what parts of the patient's care they must have help. The professional nurse must not fail to recognize her responsibility for the patient. She needs to know how closely she herself must observe him and plan to check his condition at the necessary intervals. *She is near at hand every minute for emergency care*—suctioning, administering oxygen, assisting when vomiting occurs or when the patient is in severe pain. She helps with turning and positioning. She looks for emotional problems although physical care usually makes greater demands at this point.

[5] *Op. cit.,* American Nurses Associations' Position Paper, p. 111.

While the majority of hospitals are utilizing practical nurse service as just described a few are assigning this nurse in a very different way. Patients are assigned to the professional nurses only. Under their direction practical nurses perform technical functions such as taking vital signs, keeping track of intravenous fluid levels and changing flasks. They help patients who need assistance with bathing, eating, and walking. The professional nurse performs treatments and assists with ambulation of the postoperative patient the first time these occur. Only when the patient has fully accepted the procedure and learned how to use it effectively does the practical nurse perform it. This policy permits utilization of the practical nurse's technical ability without placing upon her responsibility for which she has not been educationally prepared.

The same careful selection of patients is made for practical nurse students that is employed for the professional student. At all times consideration must be given to the patient's needs and the student's readiness to meet them.

Nurses' Aides

Although the details of the course of instruction for aides vary with the needs and policies of the hospital, it is fairly well accepted that they have been prepared primarily to do the type of work that is taught in home nursing courses with the exception that aides are not taught to give medications. Their teaching program usually consists of such activities as giving baths, afternoon care, shampoos; making occupied and unoccupied beds; taking temperatures, giving nourishments and feeding patients, recording fluids; giving enemas and other simple, unsterile treatments; getting patients up in the chair, transporting them to other departments; and performing household duties. The fact that aides are taught certain nursing procedures has never meant that they are capable of performing them for all patients. Nor does it mean that because the aide can give baths, morning and afternoon care, these activities should be considered her work. The total needs of the patient must be considered, and often these will be discovered only if the professional nurse gives his general care.

The present trend is to assign aides to assist nurses and not to give them an assignment of patients. In some hospitals aides give none of the personal care such as bathing and feeding the patient, nor do they administer treatments. Instead the aide helps the nurse when two persons are needed to turn, move, or hold a patient. She makes beds for patients who are up, prepares the unit for the nurse to give daily care, removes equipment after use, dusts and rearranges the room. The aide and the nurse synchronize their activities so the patient's care is coordinated. In these situations, the professional nurse is responsible for all activities performed by the aide. Certainly unless the aide has had considerable experience and is thoroughly dependable, she should be given very limited responsibility. The nursing team (p. 293), with little question, makes the best use of the aide's abilities.

CONSIDERATION OF PERSONAL QUALITIES IN MAKING ASSIGNMENTS

Although the preparation of the staff member, through education and experience, is the prime consideration in making assignments, personal factors play an important role. If the aide speaks the language or understands the culture of the patient, it may be advisable to have her participate in his care. She is given explicit instructions about information that is needed as well as about his physical requirements. The professional nurse assumes responsibility for the quality of personal care given, for the necessary observations and treatments.

The age and maturity of the staff member is likewise an important consideration in some instances. An adolescent patient may enjoy the opportunity to talk with a young nurse. On the other hand, he may feel a mother figure gives him more security. The middle-aged patient who is not burdened with worry often enjoys a youthful nurse. When he is troubled, however, he tends to feel a 20-year-old has had too little experience in living to understand his problems.

Although a goal of nursing is to have every staff member, especially every professional nurse, able to adapt her behavior to the individual patient, this ideal situation will probably never be reached. Some nurses relate better than others to some patients. Some nurses have more patience in caring for certain individuals. Personality, then, is a factor to be considered in assigning patients to personnel.

OTHER FACTORS INVOLVED IN MAKING ASSIGNMENTS

Six other factors help to determine the choice of patients which the head nurse delegates to a staff member for care.

The Best Time for Making Observations and Getting to Know the Patient

The best time to observe a patient, to diagnose his nursing needs, to teach is often during the process of physical ministration. The head nurse must decide when this is the case and assign herself or another professional nurse to care for the patient as long as necessary to accomplish the purposes. Even though these professional aspects of care could perhaps be accomplished at another time than during general care, the time of nursing personnel is frequently saved if both can be achieved simultaneously by assigning the professional nurse to the patient who needs this attention. On the other hand, if these activities can be performed just as well at another time, it may be preferable, because of the requirements of others, to delegate this patient's care to a nonprofessional member of the staff. The head nurse must make sure, under these circumstances, that opportunity is provided at other times for the professional nurse to give the rest of the care necessary to the patient's well being.

Amount of Supervision Available

Assignment planning is also influenced by the requirements of various staff members for supervision. A new staff member needs more supervision than a person who knows the situation; an aide who is assisting in patient care for the first time requires more guidance than would a practical nurse. If there is no one to give the needed supervision, the patient should be assigned to another person. However, postponement of learning experiences cannot go on indefinitely if a competent staff is to be built up.

Needs Within the Group of Patients

The head nurse must consider the ability of the staff member to handle the combination of needs in the group of patients to be assigned. The type of treatments to be performed, the time that they require, and the number of treatments scheduled to be given at the same time are important factors in the individual's ability to give good nursing. Impossible or impractical combinations of duties are to be avoided. It is scarcely possible for a nurse to take blood pressure every 15 minutes on one patient and to care for another who is on isolation precautions. Neither can she care for two patients at the same time who both require constant attention and are located in different rooms.

Geographic Location

The best use will be made of personnel time if patients assigned to one person are close to one another. This minimizes time for walking. Four patients in one room can be cared for more quickly than four patients in each of four rooms. When patients are close together it is possible to see them more frequently, which is especially important if they need close observation. Changes in condition and the need for attention can be noted more promptly, and the patient has a greater sense of security when he sees his nurse often. It is necessary, however, to balance the factor of location against the need for continuity of care. When patients are moved about the division as their conditions change, location may be of less importance than keeping the same assignment.

Needs of All Patients on the Division

It is well recognized that assignment planning is not as simple as matching the patient's needs with a staff member qualified to meet them. The head nurse must consider the requirements of all patients on the division in relation to the staff that she has. There is seldom available the exact combination of personnel needed to give care to each patient at the level considered desirable. For example, it is unnecessary for a professional nurse to give general care to a patient if a practical nurse, in doing so, can meet his needs in a highly satisfactory manner. The reverse of this situation is true of course. If the patient's needs call for a professional nurse to meet them adequately, under ideal circumstances he would not be assigned to a practical nurse and certainly not to an aide. It can be seen, then, that it is possible to have a staff, adequate in number but out of line in composition.

How then shall the head nurse handle the assignment? In deciding how assignments shall be made the best method is, first, to consider the needs of individual patients and the person qualified to care for him, without regard to the needs of other patients. Thereafter, if the nursing load for the various staff members is not balanced (and seldom will it be), the nursing requirements of all patients are weighed and the best possible assignment made. The first step should not be omitted, for serious errors in judgment may be made unless the total needs of each patient are considered.

When the requirements of all patients have been assessed and the competency of available staff members determined, sometimes it will be discovered that there are not enough professional nurses. On these occasions a practical nurse must be assigned to patients who need professional nursing care. The head nurse does all in her power to see that patients receive safe, effective, comforting care. A professional staff nurse, if there is one in addition to the head nurse, may have no patient assignment but be free to circulate among all patients to observe their condition and the care they are receiving. She sets a schedule for the frequency of her visits to certain patients, especially those whose condition is critical or uncertain, and those who seem to have unidentified problems. She arranges with the staff members to assist them with certain parts of care where two persons are needed or where special observations are to be made. Patients are instructed by the nurse in ways to help with their own care such as watching the alignment of a fractured leg, recording their own intake and output. In the presence of the staff member caring for him, she tells the patient the things he should report. Practical nurses, and aides, if they have a patient assignment, are given a card for each of their patients listing the things to be done for him, the observations to be made and reported. They also receive an oral report on each patient so there will be no question of their understanding their responsibility. The nurse suggests they plan their work, then tell each patient the approximate time he can expect his care. In the meantime he should be made comfortable.

When, during the day, there is but one professional nurse, in addition to the head nurse, for a division with acutely ill patients, assignment planning is a grave responsibility. There appear to be several possibilities, the choice depending upon the situation. *First,* use the above plan of having the nurse free to observe and assist with all patients. *Second,* assign the staff nurse to care for the acutely ill, leaving other patients to the care of the nonprofessional staff member with whatever help and supervision the head nurse can give. *Third,* assign an aide to work with the staff nurse in the care of the acutely ill, the aide helping with such duties as bedmaking, gathering equipment, and cleaning. The decision depends partly on how ill the patients are, the amount of care needed by all patients, the census, the ratio of staff members to patients, and the responsibilities of the head nurse in addition to those directly related to patient care. Someone has to give medicines and treatments. The head nurse may be able to do this most easily, or she may be the nurse to circulate and assist, in which case the staff nurse gives the medications and treatments. None of these plans gives the patient the kind of care he has the right to expect. The head nurse, however, uses her best judgment in delegating the work and helps her staff establish priorities. Remembering that the nursing service administrator, if she and her associates employ and allocate staff, is ultimately responsible for the quality of nursing care, the head nurse makes sure unfavorable staffing situations are reported to the department administrator. If the head nurse, as in the conceptualized role, employs her own staff she is accountable for nursing care to hospital administration through the unit director. Should she be unable to obtain necessary additional personnel, other steps must be taken to provide adequate nursing. In conference with the unit director and the chief of service, arrangements may be made to lighten the nursing load by refusing further admissions to the division and perhaps sending patients home a day early if they can be prepared, and the family can make the necessary adjustments.

Continuity in Patient Care

Another factor to be taken into account in delegating responsibility for the care of patients is the desirability of continuity in care. The meaning of continuity has been spelled out previously. If it is to be achieved the assignment of patients should not be changed any oftener than is absolutely essential. Additions and subtractions are made as patients are admitted and discharged. When assignments are made for extended periods the patient is happier because his care is consistent. The nurse's learning is better because she is able to follow the patient's progress and to know him as a person. The unit runs more smoothly because each person is familiar with her assignment and develops, after a day or two, skill in its performance. Nursing care is of a higher quality because a plan can be made, and the time which is saved in not having to adjust to a new assignment every few days can be spent in getting to know the patient, instructing him, and planning diversional therapy.

Without doubt the patient method of assignment is the best means of providing continuity of care. In this method, one nurse gives the entire care to a group of patients and when she leaves, she transfers their care to another nurse. Unfortunately this method is now seldom used except in hospitals which still have an all professional staff, or where private duty nurses or students care for one patient. Because nonprofessional personnel cannot give medications or complicated treatments, the patient method of assignment is no longer possible in most circumstances. Many hospitals reverted to the functional method of assignment when practical nurses and aides joined the nursing staff.

The functional or "efficiency" method of assignment is the greatest known deterrent to continuity of care. In this method, staff members are assigned not to patients but to special functions such as giving medications, taking temperatures, or giving baths. It has the advantage of fewer interruptions. Its great disadvantage is that patient care is fragmentized and often uncoordinated. The patient can identify no one as "his nurse" and feels he "belongs" to no one. Once his morning care has been completed seldom does any one take any special responsibility for him. This system is especially difficult for a patient when a different person every day or two is assigned to give him general care.

How can continuity of care be achieved when the patient needs the ministrations of a professional nurse for a period following surgery or during acute illness after which his physical care may have to be given by a practical nurse, or a young student? How can the functional method be avoided when nonprofessional personnel is assigned to patients, yet unable to give certain parts of the patient's care such as medicines and complicated treatments? These are important questions. If the patient is to be well-nursed, ways must be found to overcome the ills of the functional method and to provide for continuity in care within the existing situation. Many hospitals which give excellent nursing care have found the solution to these problems in the team method of assignment.

TEAM NURSING

When we speak of *team nursing* just what is meant? There are many answers to this question. Team nursing is said to be a philosophy rather than a way of working. Perhaps it is both, for patients are assigned and staff is organized in special ways when team nursing is practiced. Yet as a philosophy, team nursing expresses beliefs about patients, personnel, leadership, and relationships.

The Philosophy of Team Nursing

The concept of team nursing is based on the philosophy that a group of personnel working together in a coordinated, cooperative way can carry out the full functions of a nurse in giving individualized nursing care.[6] Team nursing is based on the belief that every member of the nursing staff has a contribution to make in planning and giving nursing care; that motivation is greater when responsibility is felt; and that individuals are happier when they feel they are making important contributions to the achievement of group goals. Team nursing assumes that when an individual's potential is taxed, ability tends to increase; that when persons work as a team they complement one another with the result that resources are more fully used; that latent leadership ability can be developed by the delegation of management and supervisory responsibilities; and that nursing care can be enhanced by team planning, group effort, and high staff morale. This is the philosophy of team nursing. Upon it is built a method or procedure by which the philosophy is implemented.

Team Nursing as a Method of Assignment

In team nursing two or more members of the staff, one being designated leader, are assigned to work together in giving care to a group of patients. If the head nurse, as portrayed in Chapter 6, is responsible for only 12 to 15 patients she will probably have but one nursing team. In larger divisions, however, two or more team leaders function under the head nurse whose role is therefore somewhat different. Since many head nurses will be concerned about their responsibility for organizing nursing teams and giving counsel to team leaders, discussion in this chapter will deal mainly with the head nurse's responsibility in her traditional role.

The team leader, always a professional nurse, maintains continuity. Along with the head nurse she is responsible for diagnosing and meeting the needs of all patients on her team. In making assignments, she retains for herself the care of some patients, but keeps in close enough contact with each patient that he identifies her as his nurse. He also knows the other members of the team and relates to them. The fact that the team leader gives medications and the practical nurse bathes him matters little under these circumstances because he understands the functioning of the team and is aware of the interest of each member in his welfare. Still, he is usually more comfortable when he can count on the same team member giving his general care each day. When a change is necessary, he feels better to be told ahead of time and to know that the next person is familiar

[6] For this definition the writer is indebted to Virginia Earles who was a graduate student at the time the definition was formulated.

with the way he likes things done. Good planning assures that the new nurse will assist with the patient's care the day before she is to take over the responsibility.

When the team leader is the only professional nurse on the team she must be relieved for her days off by a nurse who is not a member of the team (see time plan for nursing team, Figure 11, p. 187). The relief nurse probably knows the patients, however, through having relieved on evenings or nights. It is to be hoped the team leader is replaced by the same nurse each week. This, however, may not be possible since many factors must be taken into account in planning time (see p. 176). Under any circumstance the relief nurse needs a full report from the team leader the preceding day. If circumstances prevent this, comprehensive nursing care plans are of great help in achieving continuity. Written reports and records while useful are a less effective way to provide this carry-over of information.

The team leader should not fail to make the assignment to team members for her first day off. The rationale of the assignment should be explained to the nurse who will relieve her so that continuity in care will not be unwittingly broken if changes are necessary. It is obvious that continuity in care for patients can be provided only when the members of the team remain relatively constant and when the team keeps the same group of patients. Nurses who get to know and care about their patients are reluctant to change to another group. Knowledge of all patients on the division by the entire staff is far less important than providing continuity. Other ways can be found to acquaint the staff with patients on other teams.

Team assignments. Some hospitals which are committed to the philosophy of team nursing have built new wings or reconstructed old ones to facilitate team functioning. The unit is divided into geographic sections in each of which a nursing team operates. In the central nurses' station each team has its own assignment sheet, cardex, medicine card holder, chart rack. A completely stocked medicine cupboard is available for each team. In these situations a patient is cared for by the team assigned to the section in which his room is located. As a result of assigning patients according to location the nursing load may be heavier for one team than for another. If the difference is fairly consistent the matter may be handled by having more members on the team with the heavier assignment. However, if the load varies frequently it may be necessary to have one staff member free to float among the various teams. This plan militates against some of the values of the team method, namely, continuity in care for patients and satisfactions for the staff member.

When the head nurse is responsible for a large division and has two or more teams to care for patients, she may find it more appropriate to assign patients according to their needs rather than by geographic areas. The team leaders help her decide the team in which patients shall be placed. They take into account the degree of illness of the patients, the number and types of operations, treatments, and tests together with the composition of the team in determining the assignment. They should as far as possible consider the location of patients for each team and not have them widely scattered. As indicated several times in these pages continuity in patient care with all its values is enhanced when the composition of the team is stable in both personnel and patients.

Some hospitals operate on the team plan during the day period only. However, any staff composed of a professional nurse and one other individual can work as a team. During the evening and night periods the number of teams may have to be reduced. The charge nurses should have full understanding of the philosophy of the team and ways to implement it.

Composition of the nursing team. A nursing team is usually composed of professional and nonprofessional members although there is nothing in the philosophy of the team to preclude two or three professional nurses from working as a team in the care of one or more acutely ill or postoperative patients. The manner in which the team functions is the same regardless of the individuals who compose it. A competent professional nurse is appointed team leader. This responsibility is not one to be passed around to any staff nurse who happens to be working on a given day. The individual chosen as team leader should be a nurse who gives individualized, comprehensive nursing care. She should have knowledge of the objectives for patient care on the division and believe in the values of continuity. Understanding and acceptance of the philosophy of team nursing and knowledge of the responsibilities entailed in team leadership are essential. The team leader needs to be familiar with the capabilities and limitations of practical nurses and aides, with the experience needs of students and staff members. An inservice program for the preparation of team leaders is extremely helpful. In its absence, the head nurse must select the team leader carefully, teach, and supervise her until she is proficient. A new nurse, unfamiliar with the division, cannot possibly function as a team leader except in name.

Experimentation is needed to determine the composition of the team which is best for the individual unit. An analysis of the proportion of time necessary for activities which require professional competence and those which can be performed by nonprofessional nursing personnel will indicate whether the team should be composed of an equal number of professional and nonprofessional members or whether the proportion should be one to two, one to three, two to one, or some other ratio. When there is more than one nursing team on a division and staffing does not permit a safe or effective proportion of professional to nonprofessional personnel in any one of them, it is probable that the number of teams should be reduced, to one if necessary, if this will make for maximum use of professional nurses for patients who most need their care.

It is desirable for student nurses, professional and practical, to have experience working in nursing teams, and senior professional students need to serve as team leaders for at least a short period. They must be closely supervised by either the clinical instructor or by the head nurse both to safeguard the patients and to assure the students a valuable learning experience.

Functioning of the nursing team. In establishing the nursing team, it is important to define clearly the extent of the responsibility of the team leader and the patient care activities she is to assume in relation to those which the head nurse will retain. Three points are important. *First,* the head nurse must know at all times the condition of the patients and the plan for their care and must be assured that assignments and workmanship contribute to quality nursing. *Second,* the team leader must have freedom to use her initiative and the opportunity to nurse, to supervise, and to teach unencumbered by the responsibility for details of nursing administration. *Third,* in all instances it is essential that the head nurse and team leader work closely and cooperatively.

Responsibilities of the team leader. The leader and her team members, with the participation of the head nurse, *analyze their patients' problems and nursing needs, plan their care,* write patient portraits and nursing orders, changing these as necessary. For this purpose the team leader *holds a daily team conference.* She *plans assignments within the team,* the head nurse giving close supervision until the leader thoroughly understands the principles involved and gains judgment in making assignments. It should hardly be necessary to say that emphasis is focused on individualized care and the concept of the patient as a person only if patients are assigned by name. When room numbers are used personnel tend to think in terms of rooms, not individuals.

The responsibility for the care of patients assigned to the team is delegated to the team leader who is also charged with the *supervision and informal instruction of her team members.* At all times the leader must be aware of the condition of her patients and the activities of the team members. For this reason the team leader, not the head nurse or secretary, informs the team members of new orders for their patients. Whenever possible, she *accompanies physicians* and the head nurse to see patients on her team. Unfortunately this is not always feasible for by the time the team leader is located the doctor has often visited the patient and left the floor.

However, when new plans for patients need to be made, the team leader keeps the secretary informed of her whereabouts so she will not miss the doctor's visit. If the team leader has not seen the physician, the head nurse reports to her any new developments. Needless to say the *head nurse is kept informed* at all times about the patient's condition and problems so that she is prepared to confer with the doctor should the leader not be available. It can be recognized that frequent reports and conferences between the head nurse and team leader are essential to proper team functioning. The *report to the evening team or teams* should be given by the team leader, the head nurse, of course, being present. If the entire staff is present for the afternoon report, each nurse has an opportunity to learn about the patients who are not assigned to her team.

Under ideal circumstances the team leader has a patient assignment. The importance of bath time in getting to know the patient has been pointed out earlier in this chapter. Some team leaders regularly assign new patients to themselves the first day in order to become acquainted, to study the patient's needs, and to explain the team method of assignment to the patient if it seems advisable. Assigning new patients to herself may not always be a wise policy, however, particularly if a student nurse needs experience in planning for a new patient or if the patient is to be operated his first day and the team leader should not be tied up with postoperative care. Important as it is for the team leader to have a patient assignment, she should guard against getting so involved with one patient that she has no time left for supervision.

Unfortunately there is a tendency for some team leaders who enjoy a managerial role to assign all patients to team members and spend their own time in other ways. When a team has more than 12 or 15 patients, the leader can easily keep occupied in giving medicines and treatments, checking orders, charting, making rounds. Some team leaders rarely see their patients except to administer a drug. The concept of team nursing is thus defeated. With a large number of patients assigned to the team it may be necessary for the team leader to omit assigning patients to herself. However, it is very important that she plan her activities carefully, providing time to assist and supervise team members, observe, teach, and especially get to know patients well enough to diagnose their needs and give leadership in planning their care.

The team conference conducted by the team leader is the greatest single distinguishing feature of the nursing team method of assignment. Without it, the assignment is no different from the patient or functional method except that the team leader instead of the head nurse delegates the duties. The heart of the team concept is group planning.

At some time during the day after the patients have received their morning care, the team members sit down together in conference. A quiet place where the group can be free from interruption should be found, if possible. Late morning or early afternoon when the patients have been settled for rest hour is often a good time to meet. Since someone must be available for patient calls, however, it is well that the various teams hold their conferences at different times. One team can then relieve for another. If well planned and conducted the conference requires no more than half or three fourths of an hour. The team leader assumes the role of chairman. Informality is maintained with each team member contributing freely.

In general, there are three parts to the conference: 1) reports on patients, 2) planning care for new patients and changing plans as needed for others, and 3) planning the next day's assignment. Team members, particularly nurses' aides, practical nurses, and young student nurses need help in knowing what to report and in making their reports concise, complete, and interesting. It is usually neither necessary nor possible, in the time available, to have a report on all patients. Team members bring up for discussion those patients they wish to present. The leader supplements reports as indicated. Members are encouraged to ask questions of one another in order that all may be fully informed relative to each patient's symptoms, progress, problems, the results of care, and suggestions for meeting the patient's needs. Minor changes in the plan for patient care can often be made by the team leader during the conference. Major changes and new plans are written later when there is time to organize them properly. If the patient is assigned to a professional nurse, graduate or student, she makes notes during the conference of the plan evolved by the group, and following the conference writes up the portrait and nursing orders. The team leader gives whatever assistance the nurse needs, reviews and approves the plan. The leader herself or another professional team member writes the portraits and orders for patients assigned to nonprofessional members. The latter contribute to the making of the plan but usually do not have the command of English or ability to organize material sufficiently to write it in useful form.

The assignments for the following day are made in relation to the condition of the patients and the time required for their care. Each team member knows for which patients she is to have full responsibility, any parts of the care which will be given by someone else, the way these activities are to be coordinated, whether she is to assist another team member with any of her patients.

Since patients are frequently admitted after the conference has been completed, all individuals recognize that changes in assignment may need to be made. Since some changes are inevitable, the team holds a short conference to make necessary adjustments the next morning following the report of the night nurse or while the patients are eating breakfast. New patients are briefly discussed at this time. (See Special Reports, Chapter 19.) Some team leaders assign themselves the taking of morning temperatures. This gives them a chance to converse with each patient and to see his condition at the beginning of the day. The other members of the team prepare patients for the morning meal. Each member cares for her own patients and those of the team leader are divided among the other members. A breakdown in individualized care is not usually objectionable for this brief period.

A variation in the team conference is used in some hospitals. Because time is limited, only 10 to 15 minutes are spent in the conference. Rather than consider all patients superficially or several briefly, the team spends the time in discussion of one patient attempting to discern his needs and make a plan for his care. If a conference is held each day, there is usually opportunity to discuss those patients who have obvious problems. Unfortunately, the abbreviated conference provides no time for a follow-up report on results achieved by the nursing care plan evolved by the team. The responsibility for evaluation, therefore, rests with the team leader who should work with the team member assigned to the patient in revising the plan, if necessary.

Responsibilities of the head nurse in team nursing. The head nurse gives the team leader as much guidance and help as she needs, recognizing that when this is a new experience the leader needs a great deal of assistance. Together they discuss the patient's progress, effects of nursing care, his problems and needs, the plan for his care. The head nurse stimulates the leader to study and to think. Until the leader has become very proficient in delegating responsibility the head nurse reviews assignments and discusses the capability of team members for providing the care needed by the assigned patients. Most new team leaders wish help in planning team conferences—points to discuss, methods of conducting them. The head nurse attends the conferences after which she and the team leader together evaluate them. Although the head nurse is careful not to take over the meeting she is helpful to the team leader by participating with questions and comments. Another point at which the inexperienced team leader needs assistance is in supervision. (See Chapter 13.) The head nurse can never shift the entire responsibility for supervision of patient care and personnel to the team leader yet she has an obligation to help the leader develop her judgment and increase her skill in all areas of delegated responsibility.

The head nurse should make very clear to the team leader her obligation to adhere to the principles of good nursing, to keep the head nurse informed of difficulties related to patient care, and to report problems with personnel and equipment.

The head nurse or clerk usually transcribes doctors' orders to the cardex and calls for any equipment needed for the patient's care. The head nurse keeps the leader informed of changes in doctors' orders, thus obviating the need for the leader to check the order book frequently for new orders during periods of heavy activity.

The head nurse should know how the team leader is spending her time. If any responsibilities are being neglected the head nurse and team leader together should review objectives and consider obstacles preventing their achievement. The head nurse needs to remember that patient care and growth of team members are to be evaluated rather than the team leader's actions, per se.

Outcomes of the team method of assignment. In addition to the improvement in nursing care which has resulted in situations where the nursing team has been instituted, other outcomes have been evident. These outcomes have in turn contributed to better patient care. Nurse administrators and head nurses have noted marked growth in the staff nurses who were made team leaders—growth in their ability and willingness to assume responsibility, in their ability to organize work, to analyze patient needs, to plan patient care. There is much greater interest in patients and understanding of their behavior by the entire staff as a result of group effort to think through nursing problems. Because of the increased responsibility given to staff nurses they have been happier, and more satisfied with their jobs. Likewise, nonprofessional team members have a greater sense of importance and of belonging because their contributions are recognized as valuable, and because they receive more supervision and instruction. When an individual feels she is important to the team, she is less likely to take an unscheduled day off when some personal pleasure or problem presents itself.

Another important outcome of the team method of assignment is the freeing of the head nurse for over-all planning for improved patient care and for staff development. By transferring the details of supervision to team leaders the head nurse need no longer feel the full weight of responsibility for the well-being of the patients assigned to practical nurses and aides. When these individuals are given direct assignments by the head nurse it is she who must be continuously aware of the specimen that is due to be collected, the side bars that must be kept up, and all the other measures that need to be carried out in a safe and satisfactory way. With these responsibilities turned over to the team leader for immediate supervision the head nurse is less harassed. She has time to think. Thinking is essential to long-range planning; long-range planning is essential to progress.

Nursing service administrators and head nurses alike have had the erroneous idea that all staffing problems could be solved by the team method of assignment. Nothing is further from the truth. As a matter of fact, the team cannot function unless there is a stable staff. The very term *team* implies that the same group is working together consistently. Nor does the team method require fewer nurses than other methods. The nursing load on a division is the same regardless of the method used to divide up the work. If administrators are concerned with quality nursing, they will realize that the team is a better way to achieve the chief objective of the hospital, good patient care, but that it cannot be accomplished without adequate personnel.

In the beginning, when the team method is being started on a unit, a larger staff may be required. The team leader must learn to organize for a group instead of just for herself. She must give thought to planning for conferences. She must learn to supervise. These activities have not been hers before. Time is required to develop skill in their performance. Time thus spent by the leader is not available for direct patient care. Likewise, if conferences for planning patient care have not been held previously, time will need to be allowed for them. It is possible that once the nursing team is a going concern on a unit, no more staff will be required than was necessary under former methods, provided, of course, the patient care previously given was of good quality. In other words, although the number of a staff cannot be decreased by the use of team nursing, a better quality of care will be possible with the same number of personnel (if there were previously enough to carry the nursing load) due to the fact that morale is higher, interest greater, and the staff more competent.

Instituting team nursing. Since team nursing is not practiced in all hospitals, the head nurse may wonder how to go about instituting it on her division. It cannot be done overnight. Success is probably directly proportionate to the care with which planning is done. In the first place, the head nurse does not try to start the team method without the consent and cooperation of the departmental and nursing service administrators. Staffing is usually controlled by the nursing office, and, as has been pointed out, team functioning is dependent upon a stable staff. Likewise, important undertakings need the active support and interest of all who are concerned. The nursing and hospital administrators are vitally concerned with patient care.

Every member of the division staff should participate in the planning for team organization. Professional nurses will wish to learn through reading how other institutions have proceeded when establishing the team method. They will need to think through, as a group, their objectives, the organization of the team, lines of responsibility, the functions, and relationships of all staff members. Consideration must be given to time planning and to relief for team members (See Chapter 8). Every detail should be thought through and decision made as to whether the present staff is sufficient or whether additional members will be needed to insure success. Only after plans are made in detail and every person who is to function in the team has been thoroughly instructed in the part she is to play, only when the medical staff of the unit has been informed of the plan, only when the time for starting is known to all personnel and all is in readiness, should team nursing be instituted. Continuous evaluation and frequent adjustments will be necessary, but if the nursing administration and the division staff, both, are convinced of the values to be gained, the method will succeed.

PRIVATE DUTY NURSING

Another individual to whom nursing care is delegated is the private duty nurse. Although the head nurse neither selects her nor determines which patients shall have private nurses, she has obligations to both the patient and the nurse. For many years it has been customary to engage "special nurses" to care for the critically ill patient who requires constant observation and a great deal of physical care. Many lives have been saved by the ministrations of these nurses. Today some hospitals are recognizing their responsibility to provide all the care needed by a patient regardless of the severity of illness. Progressive patient care (see Chapter 3) makes it possible for the acutely ill individual to receive the intensive care he requires, without having to employ private duty nurses.

It is unfortunate when patients and families who can ill afford even the hospital charges find it necessary to assume extra expense for private nurses. Many patients assume that following surgery private nurses are essential. When questioned by the patient or family about this need the response of most nurses is that "of course the patient will be more comfortable." Perhaps the day will come when it will be a challenge to the nursing departments of all hospitals to satisfy the patient's needs without his having to employ his own nurses. However, there will no doubt always be some patients who are willing and able to pay for companionship and additional care beyond their real needs. Some families will be more at ease to know the patient has a nurse in constant attendance during periods when he is acutely uncomfortable. It is likely, therefore, that within the forseeable future, there will still be a place for the private duty nurse.

The hospital is responsible for the nursing care of all its patients. Although not employed by the hospital, the private duty nurse is considered to be a definite part of the nursing staff and is responsible to and under the guidance of the nursing department. In this capacity she is entitled to the same privileges and expected to abide by the same rules and regulations as other staff members. The head nurse should know as much about the patient nursed by a private duty nurse as she does about every other patient on her unit. She also needs to know the type and quality of care which he is receiving and to assure herself that the nurse appreciates the patient's nursing needs and knows how to meet them, that she understands the doctor's orders for the patient and the procedure methods approved by the hospital.

If the nurse is new to the hospital the head nurse sees that she is introduced to all members of the floor personnel and to the arrangement of the unit. Whatever assistance she needs in caring for the patient and in relief for meals the head nurse provides. The fact that the patient has a private duty nurse does not bar him from all the additional care which he needs. Hospital and division policy should be interpreted to the nurse. Doctors' orders are transcribed and all administrative detail handled by the unit secretary just as for other patients. Equipment is made available. The head nurse helps the private duty nurse grow professionally when she keeps her informed of new treatments, drugs, procedures, and equipment. She should make a point of notifying the nurse of lectures, exhibits, and demonstrations which are open to all nurses.

The private duty nurse, in turn, has certain obligations to the hospital and to the head nurse. She is expected to follow division and hospital policy, to see that records are properly kept and that verbal orders are not accepted. She is expected to give good nursing care and to follow orders accurately. The head nurse must see that the nurse gives her a report when she goes off duty and receives a report when she arrives on the division. It is not sufficient for the private duty nurse to report to another nurse who is relieving her. She should keep the head nurse informed throughout the day of the condition of her patient and problems in his care. Under no circumstances does she leave the floor for meals without reporting to the nurse in charge and having assurance that her patient will receive the necessary care. Her meal hours are arranged to accord with the program of the unit if her patient will need attention during her absence. The special nurse should not hesitate to ask for assistance when it is needed. She is expected to use supplies including linen economically, to take prompt and proper care of equipment which she has used, to maintain a clean and orderly environment, and to set a good example of professional nursing.

SUMMARY

A division nursing staff may be made up of professional nurses, both graduate and student, practical nurses, practical nurse students, and nurses' aides. Among the groups and within each category of personnel there are wide variations in education, experience, and personality. The head nurse and the staff nurses who relieve her for days and hours need to be well informed concerning these differences, in order that patients may receive safe, effective care. In general, graduate professional nurses who have been on the staff several weeks should be able to care for any patient assigned to the division. Licensed practical nurses are prepared to nurse patients in situations free from complexity and to assist professional nurses with those whose care is more complicated. When the practical nurse is assigned to the acutely ill, a professional nurse must always have the patient in view and should observe him closely at frequent intervals. In recent years, job demands on practical nurses have approximated those of the registered nurse. As a result, it has been suggested by some nurse leaders that practical nurse schools gradually be replaced by associate degree nursing programs in community colleges. In contrast to these developments, a few hospitals today, instead of assigning the practical nurse to patients, keep control of her activities by making her responsible to a professional nurse for performance of specific technical procedures. Nurses aides preferably assist professional nurses rather than give direct care to patients.

Assignments are made on the basis of the patient's needs and the competency of the staff member to meet them. Several other considerations need to be kept in mind: namely, the best time for carrying out the parts of the patient's care which must be given by a professional nurse; the amount of supervision available for the less able staff members; the needs of all patients which are to be assigned to one staff member; the geographic proximity of patients to be cared for by one person; the needs of all the patients on the division in relation to the availability of "ideal" persons to care for them; and the importance of continuity in care.

The use of nonprofessional personnel for direct care makes the patient assignment method impossible. The functional method defeats any attempt to provide continuity. Team nursing which is both a philosophy and method of assignment is probably the best known way to maintain continuous care for the patient. In this method, a group of staff members with a professional nurse as leader work together in a cooperative, coordinated way to provide individualized care for a group of patients. In the usual pattern today one or more nursing teams with their leaders function under the head nurse who is the coordinator, administrator, and supervisor of nursing care. The head nurse teaches, guides, and helps the new team leader in every aspect of leadership. She assigns members and patients to the team. The leader assigns team members to individual patients. Values are lost if continuity is not maintained by means of stability in team membership and patient assignment. The team leader through the team conference, in which the head nurse participates, sees that members are kept informed about the patients. Together they study patients' needs and develop nursing care plans.

Values of team nursing are many for both patients and staff. The method can succeed, however, only if plans for instituting it are carefully laid and the team leader is a good nurse, well prepared for her responsibilities.

Another person who gives direct patient care is the private duty nurse. Although employed by the patient, she is responsible to the nursing service for the quality of nursing care given to her patient. The head nurse in other words does not surrender her responsibility for the patient. She must know his condition, the kind of care he is receiving, its adequacy, and is obligated to the patient and the nurse to give all the assistance and instruction necessary. The special nurse is expected to fit into the program of the division and to adhere to its policies.

QUESTIONS FOR DISCUSSION

1. If the nurses' aides in your hospital are assigned to give routine care to assigned patients, what would be the effect of changing their role to that of assisting the professional nurse as suggested in the text?
2. In your opinion are nurses' aides given too much responsibility? If so, give examples. What do you see as the solution?
3. What are the distinctions in activities performed by the practical and the professional nurse in your hospital? It would be helpful to list things each does that the other does not do, and those things which both do. In the latter, is any distinction made concerning which personnel category is selected for the task?

EXERCISES

1. *First*, roughly classify the 1) physical, 2) observational, 3) emotional and psychological, and 4) teaching needs of all patients on your division for any given day. Use a scale of high, medium, and low for each need area. An article, Criteria for assignment of the nursing aide, in American Journal of Nursing, Volume 49 (May 1949) pp. 311-314 will be helpful in classifying.

Second, through study of the assignment sheet for the day, through observation, and if necessary, diplomatic questioning, determine the category of personnel who gave care to each patient that day.

Third, analyze your findings to determine whether the staff member was competent through *training, experience,* and *personal characteristics* to meet the patients' needs. What changes in the assignment would appear to have been advisable?

2. Question an experienced head nurse about the responsibility she assumes for patients cared for by private duty nurses. Does she have any problems in meeting her responsibility? If so, what are they? Suggest a solution to the problems.

3. Study two or three weeks' assignment sheets for one division. Were patients assigned by name? Were they assigned to specific staff members? Was this true for all periods of the day? How many patients had the same person assigned to give him morning care for five consecutive days? for more than five days? What was the maximum length of time one staff member took consecutive care of any patient? How many patients had more than two nurses (day shift) in five days? more than three? In general how would you evaluate the way assignments were planned?

4. If you have had experience in team nursing, compare it with the description of team functioning found in this chapter. Evaluate your experience. How could it have been improved?

5. If you have not had experience as a team leader make a plan for preparing yourself for the role. Indicate the specific help you would wish from the head nurse.

REFERENCES

American Nurses' Association's first position on education for nursing, Amer. J. Nurs., Vol. 65 (December 1965), pp. 106-111.
    Members of the A.N.A. Committee on Education, composed of an illustrious group of nurse educators, prepared this statement of position which was adopted by the A.N.A. Board of Directors in September 1965.

Brackett, Mary E., and Fogt, Joan R. Is comprehensive nursing care a realistic goal?, Nurs. Outlook, Vol. 9 (July 1961), pp. 402-404.
    These nursing service administrators believe comprehensive nursing is attainable if team nursing is used, team leaders are given help in establishing priorities, and if nurse educators prepare nurses for realistic practice. An excellent article, practical in approach, lofty in its ideals.

Brooks, Ethel A. Team nursing—1961, Amer. J. Nurs., Vol. 61 (April 1961), pp. 87-91.

Ten years of experience with team nursing at Hartford Hospital finds continuing enthusiasm for the idea and the method. The discussion of methods used to prepare team leaders and to spread the use of team nursing through the entire nursing service makes this article of special interest to head nurses. A basic pattern for the nursing team gives a concise picture of its functioning.

Corona, Dorothy F., and Black, Eunice E. One hospital's approach to team nursing, Nurs. Outlook, Vol. 11 (July 1963), pp. 506-507.
A description of the way a hospital in which team nursing was failing studied and improved the method.

Crumpton, Evelyn, and Rogers, Eileen P. Some effects of team nursing on a psychiatric ward, Nurs. Res., Vol. 12 (Summer 1963), pp. 181-182.
In most respects the effect of team nursing was favorable in the situation tested.

Fritz, Edna, and Murphy, Marion. An analysis of positions on nursing education, Nurs. Outlook, Vol. 14 (February 1966), pp. 20-24.
Two leading nurse educators compare the positions of the N.L.N. and the A.N.A. on nursing education.

Godard, Jean R., and Douglas, Jean. Is team nursing the answer? Canad. Nurse, Vol. 61 (July 1965), pp. 546-548.
To answer the question: Miss Godard says, "No!"; Miss Douglas, "Yes!"

Hershey, Nathan. A nurse's liability for negligence in supervision, Amer. J. Nurs., Vol. 62 (May 1962), pp. 115-116.
Because job titles (ie, practical nurse, aide) do not indicate an individual's preparation nor competency, the professional nurse who is responsible for assigning activities and for the outcome of their performance, must make sure the person is competent to perform the task.
Every head nurse should read this article for her own protection.

Improving clinical proficiencies of private duty nurses, Amer. J. Nurs., Vol. 64 (August 1964), pp. 92-93.
Innovations in a number of states regarding private duty nurses include self-evaluation forms, periodic evaluation by hospital nursing service, and educational programs—compulsory and voluntary.

Kron, Thora. Nurses' aides need clearer directions, Amer. J. Nurs., Vol. 63 (March 1963), pp. 118-119.
Many illustrations are given of the misunderstandings which result when the nurse, who is responsible for care given by nonprofessionals, fails to make sure her instructions are clear.

——— Nursing Team Leadership, Philadelphia, W. B. Saunders Co., 1961.
A concise, very useful presentation of the functioning of the nursing team and the role of the leader.

Lambertsen, Eleanor C. Nursing Team Organization and Functioning, New York, Bureau of Publications, Teachers College, Columbia University, 1953.
This manual resulted from a study of the nursing team in action. It clearly describes the philosophy and functioning of the team, the duties and responsibilities of the team leader and head nurse. The last part of the manual suggests methods for organizing a hospital nursing service on a team basis.

New, Peter Kong-Ming, and Nite, Gladys. Staffing and interaction, Nurs. Outlook, Vol. 8 (July 1960), pp. 396-400.
Annotation in Chapter 8 reference.

Nurse's aides as aids to nursing, Nurs. Outlook, Vol. 10 (August 1962), p. 505.
Nurse's aides are *not* nurses. They should not be prepared in the same manner as nurses but as apprentices, on the job, to perform certain tasks.

Private duty nurse role presents some paradoxes, Hospitals, Vol. 39 (January 16, 1965), p. 78.
The hospital may be held liable for negligence of a private duty nurse. Her rights are similar to those of the doctor who is not in the hospital employ. The hospital does have the right to regulate its internal activities although it has little authority over the private duty nurse.

Rasmussen, Etta H. Preparation for supervising licensed practical nurses, Nurs. Outlook, Vol. 10 (July 1962), pp. 472-475.
Since professional nurses are responsible for supervising practical nurses the professional nurse needs considerable knowledge about the preparation of the L.P.N. and practice in supervision of this group. Such content should be included in the curriculums of professional nursing schools.

Sorensen, Gladys. Dependency: a factor in nursing care, Amer. J. Nurs., Vol. 66 (August 1966), pp. 1762-1763.
As a result of her experience with one patient during various stages of dependency, the writer raises some very interesting questions relative to assignment and time planning for staff.

Statement of functions of the licensed practical nurse, Amer. J. Nurs., Vol. 64 (March 1964), p. 93.
The statement which was approved by the A.N.A. Board of Directors in January 1964 serves as a guide in delegating responsibility to members of this group.

Stevenson, Neva M. Perspective on developments in practical nursing, Nurs. Outlook, Vol. 8 (January 1960), pp. 34-37.
The history of practical nurse education is traced up to the present when it is now expected that the practical nurse will be prepared 1) "to nurse the patient in situations relatively free of scientific complexity under the direction of the nurse or physician, with a minimum of on-the-spot supervision"; and 2) "to assist the professional nurse . . . in more complex nursing situations."

————— Roles of the licensed practical nurse should determine curriculum design, Nurs. Outlook, Vol. 10 (January 1962), pp. 30-31.
The practical nurse has two roles. The limits of each should be clearly defined and interpreted to both practical and professional nurses. These limits in no way lessen the L.P.N.'s value.

————— The better utilization of licensed practical nurses, Nurs. Outlook, Vol. 13 (July 1965), pp. 34-37.
Miss Stevenson's logical, down-to-earth description of the legal and educational limits on practical nurse activities should be read by every nurse—professional and practical. The responsibilities of the professional nurse are compared and contrasted with those of the practical nurse.

Williams, Margaret Aasterud. The myths and assumptions about team nursing, Nurs. Forum, Vol. 3 (No. 4, 1964), pp. 61-73.
Just because a hospital or a division says it has team nursing, just because there are team conferences and some kind of nursing care plan—these facts do not indicate that team nursing (which is a philosophy, not a method) is actually in operation.

Wyatt, Lalla J., and Hannah, Helen D. Does team nursing work in a psychiatric hospital?, Amer. J. Nurs., Vol. 64 (June 1964), pp. 132-133.
An experiment showed that patients received better care and team leaders and members have been working "even harder to give patients the support they need."

chapter 13

SUPERVISION AND EVALUATION OF NURSING CARE

The objective of the hospital and, therefore, the objective of the head nurse and her staff for their division is to provide a high quality of care for each patient in accordance with his individual needs. Supervision is essential if this objective is to be achieved. The head nurse is the supervisor of patient care on her unit.

In the broad sense supervision of nursing care involves several facets of responsibility which have already been discussed—diagnosing the patient's needs, planning his care, implementing the plan through written nursing care plans and through delegation of responsibility. However, supervision of nursing care pertains to patients as a group as well as to patients as individuals. The over-all supervisory process may be said to have four elements in addition to establishing long-range objectives for nursing care of patients on the unit. (See Chapter 11.) *First,* making an assessment to obtain a comprehensive picture of the situation and to determine the condition of patients and the effects of medical and nursing care; *second,* implementing or directing nursing care; *third,* evaluating the quality of care given, to determine changes which might improve it; *fourth,* planning, putting into operation, and evaluating the revised methods. Thus it can be seen that supervision is a continuous process. Another aspect of supervision entails teaching and the further development of individuals who participate in giving care. This educational responsibility of supervision will be considered in Part 3.

ASSESSMENT OF THE SITUATION

To make an accurate assessment the head nurse must assemble information which will affect the administration of nursing care. Included in this category are the bed occupancy, the number of acutely ill patients and others requiring unusual amounts of nursing time; new patients, patients to be discharged, and those with changes in medical orders. She will also check on staffing, illness and absence, difficulties experienced by the staff during the head nurse's absence, and any unresolved problems. Information of this nature helps the head nurse establish priorities for her attention as well as priorities in patient care.

Making an assessment of the patients who are under the head nurse's jurisdiction should be a planned orderly process carried out by the head nurse, or by the nurse in charge of the division, at least once on each tour of duty. Such assessment takes place during nursing rounds. To assume the responsibility the nurse needs to be equipped with sound clinical knowledge and information about patients which has been updated through reports from her staff. Of what does this necessary knowledge consist?

First, the head nurse must know the signs and symptoms associated with the various disorders found on the service. For example, it is important that she understand the sigificance of imbalance between fluid intake and output and of a decrease in either in relation to the patient's clinical condition and symptoms. An awareness of the implications of changes in blood pressure and the importance of periodic checking of these signs is essential. The head nurse needs also to have knowledge of the effects of drugs, both favorable and unfavorable, and to be aware of their symptoms. She must be able to recognize physical and emotional danger signals, to understand their implications and seriousness.

Second, the head nurse must know of what good nursing consists for patients on the service. In many respects this varies with the age, degree of illness, and the disorders of the patients assigned to the floor. Although good nursing in the various specialties differs in some ways, certain principles apply to all nursing. Patients need sleep and rest. Insofar as possible they should be comfortable, happy, and satisfied with their care. They must be protected from harm and their therapy must be carried out in a way to be effective and safe.

Third, the head nurse needs information about individual patients including age, condition, diagnosis, and disabilities or special problems. Only when she is so informed is the head nurse in a position to determine the patient's nursing needs and his progress.

Fourth, the head nurse needs knowledge of the total program of medical care for the individual patient and the nurse's responsibility in relation to it, preferably from having participated in the formulation of the plan. Without knowledge of the purpose, expected results, and accompanying effects associated with x-ray, various diagnostic tests, physical, occupational, drug, and diet therapy, surgical and other therapeutic procedures, the head nurse cannot intelligently observe the patient or direct his nursing care. Important symptoms may go unnoted, patients may lack proper instruction and reassurance, errors of judgment may be made and necessary nursing measures omitted. The head nurse also needs to be aware of fatigue and irritability in patients resulting from a continual round of medical treatments and tests. Sometimes there is little opportunity to carry on such nursing measures as turning the patient, giving skin and mouth care, providing general comfort measures, because the patient is continually being tested, examined, or treated by the doctor or by the nurse on the doctor's order. The physician is not always cognizant of the fact that the patient's rest is being seriously interrupted and that he is failing to receive supportive nursing care. The tests or treatments may be paramount to the patient's welfare, but the head nurse must know the relative importance of rest, nursing care, and medical care in the particular situation and should keep the physician informed of problems.

Assessment by the head nurse of the situation on her division involves purposeful observation of each patient's changing condition and needs, his environment, the process of giving care, the effects of the care on the individual patient, and the interaction between the patient and the personnel. No exhaustive account of observations the head nurse should make is either possible or necessary here. An attempt will be made, however, to enumerate general areas in which assessment is needed and to give a few illustrations in each.

The Patient's Condition and Needs

In assessing the situation which influences the patient's well-being the head nurse needs to note his general condition, whether he is gaining strength from day to day, whether his color is improving, his dyspnea decreasing. Are his vital signs changing? What do his laboratory, x-ray, or operative reports show? What is their significance? On the basis of the patient's diagnosis and therapy are the anticipated symptoms appearing? disappearing? Is his abdomen distended? his Foley catheter draining? his suction working properly? Does the patient show any tendency toward pressure sores? If he does, has he been receiving the care which has been prescribed? If he is showing such tendencies in spite of this care, perhaps a change in method is indicated.

The head nurse will wish to observe the condition of the mouth of all patients who are very ill, febrile, dehydrated, helpless, debilitated, or who for any reason are susceptible to mouth lesions. She should know the care which the patient is receiving and institute new methods if good results are not observed. She will note whether there is a tendency to orthopedic deformities and institute protective measures to prevent foot drop, rotation of extremities, muscular contractures. She will recognize need for support to help the patient maintain good posture and muscular relaxation and the desirability of exercise, either active or passive, to maintain muscle tone. She will note the need of the patient for remedial or preventive care on which the physical therapist might give advice. The condition of perineal sutures and the wounds of patients whose dressings are changed by the nurse will be observed and the character of drainage and discharge noted.

The head nurse will wish to visit the bedside of critically ill patients many times a day to observe change in condition and note whether the care he is receiving is adequate and effective. She should see all postoperative patients as soon as they return to the floor and frequently thereafter until the vital signs are stabilized and the patient is conscious. By her visits she not only assures herself that the patient's condition is satisfactory but she is able to observe whether the nurse caring for him is able to give all the attention that is needed. Likewise patients who have had painful treatments or examinations following which reactions frequently occur should be visited by the head nurse during and soon after the treatment is completed. Not only will her visit bolster the patient's confidence but it will indicate to her whether the treatment is progressing as it should, whether the patient's condition is satisfactory, and whether he is receiving sufficient care.

The head nurse should be very conscious of the safety of her patients. Are those who are critically ill and irresponsible being observed closely enough? Do patients who need them have side bars on their beds and are they tightly locked? Are restraints correctly applied? Are patients securely fastened on stretchers and in wheel chairs? Are they warm enough, do they look presentable?

The patient's mental outlook, orientation, and state of consciousness should be compared from day to day by the head nurse. Is he more cheerful and optimistic as the days go by or is he becoming more discouraged and despondent? How much interest is he taking in his appearance and surroundings, in other patients? Is he understanding and accepting doctors' orders and nursing care or merely tolerating them? How well is he accepting his disability or prognosis? Does he need or wish help from his doctor or clergyman? Is he unduly concerned about what he considers to be lack of progress? Is the patient excessively apprehensive or too placid about his impending operation or a treatment he is to undergo? With either of these patients the head nurse will plan to spend time later. Perhaps she can manage to administer part of his care herself. Through ministering to his physical needs, she may make it easier for the worried patient to express his fears. On the other hand she will try to help the individual who is not facing up to an impending dangerous or painful procedure to understand something of what he is to undergo and how he will feel. Otherwise he will receive a severe shock for which he is quite unprepared.

How does the patient feel about his room, about being alone or sharing a unit with another patient? Does he have visitors? Does he enjoy them? Is he lonely or rejected by his family, other patients, or the personnel? Is he worried about finances, family affairs, or business? Does he wish help from a medical social worker with these problems?

The head nurse who is sensitive to the patient's need for religious counsel will suggest to him the ease with which a minister, priest, or rabbi can be called and the desire of these clergymen to be summoned to serve the sick. There are times when the soul is sick and a religious advisor may do more to aid recovery than either doctor or nurse. The head nurse who has a sense of spiritual values will recognize when this is true and question the patient to make sure her interpretation is correct and that he does wish to see a clergyman.

It is important that the head nurse note whether the patient seems satisfied with his care. Is he relaxed and composed or does he seem irritable and upset? Does he complain about little things? If he says that he was wakeful, was it due to noise? Was there talking in the halls or was the utility room door left open? Was his sleep interrupted to take his temerature or to administer treatments to him or someone else in the room? There are many causes of wakefulness. The head nurse wants to determine whether in this instance it was due to some preventable cause or to pain, apprehension, or worry.

Is the patient bored? The day can seem endless for one who just sits hour after hour. If the hospital has no facilities for diversion perhaps it can be suggested to the patient's family that they bring him handwork, games, or a small radio. Many hospitals, through contractual arrangement with a local company, make television sets available to patients. If the patient prefers and his condition permits, he may watch television in the lounge or he may join a card game. Is it possible for his bed to be turned so he can see out the window or the door? If he is reading or writing does he have enough light? Is there a glare in his eyes, a shadow on the page?

Visitors are probably the highlight of the day for the patient. How has he been prepared for the call from his family and friends? Has he had a chance to freshen up, to shave, wash his face, comb his hair? Has his bed been straightened, his unit put in order? Is he permitted to visit with his family and friends in privacy and without interruption? Are there chairs, and, if smoking is permitted, ash trays for his visitors? How does the patient feel at the end of visiting hour? Is he unduly tired? Depressed? Did he have too much company, did friends stay too long, talk about things which upset him? Does the patient whose visitors are restricted know that this is true so he will not feel neglected and forgotten by his friends?

Needs of the Patient's Family

The head nurse is concerned not only with the patient but with the welfare of his family. Do members of his family have a chance to confer with the patient's nurse or the head nurse and with the doctor? Are they encouraged to talk if they wish? If the patient is on the danger or critical list is the family provided with a comfortable place to rest, both in and out of the room? Are they encouraged to get as much rest as possible, to eat regularly, and are they told where they can get meals in or near the hospital? Are they permitted to help with the patient's care if they wish? Are they reassured when possible, helped to accept the inevitable, put in touch with spiritual assistance if they desire it?

The Patient's Environment

A pleasant, comfortable environment does not mean the same thing to everyone. It is therefore difficult to arrange the surroundings to please all occupants of a multiple-bed room. Some enjoy television; others loathe it. Some like jazz and western serials; others like only classical music, news reports, and documentary films. The head nurse must do her best to see that each individual has opportunity for the rest and relaxation he needs through an enjoyable environment. Noise, whether from unpleasing radio and television shows, from loud talking in the halls, moving or dropping equipment, or from the personnel call system, can be extremely irritating to a sick or convalescing patient. Sensitiveness on the part of the head nurse is essential to detect the patient's real feelings, especially if he is not given to complaining.

The social environment is also important. Is the patient's personality compatible with that of the other person in his room or are they so unlike that neither is happy? Is the patient in the next bed irrational and noisy, disturbing his roommate's rest and embarrassing him when visitors are present? If the head nurse designates the rooms for patients, adjustments are easier to make. If she does not do so she still is responsible for the comfort of her patients and must see that arrangement is made to provide a satisfactory social environment for each individual.

The appearance of the room is also very important to the peace of mind of many patients and is to them a symbol of the hospital's standards. The head nurse, therefore, needs to make note of the general cleanliness and orderliness of the patient's unit. Has equipment from treatments been left in the room? Is the bedside stand cluttered, its contents dirty? She observes also whether the air in the room is fresh, the patient in a draft, the room too hot or too cold. Is the sun shining in the patient's eyes? Is he depressed because all he can see from his window is a stone wall?

One of the head nurse's most important responsibilities is to insure the patient a safe environment. At all times, therefore, she must be alert to dangers which might result in serious harm to a patient or visitor. On the children's division she needs to be especially sensitive to unsafe conditions, hazardous toys and equipment. Throughout the hospital the danger of infection from resistant organisms is ever present. Alertness to note carelessness in the maintenance of cleanliness and asepsis is the responsibility of all persons in supervisory positions, including the head nurse. Each head nurse must train her eye to spot and recognize danger and must teach every member of her staff to be aware of possible hazards. The unit director also has a responsibility in this area.

The head nurse must note whether emergency equipment is near at hand when there is a possibility of its being required. A tracheotomy set, suction apparatus, a respirator, oxygen tank and mask, a tourniquet, cardiac arrest set, or a syringe of adrenalin may be needed in a hurry. The head nurse checks to see that the necessary equipment is present in the patient's room or in the treatment room, that it is complete and ready for immediate use, that everyone on the unit knows where it is and knows the symptoms that might require its use.

Observation of the Work Process

In assuming her supervisory responsibility, the head nurse not only assesses the patient's condition and his environment, but also she is, at all times, very aware of nursing activities and the way in which they are being carried out. In organizing the day's work does the staff care for the most uncomfortable patients first? Are nursing measures planned around treatments which are to be administered? Are the patients who are to receive care last made comfortable with immediate needs satisfied early in the day? Are patients kept waiting for long periods to have their care completed?

The head nurse also determines whether the patient's safety and comfort are assured during a treatment, whether methods used are effective and efficient. Is the infusion flowing properly, the patient's arm supported? Is the solution infiltrating the tissues? Is there sufficient fluid in the flask? Is the nurse assigned to the patient observing him closely? Is his privacy respected? The head nurse sees that oxygen is being properly administered, that the patient is warm and comfortable, that "No Smoking" signs are on the tent and door of the room, that there are no matches present. She notes the condition of the nares when a nasal catheter is used. Drainage tubes and bottles, suction, traction—all are observed for proper functioning. Are patients using their crutches correctly? Are the crutch tips in good condition? Are ambulatory patients walking enough, receiving enough assistance? Are intake and output being accurately recorded? Are patients receiving sufficient fluids? Is there cool water within their reach?

To enjoy his meals fully the patient should be clean and comfortable and ready when the tray arrives. It is important that the head nurse know the kind of care the patient receives at meal time. Does he have help in handling his food if he needs it? Is he encouraged to eat? Are the up-patients served in the solarium or at a common table? Do the patients enjoy this sociability?

The orderliness of the patients' units and the work rooms during the period of greatest activity is noted by the head nurse. It is quite possible for patients to be comfortable and their rooms in order at the end of the morning while the process of reaching that state has been wearing and nerve-wracking to patients and nurses alike. The head nurse needs to know the type of care that is being given at all periods in order that measures for its improvement may be instituted if necessary.

The Effects of Care

Determination of the effects of care on the patient entails checking the results of treatments and nursing measures. The patient's condition is not wholly dependent upon the medical treatments and nursing care which he is receiving, nor is failure to obtain results from a treatment, of necessity, an indication that it was poorly performed. However, there is a close relationship between the patient's condition, the results of treatments, and the quality of workmanship. For example, the patient may have an increase in edema in spite of receiving a diuretic. The head nurse, however, must make certain that the medication was actually administered. She must also ascertain that the order regarding fluids was carried out, that the patient received the prescribed diet, that he did not borrow salt from another patient's tray or have something extra to eat such as a candy bar.

The head nurse should also be familiar with the results of medical therapy in order that she may report effects of treatments to the doctor. Probably many patients receive treatments such as irrigations, heat applications, or perhaps even medications for a longer period of time than is really necessary because the head nurse does not follow closely the results obtained and report when the treatment seems to be ineffectual, or the symptoms for which it was ordered no longer exist. Some physicians follow up their orders far more carefully than do others. The alert head nurse saves expense to patients and nursing time by careful observation and habitual reporting of the patient's condition in relation to the treatments which have been ordered.

In determining the results of nursing measures the head nurse, from day to day, notes whether the nursing care plan is being followed and observes its effectiveness in achieving the desired outcomes. Is Mr. Samuels doing increasingly more for himself as a result of efforts to help him become self-sufficient? Is Mr. Walker responding to the "tender loving care" which the staff prescribed for him? Is he doing his exercises regularly and is his range of motion increasing? One of the major responsibilities of the head nurse is to evaluate the results of the care given by the members of her staff.

Interaction between Patients and Personnel

Ever sensitive to the patient's behavior the head nurse analyzes factors which influence his reactions. She attempts to learn the attitudes of staff members toward their patients and to note the effects of these attitudes. Likewise she observes how the patient feels about his nurse. Does he think she dislikes him or do they relate well to one another? Is he overly dependent on his nurse or does he bypass her and discuss his problems with someone else? If the head nurse is aware of relationships between the patient and the person assigned to his care, she is in a position to help the nurse or aide understand the patient and thus better meet his personal needs. At times, it may be wise to make a change in the assignment. Under either circumstance the staff member needs help in relating to patients.

Social Climate and Physical Environment of the Personnel

It is not enough for the head nurse to observe the patients and the quality of their care. She must also look at the conditions under which the personnel function. Here may lie the cause for failure to meet the desired standards of care. The head nurse needs to be continually looking for the causes of delay, of failure to take precautions, of irritability on the part of the staff. Is there enough equipment? Is it arranged conveniently? Is it working well? Is there congestion at the medicine closet at certain hours? If so, could the time for administration be spaced differently or could the medicine cupboard be moved? Does everyone need the cardex at the same time? Perhaps members of the nursing staff or unit manager will have suggestions to remedy these situations. Is the staff working as a team? Does harmony prevail on the division? The head nurse must be ever aware of the need for improvement in relationships. She should be alert to discover factors contributing to inefficiency and poor workmanship and conscientious in a continual search for better ways of administering patient care. If wise, the head nurse will make full use of her staff in helping to find solutions to problems and in setting and upholding standards. She will also call on the greater experience of the department administrator for guidance and reassurance.

DIRECTING NURSING CARE

Implementing or directing nursing care is the part of the supervisory process usually spoken of as *supervision of nursing care*. Direct observation is indispensable to supervision. Although other methods are used to supplement personal observation, there is no substitute for the head nurse seeing with her own eyes. She cannot properly direct nor adequately assume responsibility for the patient's care unless she herself observes him. She should see and talk with every patient at least once a day. In large divisions with 50 or 60 patients, this may be all that is possible unless there is a unit manager assigned to the floor. Under any circumstances, there will be some patients the head nurse must see frequently throughout the day.

Making quick rounds with the night nurse in the morning and with the evening charge nurse in the afternoon provides opportunity for the two together to raise questions, discuss problems, make plans. Questions come to mind on rounds that might be forgotten if reliance were placed wholly on the report. These rounds at the beginning and at the end of the day also provide the head nurse with an overview of the nursing situation on the division.

In addition to short rounds at the time charge nurses are changed, the head nurse sets aside time each day for purposeful rounds to observe all patients carefully. She should plan her visits to see the patients at different times of day, that is, sometimes right after the night report, on other days midmorning or after lunch. Beginning her rounds in different parts of the division also gives her opportunity to see patients under varying conditions. The head nurse will often make her rounds alone, but other nurses may accompany her. If the head nurse has a nurse assistant, they will find it valuable to make rounds together when time permits. For a young assistant this can be a valuable learning experience. At times the department administrator may wish to accompany the head nurse.

If the pressures of administration prevent this organized type of rounds, the head nurse will need to make her observations as she goes about the unit during the course of the day. In hospitals where the head nurse is free from nonnursing administrative activities she has time to organize her supervisory program.

Another highly valuable method of supervision is the short informal conference with individual members of the staff. There is no specific or regular time for holding these conferences, but the head nurse needs to be aware of their value and to make opportunities for them. As she goes around the unit while nurses are in action she can raise questions about the condition and treatment of the patients, encourage the nurses to make suggestions, and assist them in working through difficult procedures. The latter will help the head nurse understand the problems involved in the care of these patients, and this, in turn, will make it possible for her to plan assignments more intelligently. The head nurse can also give suggestions and share ideas with staff members as she transmits new orders or takes the nurse's report. The head nurse sets an example by the reports she gives and by the kind of reports she expects from her staff.

Brief conferences with students, practical nurses, and new staff nurses to plan patient care are a necessity if the patient is to be well-nursed and the staff is to learn. The purpose of this conference, which is held before the day's work begins, is to make sure the staff member understands the patient's needs and the plan for his care, to assist her in organization of the day's work, and to determine the help she needs.

To some extent staff members are the head nurse's eyes and ears. She performs her supervisory function in part through them. The head nurse, knowing the information which she needs, questions the patient's nurse relative to his symptoms, attitudes, problems, behavior. The degree to which the head nurse can rely on the staff member's observations depends on the individual's competence to make judgments, her understanding of the objectives for the care of the patient, her motivation to provide the best possible nursing. When a professional staff nurse is responsible for the patient and has these qualities developed to a high degree, the head nurse does not need to make such frequent visits to see the new post-operative, the unhappy, or the uncomfortable patient. On the other hand, if a nurse of limited experience is assigned to patients who have these problems, the head nurse feels responsible for observing the patients very often and gives close attention to the details of their care. In other words, personal observation by the head nurse is essential in administrative supervision but it may be supplemented by the observations of a competent professional nurse. Under these circumstances the amount of direct observation by the head nurse is lessened.

EVALUATION OF THE QUALITY OF NURSING CARE

Evaluation is indispensable to the maintenance of high standards, to progress, and to the growth of individuals. Evaluation of any undertaking should be made in terms of the desired outcomes; that is, of the objectives it is hoped will be achieved. It is important to establish realistic goals for an undertaking and to state them in specific terms so it is possible to know whether the objectives have been reached.

Establishing Objectives

The over-all objective on a hospital division, as previously stated, is to provide high quality care to each patient according to his individual needs. Since "high quality" may mean different things to different nurses, the head nurse, with her staff, needs to determine what is entailed in good patient care for the types or degrees of illness represented on the unit. Meeting basic human needs for compassion, understanding, empathy, and acceptance are objectives for all patients. But the objectives for medical therapy and physical nursing care differ for the new mother and for the acutely ill; objectives for the patient with coronary artery disease are different from those for a person who has had an appendectomy. Attainment of the objective—good nursing for each patient according to his needs—is determined by criteria or standards against which the quality is measured.

Developing Criteria

It might be said that criteria are the conditions which will presumably exist if the objectives are met. Examples of criteria by which to evaluate nursing care are listed below. Some relate to specific conditions but many are appropriate in every situation:

Patients seldom find it necessary to use their signal lights or the "intercom" to get attention for physical, emotional, or environmental needs. (This judgment may be difficult to make. The key words are find it necessary.*)*[1]

Families feel comfortable in leaving their loved ones in the care of the staff.

Patients are composed but not unduly placid when going for surgery, delivery, special treatments, or diagnostic tests. They require no unusual amount of sedation.

Postoperative patients understand the need for coughing, turning, and ambulation and try to follow instructions.

The public health nurse reports a quick, easy home adjustment for discharged patients.

Incontinence is rare.

The skin and mouths of patients are in good condition.

Patients have no preventable contractures or deformities.

Patients convalesce rapidly to optimism, good spirits, and self-dependence on the basis of predetermined expectations.

Other criteria indirectly indicate that good nursing care is given in the division:

[1] Marjorie C. Hogan. *Relationships Between Patients' Needs and Requests Made Via the Inter-com System.* Masters' Report, Yale University School of Nursing, New Haven, 1966.

The number of errors and incidents which require a report is negligible.

Doctors request that their patients be sent to this unit.

Few requests are made for private duty nurses except when the patient is in critical condition.

Few patients discharged from the division return because of inadequate teaching or lack of referral for follow-up care.

Few complaints are received from doctors, patients, or families about the quality of care; the care is frequently praised by these individuals.

Questionnaires filled out by discharged patients indicate a high degree of satisfaction with their nursing care.

Former patients and their families express satisfaction in being placed on the division.

Each of the criteria listed above represents a desirable state or condition and is, therefore, an objective to be attained. Each is sufficiently specific that the extent to which it is being met may be determined. Records can be kept of the instances when the care does not meet the criterion, for example, the patients who remain incontinent, those who have breaks in the skin. Causes or extenuating circumstances are recorded in each case. A record of favorable incidents is also kept, as, for example, commendation for the care given, by whom it was made, and the circumstances. Doctors' criticisms both favorable and unfavorable are especially valuable if they are recorded at the time of occurrence. When reviewed at intervals they may show a pattern which will be useful in evaluation of nursing care.

The development of criteria is not an easy undertaking. Thinking of instances of care considered especially good and those which were of poor quality is one way to facilitate the undertaking. The *critical incident technique* is another useful means for developing criteria for nursing care. This technique calls for the recording of instances of human activity which are sufficiently complete and of such significance in relation to objectives that inferences about the quality of care and about the person performing the act can be drawn. To be *critical* the purposes of the action must be clear to the observer and the effects or outcomes fairly definite.[2]

The following is an illustration of a critical incident:

Miss G. refused to sign the permission for operation, which an aide had brought to her for signature, until she had seen her doctor. The patient had been admitted two days earlier with a fulminating infection of one eye. Her doctor hoped to save it with intensive therapy but feared he

[2] Elizabeth Hagen and Luverne Wolff. *Nursing Leadership Behavior in General Hospitals,* New York, Institute of Research and Service in Nursing Education, Teachers College, Columbia University 1961, pp. 25-28.

might have to do an enucleation to save the other eye. When after two days he decided that surgery was necessary, he wrote preoperative orders but failed to discuss developments with Miss G. The assistant head nurse who was handling the doctor's orders sent the aide to obtain the operative permit. Miss G. felt the doctor, or at least the head nurse, should have talked with her about her condition and the need for such drastic action; that this devastating news should not have come to her casually through an aide.

The inference to be drawn from this incident is obvious. The patient had no part in the planning of her care and had a psychologically traumatizing experience by being tacitly informed by a nurses' aide that therapy had been unsuccessful, that she would have to lose her eye. The purpose of the action was to get the operative permit signed and thus comply with hospital policy. Effects of the action were clear. Miss G. was thoroughly upset and would not sign the permit until she had talked with her doctor.

In this instance the patient provided the facts concerning the critical incident. Patients and their families are probably the richest and least tapped source of information about the quality of their care albeit they are more accurate in their judgment when they think the care is poor than when they think it is good.[3] If nursing care in a division were to be evaluated by the critical incident technique, patients and their families, when the day of discharge nears, might be asked such questions as: What was the best care you received in the hospital? The worst care? What was your reaction when you were admitted to the division? How did you feel about going to the operating room? about having a cardiac catheterization? Answers by many patients to a series of nonevaluative questions like these identify criteria of good nursing care and provide data for evaluation.

Other persons besides patients, however, may recount critical incidents. In one extensive study made some years ago in which this technique was used,[4] doctors, head nurses, and nurse instructors as well as patients were asked, in response to specific questions, to recall important nursing care incidents which they had recently observed. If this technique were to be adopted by our hospitals as a means of developing criteria for evaluation of nursing, who should collect the critical incidents? Unless they are to contain a good deal of subjectivity, an observer, not in the administrative line, who is skilled in interviewing and clinically competent, should be assigned to make periodic, systematic appraisals of nursing on each

[3] Mark S. Blumberg and Jaqueline A. Drew. Methods for assessing nursing care quality, Hospitals, Vol. 37 (November 1, 1963), pp. 72-80.
[4] June Teig Bailey. The critical incident technique in identifying behavior criteria of professional nursing effectiveness, *Nurs. Res.*, Vol. 5 (October 1956), pp. 52-64.

nursing care division. It has been suggested [5] that nursing service or hospital administration employ professional nurses whose specific job would be to improve the quality of care in the patient care divisions. These nurses would not only interview patients and their families and the staff but would observe nursing in action and keep records of critical incidents. Characteristics of nursing care to be noted would be much the same as those the head nurse observes on rounds. Having such an observer would in no way absolve the head nurse of her responsibility for being mindful of the same things and taking necessary action. A policy of placing qualified independent observers in the hospital to help improve nursing care—not to blame or find fault—is one which, if instituted, should have far reaching effects on the quality of care.

Since it is probable that at present, few if any, hospitals employ observers, the head nurse, particularly if she is free from unit administration and has time to nurse, and the team leader would find it useful to keep a record of critical incidents. They could note their personal observations and could also have in mind a list of questions to ask patients, families, doctors, and staff nurses. The record would need to be analyzed from time to time to determine whether the incidents were critical in nature, and to formulate criteria for the evaluation of nursing care.

At regular intervals the head nurse and staff should review the criteria and any records which have been made. They judge to what extent patient care meets the objectives, wherein improvements have been effected, and steps which need to be taken to bring about still better nursing care.

PLANNING A PROGRAM FOR THE IMPROVEMENT OF PATIENT CARE

This is an area which will test the leadership ability of the head nurse. There should be no problem in maintaining staff interest if members have participated wholeheartedly in thinking through the characteristics of good nursing for patients on this division and in developing the criteria for evaluation. It is, however, the head nurse's responsibility to keep objectives clearly before the staff without their feeling she is imposing them. The staff members must always feel these are "our" goals, it is "our" responsibility to meet them. Each person needs to realize she has something to contribute and much to gain from concerted effort to give patients the very best of care.

[5] Blumberg and Drew, op. cit.

In reviewing criteria, the staff will find that some are being met less well than others. They will strive to improve in all deficient areas, but it is wise to select one or two on which to concentrate attention. The staff should make the selection, but they will look to the head nurse for guidance. She will do well to suggest a pressing problem which she knows is of concern to the entire group. She can stimulate interest and gain cooperation if she invites the staff (as many as can be spared from the unit) to meet with her to try to find a way by which the objective can be met. She must sincerely believe that there is power in group thinking and action. It may be difficult to find time for such a meeting. It need not take long if the staff gives some thought to the matter before coming together. Staff members have been known to have sufficient interest in improving patient care to spend an evening on their own time developing a plan of action. It could be considered by the individual to be a part of her professional responsibility to spend a few hours a month making a contribution to nursing and increasing her own insight into patients' needs.

Perhaps the problem which is selected for study is an increasing incidence of bedsores. The staff is concerned because several patients have developed skin lesions recently. The division has been unusually busy and back care has not been given regularly. Some patients are hard to turn and it has been difficult to find someone free to help. Sometimes there has been no lubricant in the bedside stand so its application has been omitted when time was short. There may be other problems, also, which the staff can enumerate.

The staff members will set as their objective: To decrease the incidence of skin lesions. Their next step will be to outline the procedure for achieving the objective. In this instance it may involve:

Turning helpless patients every hour.
Each time the patient is turned, washing and rubbing well with a lubricant the back and buttocks of those who are incontinent, edematous, or obese. Providing this care for other bed patients at least three times daily.
Use of sponge rubber mattresses or pads for patients predisposed to bedsores.
Systematic bi-daily observation of the skin over the back and all bony prominences of patients predisposed to pressure sores. Recording of these observations whether findings are positive or negative.

The group should not forget, in setting up the procedure for attainment of this objective, the importance of personalized care for patients. A functional assignment in which one or two nurses or even aides would make rounds every hour to turn patients might keep the patient's skin from breaking down. However, it would hardly keep him happy if his care were so routinized that his personal needs were disregarded. The values of continuity and individualized care would be lost and his nursing could not be considered good. No one yet knows the degree to which the patient's freedom to make choices in relation to his care, and his sense of personal worth have to do with healing, but at least one nurse[6] is convinced by her experience that these factors have a bearing on recovery. It is, therefore, important to determine how time can be arranged so the nurse assigned to the patient can carry out the necessary procedure for the prevention of bedsores. The answer would appear to lie in the number and type of patients assigned to each nurse, the use of the nursing team or the assignment of staff members to work in pairs; the scheduling of treatments and medications to avoid interference with the program of turning; perhaps devising a method of turning and cleansing which will be simple and will require a minimum of time, and setting up a plan for having at hand the necessary supplies and lubricants.

To determine the success of the program in decreasing the incidence of skin lesions, records are kept of all patients who develop them. Ideally data regarding the incidence and severity of decubiti which developed during one or two months preceding institution of the plan should be tabulated for comparative purposes. The head nurse is responsible for knowing that the procedure designed by the group is being followed. It should be reviewed by the staff frequently, especially in the beginning, to determine whether it is practical. If not, it can be changed by the group. If, after a reasonable period of trial, the procedure is found to be unsuccessful in preventing bedsores, reasons need to be sought and steps taken to revise the methods used. Continual evaluation under the leadership of the head nurse is necessary. Likewise each new staff member coming to the floor must be oriented to the procedure or it will soon fall into disuse. The evening and night nurses are, of course, involved in the original planning.

When one problem has been solved by instituting measures to meet an objective, another criterion which is not being met is selected for the same kind of group planning and action. Evaluation must be carried on continuously if the patient is to be well nursed. Ways of meeting needs should be reviewed from time to time and experimentation carried on to find better methods. Periodic re-examination of goals and acceptance of new ones are necessary. Objectives are never met and discarded. They are continually enlarged upon.

[6] Lydia E. Hall, Director, Loeb Center for Nursing and Rehabilitation of Montefiore Hospital, New York City.

Values of Group Participation in Evaluation

There are two outstanding values attained when the staff actively participates in formulating objectives or criteria, evaluating patient care, and planning ways to improve it. The *first* value lies in the improvement in patient care that is achieved. People, as a rule, have much more interest in plans they make themselves and interest contributes greatly to success. It is probable, therefore, that cooperative planning will bring better results than a brilliantly conceived plan formulated by the head nurse alone and presented, ready made, to the staff. Sometimes the staff will cooperate wholeheartedly with the head nurse's plan if she is a leader, but they miss the satisfaction of participation and, more important, the patients lose the benefit of their ideas. The *second* value of group participation in evaluation of patient care is the development of the staff which results. This will be discussed in Part 3.

SUMMARY

Since the head nurse is responsible for providing good nursing to the patients on her division, one of her chief functions is the supervision of patient care. Administrative supervision involves assessment of the patient's condition and environment, directing and overseeing his care, evaluation of his medical and nursing care, and implementation of measures designed by the staff to improve the care of patients.

Informal conferences, short rounds with night and evening nurses, and daily, planned, detailed rounds are methods by which the head nurse carries her supervisory responsibility. As she goes about the floor she has specific observations she wishes to make regarding each patient and his care. She is alert to any hazards which might harm patients, visitors, or personnel and is consciously aware of the social climate.

Critically ill and new postoperative patients need to be seen often by the head nurse. Their families also need special consideration. To some extent the head nurse relies on the observations of competent nurses, but their reports do not relieve her of responsibility for personal observation.

In evaluating patient care, it is important to have criteria or standards by which to measure. Analyzing the characteristics of good nursing for patients on the division leads to improvement. Under the leadership of the head nurse this analysis can be made and criteria stated for use in evaluation. When this is done records need to be kept of instances when the criterion is not met. Review of the records will show areas in which patient care fails to meet the standards. The staff then studies reasons for the failure and plans a program for improvement. It is usually best to concentrate attention on one or two areas of weakness at a time. Continuous evaluation is essential, as is the frequent review of objectives to see whether they need to be enlarged.

Joint effort based on strong motivation stimulated by the leadership of a good head nurse brings rewarding results in better patient care.

QUESTIONS FOR DISCUSSION

1. If you were the head nurse how would you handle the following problem? The permanent evening practical nurse and aide consistently refuse to give back care to incontinent patients. The evening charge nurse seems powerless. You are planning a campaign to reduce the incidence of decubiti.
2. If the permanent night nurse on a division consistently fails to carry out nursing care plans what measures can the head nurse use to solve the problem? Be specific.
3. A patient complains to the head nurse that an aide has been "mean" to her. What are possible satisfactory ways of handling this situation? Is a conflict of loyalties involved for the head nurse?

EXERCISES

1. For a group of six to eight patients on your division make a list of the observations the head nurse should make in relation to their condition, needs, environment, and the desired effects from drugs and treatments the patients are receiving. Make rounds on these patients observing all you can remember of the items on your list. It may be necessary to take a second look if many points were forgotten. From the observations you have made assess the condition of each patient and evaluate his care. Decide what changes in the plans for care you will suggest to the staff and the patients. What over-all problems should be discussed with the nursing staff? the medical staff?
2. Make rounds on your division paying special attention to the patient's mental and emotional state. Be familiar with comments made previ-

ously in doctors' and nurses' notes and in oral communication. Try to validate your observations with the patient and if indicated suggest or have him suggest a plan for dealing with a problem. (Ernestine Wiedenbach's book, *Clinical Nursing: A Helping Art* may be useful in carrying out this exercise.)

3. Make rounds on your division noting and listing a) health hazards in the environment, b) precautionary nursing care measures indicated. Suggest ways for handling both.

4. Observe staff members as they are giving patient care. Is there a difference in the orderliness with which different ones work? Consider the most orderly and the least orderly working environment you found and for both situations identify with each of the following in turn: the patient, his doctor, his wife, his boss, the nursing service administrator. What reaction did you have to the most orderly? the least orderly?

REFERENCES

Bailey, June Teig. The critical incident technique in identifying behavior criteria of professional nursing effectiveness, Nurs. Res., Vol. 5 (October 1956), pp. 52-64.
An interesting and informative article of value to head nurses as well as to nurse The purposes of this study were to identify behavior criteria of effective staff nurses and to determine to what extent judgments of effectiveness vary among nurses, doctors and patients. Of particular value to head nurses is the list of criteria of nursing effectiveness.

Blumberg, Mark S., and Drew, Jacqueline A. Methods for assessing nursing care quality, Hospitals, Vol. 37 (November 1, 1963), pp. 72-80.
An interesting and informative article of value to head nurses as well as to nurse administrators. The need for a system of continuous reporting on the quality of nursing care together with methods for gaining information are described.

Brodt, Dagmar E., and Anderson, Ellen H. Validation of a patient welfare evaluation instrument, Nurs. Res., Vol. 16 (Spring 1967), pp. 167-169.
An instrument for measuring patient welfare reflects quality of nursing care. The instrument used in this study compared patient welfare on a "service managed" (unit manager) and on a traditionally managed unit.

Brown, Esther Lucile. How hospitals can evaluate causes of patient discomfort, Mod. Hosp., Vol. 106 (March 1966), pp. 112-113.
Three causes of inadequacy in care are 1) limited preparation of most personnel in handling interpersonal relationships; 2) rigid hierarchical structuring of staff relationships, especially between nursing and medicine, and 3) lack of facilities symbolic of normal living at home. The insert on page 113 graphically describes the way in which the hospital admission procedure increases patients' anxiety.

Estes, M. Diane. Introducing the nursing audit, Amer. J. Nurs., Vol. 64 (September (1964), pp. 91-92.

The method used to introduce the nursing audit in one hospital is described. It includes the items which were evaluated.

Hall, Lydia E. A center for nursing, Nurs. Outlook, Vol. 11 (November 1963), pp. 805-806.
Annotation with Chapter 10 reference.

Hogan, Marjory C. Relationships Between Patients' Needs and Requests Made Via the Inter-com System, Masters Report, Yale University School of Nursing, New Haven, 1966.
This study of mothers on the maternity division showed they were highly satisfied with the intercom system. However, they used it mainly for physical and environmental needs. Emotional needs were not expressed. The study revealed that requests patients make of nurses—especially those over the intercom—may not always indicate the need the patient is experiencing.

Hospital noises disturb U. S. patients also, Mod. Hosp., Vol. 105 (December 1965), p. 85.
This is an insert on a report of a British study on noise. Interestingly, more preventable noise caused by nursing personnel was reported in the U. S. study. There are implications for head nurses here.

Lambertsen, Eleanor C. These 19 questions can be used to evaluate emergency service, Mod. Hosp., Vol. 106 (January 1966), p. 124.
"The nurse in charge of the emergency unit frequently encounters problems because of the absence of clearly defined policies and procedures." The questions listed are pertinent for the nurse as well as for administration.

Paulsen, F. Robert. Nursing goals beyond commitment, Nurs. Outlook, Vol. 14 (December 1966), pp. 57-58.
Although quality nursing care is an ultimate philosophical objective, as a concept it does not establish the means for achieving it nor the actuality itself. The author emphasizes the need for measures of quality care and of the success of this care in bringing about patient recovery.

Phaneuf, Maria C. A nursing audit method, Nurs. Outlook, Vol. 12 (May 1964), pp. 42-45.
Evaluation of nursing service by means of a nursing audit.

Raphael, Winifred. Nurse, nurse, for better or worse, Nurs. Times, Vol. 61 (December 10, 1965), pp. 1686-1687.
In the third of a series of articles a research consultant found patients' comments regarding their care centered around two matters—nurse-patient relationships and skill. Relationships were mentioned much more than skill.

Simon, J. Richard. Systematic ratings of patient welfare, Nurs. Outlook, Vol. 9 (July 1961), pp. 432-436.
As part of a research study four rating scales to depict patient welfare were developed: 1) mental attitude, 2) mobility, 3) physical independence, and 4) skin condition. Should be helpful in analysis of patient care and result in its improvement.

———— and Chastain, Sally S. Take a systematic look at your patients, Nurs. Outlook, Vol. 8 (September 1960), pp. 509-512.
A code for recording patient activity, devised to test quality of patient care, has proved to be a reliable measure. It can be used for systematic appraisal of nursing before and after efforts to improve care and is of value also to the individual nurse in determining a patient's progress toward health.

Sister Mary Luke. How the operating room nurse can help to personalize patient care, Mod. Hosp., Vol. 105 (December 1965), pp. 90-92.

The operating room nurse is the most knowledgable nurse to talk with the patient prior to surgery. To be effective she needs psychiatric nursing skills. A follow up visit to evaluate the patient's response to her previous visit will help her improve her skill.

Smith, Christine S. We asked the patients, Nurs. Outlook, Vol. 6 (August 1958), pp. 458-459.
Report of a very interesting study in which obstetric patients were asked to answer a series of questions relative to their care. The study resulted in many changes in old routines and an emphasis on teaching patients in the area of family living. Excellent.

The DHN forums on administration of nursing services in hospitals, Nurs. Outlook, Vol. 14 (March 1966), p. 31.
Forums are assisting administrators of nursing services in hospitals to study their problems, to experiment with solutions, and to evaluate their efforts. Some of problems being studied are listed.

part 3 THE HEAD NURSE'S RESPONSIBILITY FOR STAFF DEVELOPMENT

The head nurse has two major responsibilities, each of which is inextricably involved with the other. Part 2 dealt with the first of these responsibilities—patient care. Part 3 will consider the head nurse's obligation to help members of her staff develop to their highest potential. Changes in nursing practice are constantly occurring as better diagnostic and therapeutic methods are developed and more is learned about human physiology and psychology. Many nursing methods used only a few years ago have been discarded and replaced by new ones. The hospital which would provide the best in care for its patients is obligated to prepare its nursing staff to keep pace with modern developments. Change is so rapid and working time so short that it is no longer possible to rely on nurses developing fully through experience alone. Nor are the best nurses satisfied to drift along from day to day without the stimulation of an educational program.

Focus in this next section will be on staff members and the manner in which the head nurse influences their growth. The kind of person she is, her interest and ability in nursing, and her understanding of the ways people learn, all have a bearing on the development of the staff. The purposes of inservice education and the influence of the general practices on the division over which the head nurse has control will be taken up first. These will be followed by consideration of the more formal, planned methods which the head nurse employs in helping her staff to grow.

chapter 14

PURPOSES AND OUTCOMES
OF INSERVICE EDUCATION

There is increasing recognition by hospitals that if nursing service is to be improved educational programs for the nursing staff must be undertaken. The problems involved in giving good care to patients result partly from the fact that most hospitals today are staffed with individuals who have, at least at the professional level, widely different backgrounds of preparation. Also nurses, as do others in these times, move around the country, thus bringing about a frequent turnover in staff. Another reason for instituting inservice educational programs results from the rapid changes in medical and nursing practice. If nursing care is to keep pace with developments in the natural, behavioral, and medical sciences, an educational program is necessary. Hospitals are hopeful that satisfactions will be incurred from the educational program which will reduce the attrition rate among the staff.

Many institutions have appointed one or two nurses who devote full time to inservice education. They are responsible for conducting programs for all groups—head nurses, staff nurses, aides, and orderlies. A common procedure is to arrange for staff nurses a series of doctors' lectures on new developments in medical science. Sometimes nursing demonstrations are included in the plan. The aim is to improve nursing care through an upgrading of the staff. It is believed that by giving nurses more information they will have greater understanding of their responsibilities and will improve the quality of their nursing.

Often, however, staff nurses feel little need to be upgraded, at least by these means. Even when members of the group choose the subjects for discussion or demonstration, interest often lags. Although some programs of this type are well attended, it is to be questioned whether this is the most productive method of staff development. No doubt there is considerable learning for those who attend the lectures, but many times only a small proportion of the total staff comes to the meetings and those who need them most may never attend.

The question must be raised, then, as to whether this is the best approach for an inservice program. Would hospitals have better results if emphasis were placed on improvement of nursing service rather than on the "education" of those who give the service?

The highest type of staff education, which is probably more acceptably called staff development, results when groups of staff members work together to achieve a common purpose. In the process of working together in a democratic manner the individuals grow both personally and professionally. Staff members probably get far less "education" from hearing interesting lectures than they do from developing an orientation program for members of their group, formulating criteria for evaluation, studying and suggesting improvements in ways to deliver nursing care, working on committees to identify and solve problems of the staff in meeting objectives. Through working together morale is improved, interest in the institution and its welfare is engendered, greater loyalty results. When a staff has a sense of belonging and feels its ideas are important and valuable to others, the quality of its work, in this instance caring for patients, improves as a result. Needless to say, a program for the improvement of care can be successful only if the administration believes in its people and in the worth of their contributions, is willing to take them into its confidence regarding the problems the administration is meeting and to act upon the suggestions made by the staff. Leadership in such a program must come from the nursing service administration. If activities undertaken are of vital interest and concern to staff members, if the outcomes are important to the individual and the group, time and effort will usually be given unstintingly.

Another area in which staff nurses may be interested is the organization of the nursing team. If the hospital is considering the establishment of team nursing, graduate staff nurses might like to study the requisites for nursing team leadership since theirs is the group from which leaders would be drawn. From such a study there might well come a request for conferences to help the staff nurses learn principles and methods of organization, of supervision, of planning patient care, of making assignments. This study might lead them to a recognition of need for more clinical content, in which case this is the time to plan doctors' lectures, nursing demonstrations, conferences on nursing care.

Some of the suggestions made for staff nurse participation can be followed for the practical nurses and aides, also. For example, they may help plan the content of an orientation program for new members of their groups. They may be instructed in the way in which they are to function in the nursing team and encouraged to make suggestions. As with the staff nurse program it is essential that activities be of interest and concern to members of the group and that their suggestions be respected.

Whether or not the hospital has an inservice program for staff development, the head nurse still has an obligation to her staff for helping the members grow professionally. The immediate aim of inservice education is to have each staff member develop her nursing ability to its highest potential. This can happen only in the clinical situation. Growth occurs best when all staff members are striving toward the common goal of better patient care. It is therefore on improving nursing that the emphasis should be placed. Nurses are more likely to respond, to want to do a better job, to desire help in determining their strengths and weaknesses and in improving their work when they have a purpose in common with the head nurse and the rest of the division staff. How much more comfortable for the staff nurse to have attention focused on improving nursing care rather than on making her a better nurse! The approach to staff development is more fruitful if the emphasis is on improvement of the product, not the person.

In brief, the ultimate aim of a staff development program is to improve patient care. It is anticipated that increasing the ability of staff members will help to bring about better nursing. But it is also recognized that individuals are more highly motivated to learn when they help set the objectives of nursing care, make the plans for their achievement, and evaluate results. In striving to give the high quality care they have set as their goal, each staff member evaluates her own shortcomings. If the atmosphere is permissive she seeks help from the head nurse in evaluating herself and in making a plan for improvement. The head nurse not only helps create the desired atmosphere and stands ever ready to help, but she also plans ways to proffer assistance which will be acceptable (see Chapter 18).

PRACTICES OF THE HEAD NURSE WHICH AFFECT PERSONNEL GROWTH

Since the immediate aim of inservice education is staff development, it is important, before proceeding to a consideration of method, to review the general practices of the head nurse which affect personnel growth.

First, probably the greatest single influence in the growth of the staff is the leadership of the head nurse in setting high standards for patient care. She will stress what she thinks important and the staff will strive to achieve it if they respect her judgment. In general, the staff is not likely to give better care than the head nurse expects. If she is satisfied with mediocrity, the staff will be satisfied with this also. The quality of work which the student and aide see performed by the head nurse and staff nurses affects, for good or ill, their standards of workmanship. If patients and their families are treated with understanding and kindness, if patients participate in the planning of their own care, if a program of instruction is a part of every plan, if referrals to community agencies are consistently sent when needed, the staff member learns much better than by exhortation. The student nurse is influenced far more by these practices than by the ideals she hears extolled and the perfect performance required of her in the nursing laboratory.

Second, the example the head nurse sets in other matters also influences the attitudes of the staff. If the head nurse and staff nurses were fully conscious of the influence of their example, they would be more careful that it was of a desirable character. What the head nurse does, the way she talks with and about patients, visitors, clerks, maids, doctors, administrators are indicative of her own attitudes and have a direct effect on the behavior of the personnel. The head nurse's attitude toward hospital and nursing service administration, toward rules and regulations, and toward mistakes; her attitude toward the nursing profession, toward supervision and teaching help to determine the relationships which exist in the division and hospital. The head nurse's faith in or distrust of people has a marked effect on her success as a supervisor or administrator. Her actions speak louder than her words, and her tone of voice may belie the words she speaks. The head nurse's dignity in appearance and manner, her graciousness and warmth in human contacts, fairness in making decisions, and generosity in interpreting regulations are all examples of behavior which set the standard for the others on the division. Whether the head nurse finds joy and satisfaction in her work, or whether she displays complacency or discouragement, makes lasting impressions on her associates. In much the same way, although perhaps not to the same degree that the head nurse influences the entire unit personnel, the staff nurse affects the student nurse, and the upper classmen in the school of nursing influence the attitudes of the younger students.

Third, the social environment goes far in creating a climate for learning. The head nurse's consideration of the staff and her relationship to the members affect their desire to learn. An atmosphere in which each person is free to make suggestions or to question any other individual, be he head nurse, doctor, or administrator, is conducive to growth of the nursing staff.[1] Important is the spirit of cooperation and friendliness which pervades the unit and the personal interest in each individual shown by the head nurse.

[1] Gladys Nite. Learning every day, *Amer. J. Nurs.,* Vol. 60 (December 1960), pp. 1761-1764.

Although salaries and promotions, hours and living conditions have a decided influence on the morale of nurses and other workers, of greater importance is appreciation and recognition of effort and good work. These rewards the head nurse can control to a large extent.

Fourth, the efficiency with which the division is managed, whether by a unit manager or the head nurse, may foster learning or may hinder it. Good administration, in which reports are complete, orders accurately and promptly transcribed, equipment and supplies available and in good order, goes far to keep tension at a minimum. Learning and efficiency are inhibited by frustration whatever the cause.

Fifth, the head nurse's utilization of learning opportunities which present themselves every day rounds out the experience of her staff. Diagnostic findings and their significance, the rationale of new therapy, the return report of the public health nurse on a patient referred to the agency, these and many other developments provide opportunities to keep the staff informed. Likewise, when a patient manifests an unusual symptom or condition a learning opportunity is presented. The head nurse who recognizes and uses these occasions increases the learning of her staff in two ways: first, the staff gains new knowledge and second, their interest is stimulated by the head nurse taking time to keep them informed.

A *sixth* influence on staff development pertains to the extent to which the head nurse involves all members of the staff in defining good care for the patients, in establishing objectives and the criteria for evaluation of their attainment. This was discussed at some length in Chapter 13 and earlier in this chapter. All that need be said here is that active sharing in these activities leads to growth of the participants.

Seventh, the utilization of the special interests and abilities of members of the staff not only encourages greater development of a particular skill but also stimulates the acquisition of others. For example, a nurse especially skilled in making patients comfortable, if asked to demonstrate to others on the staff, not only studies *why* certain measures are effective in making the patient comfortable, but she also learns something about ways to demonstrate.

Other talents of nursing personnel may also be used for the benefit of the patients, the staff, or the individual herself. The head nurse may ask the evening charge nurse to teach a new staff nurse procedures for the evening tour of duty. She may arrange for the treatment room aide to explain to a group of new students the location of supplies and trays, the way in which soiled equipment is cared for, and the functions of the aide. An individual likes to be singled out for a particular responsibility. It shows that her special ability is recognized and indicates that she has the head nurse's confidence. The staff member, many times, will need help with method of presentation and when this is given in an acceptable way, the opportunities for growth of the individual are immeasurable.

An *eighth* influence on the development of the staff results from stimulation of individual and group initiative by the head nurse. Professional growth is fostered when nurses are encouraged to assume a piece of creative work which they can call their own. The night nurse, for example, might devise a sleep chart for patients and study the causes of wakefulness and methods of inducing sleep and rest. Likewise, if a nurse is encouraged to try out an idea she has for getting a patient up or helping him socialize with other patients, she feels free to make other suggestions. Thinking about ways to do things better increases learning if opportunity is provided for experimentation and evaluation.

Experimentation can be carried on by the staff as a group as well as by individuals. For example, special attention of the staff might be concentrated on a patient who is not responding to care or who for some reason is unable to participate in his therapeutic program. Perhaps he feels he cannot eat or take fluids; or he may be suffering more pain than his condition seems to warrant. It may be that a chronically ill patient has no desire to get well, no interest in anything outside himself. The staff might respond in one of several ways: they could give up trying to carry out the plan for care, they could become annoyed, or they could be challenged. The concerned head nurse may assign a particular nurse to the patient, challenging her to discover causes of the patient's behavior and to develop with him a plan he can accept. The nurse can then interpret his needs to the staff and gain their enthusiastic help in trying to meet the patient's needs in a way acceptable to him. It is often surprising what staff members can do under such circumstances. The head nurse acts as counsellor and leader. She may supply pertinent references. She calls on the nurse to give periodic progress reports to the staff. A problem-solving approach by members of the staff not only stimulates their development but also results in improved methods of care. If outcomes are evaluated as an inherent part of each project, growth ensues for those involved.

The head nurse may also help her staff to develop by means of a concerted effort to utilize the findings of nursing practice studies and thereby test their applicability in the day-to-day activity of the unit. There have always been nurses who were dissatisfied with the way nursing was given, with the results that were attained. Some of these nurses have experimented with new methods in an attempt to find solutions to problems. No doubt nursing care was improved to some extent as a result of these efforts, but there has been no way to be sure how successful they were nor whether the methods employed were responsible for the results which seemed to have been achieved. It is only within the last few years that the scientific method of analysis has been employed to study nursing care. Effort is now being made to ascertain the relationship between cause and effect in nursing, to develop measures for determining outcomes. Scientific studies of nursing practice made thus far have been limited in number and in size of patient groups included in the tests. Findings have been interesting and may prove to have considerable significance for nursing if the studies can be replicated by other researchers in other situations.

One purpose of research in nursing practice is to determine the effects of different nursing methods on outcomes as they relate to the patient's welfare, his happiness, his comfort. Only as the findings of research are tested in many situations by many people, only as the findings can be translated into practice does nursing research fulfill its mission. It is unlikely that many head nurses and their staffs are equipped to replicate research, for this takes special preparation, but they can informally test the findings of studies to see if they are workable within the framework of the usual hospital.

The first requisite for such testing is a head nurse who has leadership ability, a keen desire for her patients to receive a high quality of nursing care, an interest in finding solutions to problems, and an exploring attitude. She must be one who is stimulated by reports of research and who has imagination as to the ways in which findings can be tested with her patients. Then she must be able to inspire and challenge her staff. Some illustrations may be useful:

If the head nurse is having problems in getting plans for care, particularly of long-term patients reevaluated by the health team, the staff might follow up the study made by Doris Schwartz[1] in which analysis of the situation and careful planning of the reports to the doctor resulted in reevaluation of the case. Several other nursing studies whose findings nurses might test are also listed in reference readings at the end of chapters in this text.[2]

In one study the research nurse explored with a group of preoperative patients to determine causes for distress and ways to relieve it. Results showed that these patients had less postoperative vomiting than those for whom the research nurse had not cared. Could the staff nurses read Mrs. Dumas' study, to get ideas as to ways they might diminish preoperative dis-

[1] See reference list at end of Chapter 6.
[2] See references: Rhetaugh Dumas (Chapter 6), Roslyn Elms and Donna Diers (Chapter 10), Phyllis Tryon and Robert Leonard (Chapter 9), Angela McBride and Jean Johnson (this Chapter).

tress? This would entail record keeping and analysis of results. Would it not be an interesting endeavor for the staff? They might decide they needed help with interviewing skills which perhaps could be arranged through the director of inservice education.

Another study (Elms and Diers) indicated that a group of newly admitted patients with whose reactions, feelings, and fears the nurse concerned herself, accomplished a relatively easy adaptation to the hospital, while others not so nursed had more difficulty in adapting. Again, could the staff not read the article describing this study and themselves test the hypothesis?

In a third study (Tryon) the predelivery enema was found to be more effective when the patient had a thorough understanding of the procedure and her part in it, and when she participated fully in the measure. Surely this is something maternity nurses would be interested to test. The article tells the way in which the experiment was done. Staff nurses after reading about it could establish methods and criteria for evaluation and learn for themselves the differences which occur as a result of the full involvement of the patient in the procedure.

The study by Mrs. McBride recognized that the patient in pain has not only physical but also intellectual and emotional needs which the nurse can help to meet and thereby reduce his pain. Mrs. Johnson studied postoperative pain. The evening before surgery she visited patients who were to have a hysterectomy or cholecystectomy. This nurse concentrated on prevention of unnecessary postoperative pain, taking into account all three types of patient need (physical, intellectual, emotional). She discussed the pain and discomfort the patient should anticipate and how deep breathing and abdominal relaxation might relieve it. Might the head nurse challenge her staff to read these studies and interest them in trying out alternative ways of preparing the patient preoperatively? The staff is not prepared to perform controlled experiments but, since nurses are used to evaluating the patient's clinical course through observation of pain, vomiting, vital signs and general reaction, they would be able to make a judgment about the effect of different methods of preoperative preparation on the smoothness and rapidity of the patient's recovery. Data collection need not be elaborate. A simple record for noting results could be devised and used for the analysis of findings.

The nursing staff may also become involved in other types of studies. In institutions where clinical medical research is carried out, nurses are usually called upon to participate in some way. A great deal can be learned relative to the research by an interested head nurse who should keep her staff informed about the scientific basis for tests being done, the progress of the study, and the findings. These can be very exciting. Unfortunately, however, it is possible for nurses to learn little or nothing of the research going on about them if they are not sufficiently interested to ask questions.

In addition to stimulating the staff to undertake individual or group studies either to solve their own special problems or to discover the effectiveness of particular nursing measures, or to follow up the research findings reported by others, the head nurse may encourage certain nurses to know more about and be able to do some one thing better than others do it. Many possibilities could be mentioned; a few will suffice. The nurse might become an expert in helping patients who are to have abdominal surgery learn to relax; in supporting conscious dying patients or in comforting their families; in preparing patients for sleep; increasing patients' enjoyment of meals; convincing mothers of the value of antepartal breast care in their ability to breast feed; alleviating discomfort of perineal sutures; teaching hemiplegic patients to get in and out of bed. Almost every nurse has some area of special interest in which she might enjoy studying in depth. Becoming an expert involves, for the nurse, thinking through what she wants the measure or the skill to accomplish and the problems which interfere with its achievement. It requires reading, thinking, observing, conversing with patients and others. Eventually a plan is conceived for attaining the objectives. The plan is tested through experimentation and is evaluated. Both practice and evaluation must be continued indefinitely if the nurse is to remain expert.

We see, therefore, that the head nurse influences the growth of her staff in many ways while their continuing development has a marked effect on the quality of care given patients.

SUMMARY

Many hospitals today are employing nurses to take charge of inservice programs for the nursing service staff. The ultimate aim of inservice education is the improvement of patient care. This objective can be achieved, however, only through measures which will strengthen weak backgrounds of present personnel, orient new staff, and keep all members abreast of change. The immediate purpose of staff education, therefore, is to help each individual develop to her highest potential. Programs are more acceptable if emphasis is placed on improving the product—patient care—rather than on the improvement of the staff member. Whether or not the hospital provides a specific inservice program for staff development, the head nurse has both responsibility and opportunity for increasing the effectiveness of her staff members.

By her everyday practices the head nurse has a marked influence on the development of her staff. The quality of patient care she expects and the example she sets by her attitudes and behavior to a large extent determine the standards and behavior of staff members. Effectiveness of division management and the social environment also influence learning. In addition, staff growth is affected by the extent to which the head nurse capitalizes on learning opportunities, whether or not the staff is encouraged to participate in planning for the improvement of nursing care, the degree to which initiative is encouraged and special talents cultivated. Testing the findings of nursing practice studies is not only a fruitful means of bringing about staff growth, but also has a specific bearing on the quality of nursing care.

QUESTIONS FOR DISCUSSION

1. How does the psychological climate on your division affect the development of the staff?
2. To what extent can the quality of nursing care on your division be attributed to the head nurse? How do her standards affect the staff? Give specific illustrations.
3. If you have a staff development (or inservice education) program for nurses in the hospital in which you are employed, of what does it consist? *Specifically,* how does it affect the quality of care? staff morale?
4. What does the head nurse on your division do in the way of staff development? What more would you like to have her do? Is there anything to prevent her from developing the program you desire? If so, what?

EXERCISES

1. Read the report of one of the studies mentioned in this chapter and develop a way of nursing by which you can test the findings. Objectives of the method devised must be very clear and its use continuously evaluated to determine whether you fulfilled the objectives. This will require development of criteria. When you have perfected the method use it to see if you obtain the same results as the researcher.

For example, if you wish to see whether you can reduce the incidence of postoperative vomiting, as did Mrs. Dumas, by discovering and relieving unnecessary preoperative anxiety, you need to develop a way of nursing which will have for its purpose the reduction of preoperative anxiety. Then each time you nurse a patient in this way you need to determine whether you succeeded in your objective. You also need to think through ways by which you can be *relatively sure* you made the patient less worried. This is difficult and could perhaps become a class project. *Finally* you should keep track of the vomiting by patients you nursed in this way and those whom you did not nurse. Observation in the recovery room will be necessary since it is unlikely all instances of vomiting will be recorded. When you have observed an equal number of those whom you nursed and those you did not, compare results. Keep on trying, especially to perfect your ability to help the patient express his fears and to relieve those which are exaggerated or groundless. Mrs. Dumas' study to date shows that her nursing is effective in reducing vomiting. Is yours?

2. Evaluate your professional growth since you took your present job. What criteria did you use to make the evaluation? What *concrete* evidence of growth do you have? To what do you attribute your development? lack of development?

3. If you are a head nurse evaluate one of your more permanent staff members in the same way (as 2). What part did you have in the growth? What more could you have done?

REFERENCES

Barckley, Virginia. Enough time for good nursing, Nurs. Outlook, Vol. 12 (April 1964), pp. 44-48.
Among the many values in this fine article are 1) its portrayal of quality nursing for the terminally ill, 2) its description of the training and incentive program for nurse technicians, 3) its picture of the spirit of dedication which pervades Calvary Hospital.

Brown, Esther Lucile. Newer Dimensions of Patient Care, Part 2: Improving Staff Motivation and Competence in the General Hospital, New York, Russell Sage Foundation, 1962.
This second of three volumes describes the effects of hospital organization and operation on staff motivation and functioning. It suggests how, through orientation and continuous staff development, the staff's self-confidence and esteem can be strengthened.

Cochran, Thelma C., and Hansen, Paul J. Developing an evaluation tool by group action, Amer. J. Nurs., Vol. 62 (March 1962), pp. 94-97.
A group of nurses, dissatisfied with the hospital rating scale, developed one of their own. The entire staff was involved in the venture including the preliminary study.

Donovan, Helen Murphy. Inservice programs and their evaluation, Nurs. Outlook, Vol. 4 (November 1956), pp. 633-635.
For a successful inservice education program specific objectives and criteria for their evaluation must be identified. Once this is done many evaluative methods may be used. Active staff participation in developing the program is important to success.

Fine, Ruth Barney, and Vavra, Catherine. Content and consequences of an inservice education program, Amer. J. Nurs., Vol. 62 (January 1962), pp. 54-56.
The wide participation of many individual staff members and of staff groups in this excellent program demonstrates the value of such involvement.

Jenkinson, Vivien M. The ward sister, in relation to administration and research, Int. J. Nurs. Studies, Vol. 2 (April 1965), pp. 105-113.
The ward sister (head nurse) is not only an administrator upon whom the advantageous use of available resources depends, but she also needs to question and study nursing practice to find better ways to improve services and provide care for patients.

Johnson, Jean E. The influence of purposeful nurse-patient interaction on the patient's postoperative course, A.N.A. Regional Clinical Conferences (2), Exploring Progress in Medical-surgical Nursing Practice, New York, Amer. Nurses Assn., 1965, pp. 16-29.
Tests hypothesis that the patient who is informed about the experience he will undergo in the hospital and is encouraged to communicate his concerns will make a faster and more comfortable recovery.

Jones, Edna Mae. Who supports the nurse?, Nurs. Outlook, Vol. 10 (July 1962), pp. 476-478.
The nurse cannot support the patient unless she herself receives support—from her peers, her head nurse, supervisor, or other co-workers. An excellnt article which will give the head nurse many ideas about ways to give support to her staff.

Kane, Maureen. An inservice program for professional nurses, Nurs. Outlook, Vol. 12 (May 1964), pp. 38-39.
This article is of value in its description of the process of reorganizing an inservice program as well as for the content of the new program.

Long, Lewis M. K. Motivating personnel for inservice education, Nurs. Outlook, Vol. 7 (June 1959), pp. 333-335.
A psychologist describes eight essentials for an inservice education program if nurses are to become involved in it. Very helpful.

Mathews, B. Phelps. Measurement of psychological aspects of the nurse-patient relationship, Nurs. Res., Vol. 11 (Summer 1962), pp. 154-162.
Of special interest to head nurses is the finding that patient-centeredness tends to decrease in hospital nurses as the years since graduation increase. This characteristic also varies with the age of the nurse.
Also of interest are the ways in which the instrument—Response-to-Patient Inventory—which was designed by the researcher can be used in student and staff education.

McBride, Mary Angela B. Three Approaches to Relieve Pain, New York, American Nurses Foundation, Nurs. Res. Report, Vol. 2 (March 1967), pp. 1, 4-6.
An interesting report of a research study dealing with the relief of pain. Three approaches to the patient in pain were tested.

Miller, Mary Annice. Inservice education—are orientation and skill training true in-service education?, Nurs. Outlook, Vol. 10 (December 1962), p. 787.
The answer is "No". Staff development is true inservice education.

——— Inservice education—conceptual handicaps (Part I), Nurs. Outlook, Vol. 10 (October 1962), p. 691; (Part II), (November 1962), p. 753.
Four interesting misconceptions about inservice education are presented in these two issues in which a column on inservice education is a new feature.

——— Inservice education—what, why, where, how, when, Nurs. Outlook, Vol. 10 (August 1962), pp. 541-543.
Inservice education is an accepted practice today. Employing agencies do not expect individuals to come with preparation for the job. In hospitals the cost must be borne by the patient along with other hidden costs. Hence it behooves health agency personnel to make these educational activities result in improved services to patients.

Neylan, Margaret Prowse. The nurse in a healing milieu, Amer. J. Nurs., Vol. 61 (April 1961), pp. 72-74.
This article is so full of stimulating ideas that it should be read by every head nurse and teacher. The psychological factors in providing an atmosphere for growth, learning, and healing are clearly described.

Nite, Gladys. Learning every day, Amer. J. Nursing, Vol. 60 (December 1960), pp. 1761-1764.
A description of the way in which nurses in one hospital continue to learn as a result of the learning atmosphere which exists in the institution as well as of a structured inservice program. Excellent.

Pettus, Mary A. Staff nurses plan their own inservice program, Amer. J. Nurs., Vol. 63 (June 1963), pp. 82-84.
The story of the way an inservice program in a V. A. hospital got started and the gratifying way it developed should give other nurse administrators courage.

Pirnie, F. Anne. Why, what, and how of inservice education, Nurs. Outlook, Vol. 12 (January 1964), pp. 47-51.
The purposes of inservice education are given as 1) to help nursing personnel understand and deal with change, 2) to discover resources available to them, and 3) to find ways to solve their problems and reach their goals under current circumstances.

Ritvo, Miriam M. Human relations training for supervisory personnel in hospitals, Nurs. Forum, Vol. 2 (No. 3, 1963), pp. 98-112.
Description of many experiences with supervisory groups, the means used, the outcomes in terms of more effective working relationships.

Schwartz, Doris R. The value of small local nursing studies, Amer. J. Nursing, Vol. 66 (June 1966), pp. 1327-1329.
Miss Schwartz discusses her beginning interest in nursing research and describes several small local studies she has made.

Stevens, Leonard F. Look at your own practice, Amer. J. Nurs., Vol. 65 (June 1965), pp. 106-107.
Nurses in a V.A. hospital are expected to make studies of the care they give and measures taken to improve it.

Storlie, Frances. A staff nurse proposes, Nurs. Sci., Vol. 3 (October 1965), pp. 366-369.
The writer disagrees with the claim that nurses are returning to the bedside. Lack of status of the staff nurse role and empty verbalizing by nurse leaders are part of the reason. Six excellent suggestions for improving staff nurse morale and adding to their numbers are listed.

Stryker, Ruth P. Ramifications of a procedure investigation, Nurs. Outlook, Vol. 13 (April 1965), pp. 75-77.
Nursing staff, laundry personnel, and patients participated in the revision of the bed making procedure which resulted in marked reduction in the amount of linen used.

Talking about patient care, Amer. J. Nurs., Vol. 61 (May 1961), pp. 56-59.
"At four A.N.A. conferences across the country, nurses raised questions and sought ways to improve their practice."
Theresa I. Lynch states that "superior nursing service and nursing education are possible only when every member of the nursing department . . . participates in comprehensive inservice education." (p. 58).

Weinsaft, Paul, and Frishman, David N. Inservice training program offers continuous improvements in geriatric care, Hospitals, Vol. 39 (January 16, 1965), pp. 55-58.
The medical director and administrative assistant of a nursing home report the content and methods used in an inservice program for nonprofessional nursing personnel. Favorable results were noted in terms of better attitudes of staff, improved patient care, improved environment. Illustrations are given.

Wiedenbach, Ernestine. Clinical Nursing: a Helping Art, New York, Springer Publishing Company, Inc., 1964.
Annotation in Chapter 10 reference.

Wolanin, Mary Opal. They called the patient repulsive, Amer. J. Nurs., Vol. 64 (June 1964), pp. 72-75.
An unusually perceptive description of nurses' behavior in the face of "repulsive" behavior. Under such circumstances the head nurse has an important nursing and educational responsibility.

chapter 15

ORIENTATION

From the point of view of nursing administration, orientation of personnel is important for three reasons. *First,* efficient administration of any organization is dependent upon a well-developed program of orientation for its members. No hospital nursing care division can function smoothly unless the personnel are acquainted with the general policies of the institution, the routines of the department, the philosophy and methods of patient care. *Second,* nursing staff members must have knowledge of the institution, its purposes and organization, to be able to function efficiently and safely. *Third,* through an orientation program the nursing department hopes to start the new staff member on her way to becoming a highly competent practitioner of nursing in this hospital and this division.

The new member of the staff also has needs which she hopes will be met through a good orientation procedure. Before she is expected to assume any responsibility she wants to have sufficient information and understanding to avoid errors which might be harmful or cause inconvenience. If she is poorly oriented she is anxious and frustrated. Delays in her work are necessitated by the need to check procedure every step of the way or else risk mistakes. These delays may make it impossible for her to complete her assignment in good time. Even with a well-planned introduction, work is slow in a new setting. The second need of the new staff member, therefore, is to feel comfortable and at ease in the new situation. Her third wish is to learn, as quickly as possible, to function effectively in her job. For the professional staff nurse, this means learning to care for patients who present the kinds of diagnoses, therapy, and conditions represented on the unit. To be competent and comfortable in each role played by the staff nurse—team leader, evening and night charge nurse, head nurse relief—is important to the new nurse's sense of security and to her feeling of worth.

How are these purposes of an orientation program to be achieved? Before this question can be answered, it is necessary to recognize that the content and method of orientation are dependent upon the position the person holds. They vary also with the previous experience of the individual, especially experience in this hospital.

ORIENTATION OF THE STAFF MEMBER
NEW TO THE HOSPITAL

The staff member who has not worked in the institution previously is introduced to the hospital, the nursing department, the division, and to special experiences such as evening duty.

Orientation to the Hospital

Introduction to the hospital and the general policies which affect the particular staff member is usually handled by central nursing office personnel or the department administrator. When hiring new staff is a frequent occurrence, different categories of personnel often start their employment on different days. Professional nurses may begin on Monday every week, every two weeks, or once a month depending on the rate of staff turnover. Practical nurses begin on Tuesday, aides on Wednesday, and so forth.

A commendable practice of some hospitals is the joint orientation program conducted by the personnel department for all staff new to the institution. Included is a tour of the hospital to see its facilities and the location of the various departments. In a conference the group is helped to see that the welfare of the patient is the common objective of all members of the hospital staff and that harmonious working relationships are therefore necessary. Every effort is made to give the individual a sense of belonging to the hospital family. Questions and group discussion are encouraged. The following subjects are usually of interest and help newcomers to develop desirable understandings and attitudes:

The type of hospital and its means of support; that is, whether it is a governmental, church or other community hospital, whether it is a private nonprofit institution or one which is privately owned and operated for profit. The group should be told the services which are found in the hospital such as medicine, surgery, obstetrics, pediatrics.

The organization of the hospital. The individual will wish to know to whom he or she is immediately responsible, his or her relationship to the department administrator.

Health service for the staff and the procedure to be followed when the person is ill and unable to report for work.

Meal hours, coffee periods.

General plans for staff development.

Hospital social program if such exists.

Orientation to the Department of Nursing

Following general orientation one or more members of the nursing department meet with new nurses to instruct them in matters related more specifically to their work. This conference should cover such subjects as the following:

The composition of the nursing staff; that is, whether the services of practical nurses, aides, or students are used on the divisions; the relationship of a unit manager or clerk to the head nurse.

The aims of the hospital in relation to patient care.

The relationship of the hospital to the school of nursing and to the medical school if there is an association.

The doctors who may practice in the hospital; whether there is a teaching staff, a courtesy staff.

Professional departments other than nursing and medicine, such as medical social service, dietary, physical therapy, and their relationship to the nursing service.

Staff development program for nurses.

Content of orientation conferences for other nursing service personnel is selected according to their needs. Information regarding salary, hours, and vacations will have been given to the staff member at the time of her employment. Much of the information included in the introductory conferences may be incorporated in a policy book which can be given to individuals when they join the staff. It is well to go over the material in a conference, however, to give opportunity for questions.

An orientation program for new staff lasting for a period of a week or more is organized in some hospitals. Usually the program is given by the head nurse of the unit to which the individual is assigned. However, new personnel are sometimes placed on a division used for orientation purposes. Here new members are introduced gradually to the hospital routines and nursing procedures and are given a controlled assignment under close supervision. Following the introductory period the staff members are assigned to a unit for regular work. The problem with this system is that the new member must after a few days or weeks spend time and energy becoming acquainted with procedures and routines in her permanent assignment.

Orientation to the Division

Staff members who give care to patients may or may not be assigned a group of patients their first day. This is true whether the individual begins

her service on a special orientation unit or on the division to which she is
to be regularly assigned. In some situations the new member is given no
specific assignment. She is expected to go about the floor observing nurses
and aides at work and discovering where equipment is located. Some individuals like this method of introduction. Others either feel lost without
something tangible to do or do not know how to observe with a purpose.
If at all possible the person being assigned should be given a choice in
the way she is assigned.

A more common and desirable method of assigning the new staff
member is to have her work with another nurse or another aide for a
day or even for a week. She learns as an apprentice. In this plan, the
newcomer is first taken on a tour to see the general arrangement of the
division. Some visually minded persons find a diagram showing the location of utility rooms and offices and sections for patients very helpful in
gaining a clear picture of the unit. Following the tour, the new individual
spends her time with the staff member to whom she has been assigned. If
the new staff member is a nurse, the two obtain the patient's orders and
plan the day's work together. The new nurse assists the experienced one
and observes her preparation for medications and treatments. In this way
knowledge of procedure methods is acquired, the location and care of
equipment is learned. Policies and routines are explained as occasions arise.
Opportunity is provided sometime during each day for further explanations
and for answering questions. When introduction by this method is carried on
for a week the new employee is gradually given more and more responsibility as she becomes ready to assume it. Whether the new practical
nurse or aide observes and assists a professional nurse or whether she
works with someone in her own category depends on the type of function
performed by this group in the particular hospital. By either plan, the new
staff member will learn good attitudes and practices by the apprentice method
only if she is assigned to assist a *good* nurse or a *good* aide who has some facility in teaching and organization.

In a third method for introducing the new staff member, she is assigned
one or two patients whose care is uncomplicated. It is important that she
not be given so much to do that she feels frustrated. Preferably a new
nurse does not administer medications or unfamiliar treatments. On the
first day in a new situation no one is able to accomplish her usual volume
of work. Considerable time is consumed by the initial conference causing
the staff member to get a late start. She may have to spend time locating
equipment due to unfamiliarity with the situation. Methods may be new
to her. She therefore should not be given more to do than she is able to
accomplish easily and well in the time available. She needs to feel satis-

fied with her first day's work. A certain amount of strain is always present on entering a new position but it should be kept to a minimum by a carefully planned assignment.

The staff member who starts the first day of orientation with an assignment of patients needs a more extensive introduction to the unit than one who acts as an assistant. The specific information needed varies with the situation but certain general guidelines for attaining the objectives of orientation can be laid down. *First,* the initial conference should include only that information which is needed by the staff member for her to function safely, intelligently, and with self-confidence during the first morning on the unit. It is very difficult to retain a great deal of new information if it is given all at one time, and especially if it is only heard and is not seen or experienced. The head nurse cannot assume that information which she has given has been learned. Since a new nurse or aide may hesitate to ask for a repetition, it is essential that she be given in any one conference only that amount which she can be expected to remember. *Second,* initial conferences should be followed up with later conferences in order to clear questions and to give additional information which was not needed in the beginning. In other words, the orientation procedure should include a series of conferences. *Third,* introductory conferences should be leisurely, well organized, and free from interruption. *Fourth,* they should be an established part of the program for every new staff member who is responsible for the care of patients her first or second day. This means that the head nurse must set aside time for herself or for her assistant for the period necessary to introduce a new group or individual.

In compliance with the first guideline which aims to make it possible for the new nurse to function safely, confidently, and efficiently, the initial introductory conference for members of the nursing staff new to the hospital includes the following:

1) Introduction of the newcomers to the division personnel, including the department administrator, unit manager, secretary, clerks, aides, the house medical staff, and other individuals regularly assigned to the division.
2) Information about services represented on the unit.
3) Responsibilities of the nursing staff, unit manager, secretary.
4) Explanation of method of assignment.
5) Location of time plan; schedule for coffee break and lunch hour.
6) Outline of the patient's day—time for wakening, taking temperatures, serving meals, visiting hours.
7) Special duties of aides such as passing wash water, carrying diet trays, passing linen.
8) Method of obtaining daily assignment, obtaining orders, and charting.

9) The person to whom she should go with questions and problems.
10) Tour of the floor to give a general idea of its arrangement. Here it is necessary for the head nurse to remember not to tell the new person more than she can remember but to give sufficient information for her to feel secure and for the patients to be cared for with safety. Each individual should be told as much as possible about her own patients including their personal interests, their medical and nursing histories, and nursing care.
11) Location of equipment which will be needed for giving morning care.
12) Location of exits and emergency equipment such as fire hose and extinguishers, oxygen, emergency drugs, hypodermic equipment. (Aides and practical nurses should know where emergency drugs are kept even though they will not administer them.)
13) Sources of information such as procedure, routine and guide books.

The head nurse needs to make time available later in the day for a follow-up conference. This session gives an opportunity to acquaint the new member with the other patients on the unit and with medical personnel, and to answer her questions. In later meetings the head nurse interprets the hospital's philosophy of patient care and methods for implementing it. More details about hospital and unit organization are given. The head nurse explains policies for delegation of responsibility, discusses the functions and relationships of aides and practical nurses. Although informal, these conferences should not be haphazard. A definite body of content needs to be planned. It is important that the new member be encouraged and feel free to ask questions and discuss problems. Later conferences include introduction to special experiences such as evening and night duty.

ORIENTATION OF THE STAFF MEMBER WHO IS FAMILIAR WITH THE HOSPITAL

Introduction of the nurse or aide who is transferring from another division in the hospital calls for a different approach. Methods of assignment, time planning, obtaining orders, administering medications, and charting need not be discussed if there is a uniform procedure throughout the institution. The absence of such uniformity, it can be seen, creates a need for a long, intensive introductory process. Considerable confusion occurs in the minds of nurses, especially students who change services frequently, when different methods are used to accomplish the same tasks. When methods are essentially alike, orientation to a new division is relatively simple. Special emphasis is placed on the points of care which are most important for the patients on the particular unit. It is advisable for the head nurse to have written in a policy book the outstanding variations in patient care and the points which need special emphasis. This prevents omissions in the introductory conference due to oversight. Every nurse new to the division should be familiarized with the patients, especially those assigned to her care. She should be introduced to the arrangement of the unit and the location of equipment unless it is identical with other divisions with which she is familiar. It is essential that she know where to locate articles which may be needed in an emergency.

The content of the introductory conference for the nurse who is returning to a unit where she has previously worked will vary with the length of time she has been away. She may need a review of unit routine or the variations in procedure and of special points of emphasis in the care of patients found on the service.

ORIENTATION TO SPECIAL EXPERIENCES

Staff members are prepared through conferences for night duty, evening duty, and other special responsibilities. Preferably the conference is held within a day or two of the assignment because an individual is motivated to learn when she needs to use the information immediately. The head nurse instructs the staff members in their responsibilities, in methods of handling them, and in the limitations to their authority. Evening and night nurses are told to whom to appeal for help and advice. They are helped to understand clearly their relationships to the evening or night nurse administrator, to the head nurse, and to one another. One nurse is in charge; the other is responsible to her even though each has her own specific duties and though both are of equal status in regard to experience. The charge nurse is responsible for the entire floor. Messages and reports are cleared through her. The method of operation would be different if the evening and night nurses were responsible to an autonomous head nurse (see Chapter 6) and unit management were the responsibility of a unit director. Whatever the organizational pattern, it is important that the evening and night nurses understand the extent of their responsibility and to whom they are accountable. They must also be fully informed about the functions and responsibilities permitted the practical nurse and aide. If the nurse is to function safely and effectively this type of information is necessary as well as the reports required, routines to be followed, and the regimen for patient care. Since a considerable amount of detail is involved and there is not usually someone immediately at hand with whom the evening and night nurse can consult, it is desirable to have the information they will need written in a guide book. In the introductory conference the head nurse and staff member together go over the material making sure that all points are clear. When introductory conferences are thorough work performance is improved, there is less discouragement, the individual is happier in the initial work period. Relationships with the head nurse and nursing administrators are likely to be more satisfactory and pleasant.

SUMMARY

Orientation of nursing service personnel is essential if the administration of the division is to function smoothly, if the patients are to be safely and effectively cared for, if staff members are to feel comfortable and at ease as they begin their work. In addition, orientation is the first step in the preparation of the nurse or aide to become a competent member of the nursing service staff in the institution. Orientation to the hospital, the nursing department, the division, and to special services such as night duty are all of importance. The introductory program for the nurse new to the hospital is much longer and more extensive than for the individual who is merely changing services. Giving more information than can be absorbed and remembered is a common error. It is far preferable to give a series of well-spaced conferences as part of the orientation procedure than to spend several hours at one time telling the new member all she needs to know. The person who receives a thorough introduction makes a better adjustment with less discouragement than one who does not receive such help.

The first day on the division a new staff member may be left free to observe the personnel at work and learn the location of equipment. More desirable methods for acquainting the new member with procedures and policies are to have her work with a staff nurse or peer, assisting with the care of patients but assuming no responsibility, or to give her a small assignment which she can handle with satisfaction. Some hospitals assign all new nursing staff members to work with someone else for their first week. Individual choice in manner of assignment is very desirable.

QUESTIONS FOR DISCUSSION

1. To what extent should new nurses and aides be given a choice in the way they are to be oriented to the division?

2. Who should orient a new evening nurse—the head nurse or the present evening nurse? Give reasons for your answer.

EXERCISES

1. Outline a procedure for orientation of a new nurse to your division.
2. Confer with a nurse new to the hospital *who is not responsible to you* asking her to evaluate her orientation to the hospital and to the division to which she was first assigned. Preferably she should be given time to think about the matter before expressing her opinions. Prepare a list of the features she felt to be good and those she felt were poor or lacking. Was she reasonable in her evaluation?

REFERENCES

Clark, Louise. Individualizing hospital staff orientation, Amer. J. Nurs., Vol. 62 (October 1962), pp. 102-105.
A master plan for orientation of registered nurses was developed by the clinical supervisors and the inservice education department. Both groups share in the orientation while the nurse herself indicates her orientation and training needs on a check list.

Erickson, Janet L. How nurses feel about their first work experience, Nurs. Outlook, Vol. 12 (May 1964), pp. 62-65.
A study of twelve young graduates of collegiate schools of nursing through interviews three to four weeks after they had begun work and a second at the end of five months. Factors which helped the nurses' adjustment have implications for the head nurse.

Fogt, Joan R. Inservice concerns everyone, Amer. J. Nurs., Vol. 63 (November 1963), pp. 83-85.
In a large eastern hospital an orientation supervisor for new staff nurses is employed but no inservice education director. Instead the various categories of staff —staff nurses, head nurses, etc.—through elected committees plan and conduct their own staff development programs.

Keys, Marjorie L., and Aeschliman, Jean F., Nurs. Outlook, Vol. 15 (January 1967), pp. 32-33.
Private duty nurses participated in establishment of an orientation program for their group which as a result is no longer isolated from the nursing staff. Contains excellent ideas.

Kramer, Marlene. The new graduate speaks, Amer. J. Nurs., Vol. 66 (November 1966), pp. 2420-2424.
Report of a study of new graduate nurses at the time of graduation and three

months later. Results will be of interest to the head nurse as well as nurse administrators and educators. Lack of orientation plays a large part in dissatisfaction.

Miller, Mary Annice. Transition: student to employee, Nurs. Outlook, Vol. 10 (February 1962) pp. 84-87.
Steps need to be taken by schools of nursing, students, and employing agencies to help nurses make the transition from student to earner. A survey of new graduates showed that the head nurse through her orientation was the most helpful in the nurse's adjustment.

Swansburg, Russell C. Blueprint for a refresher course, Nurs. Outlook, Vol. 14 (February 1966), pp. 54-55.
Detailed description of course given by a district nurses association includes content, resources, planning, evaluation. Ideas are useful for orientation programs.

Turner, Norma A. Our audience is a parade, Nurs. Outlook, Vol. 12 (July 1964), pp. 53-54.
Inservice education is a necessity because of a continually changing staff. The program, which must attract attention because of its captions, "is based on the four areas of personnel needs: orientation, skill training, continuing education, and leadership and management development."

chapter 16

GUIDED EXPERIENCE

The head nurse is accustomed to student nurses having carefully planned, guided clinical experience to ensure their learning. She often fails to realize that all staff members need guided experience to learn how to assume responsibilities with which they are unfamiliar. Through a planned program the head nurse acquaints the new staff member with nursing as practiced in this institution. In like manner she helps the present staff extend their ability and keep up-to-date in their clinical understanding.

GUIDED EXPERIENCE FOR NEW STAFF MEMBERS

For new staff members guided experiences are an extension of orientation. The purposes are similar: to develop a safe practitioner who has the ability and desire to meet at her level (aide, practical nurse, or professional nurse) the expectations of patients and the nursing service administration (including the head nurse), the doctors, and herself. Obviously, for the professional nurse the latter purpose implies that she should become able to give comprehensive nursing care to all patients assigned to the division. It also includes competence to function as a team leader, if team nursing is practiced, and as charge nurse at the various periods of the day. Ability in these areas is developed through carefully planned assignments in patient care, in administration and supervision of nursing care, and in conducting team conferences. Through similar planning the practical nurse and aide improve their skills and become better team members.

Variations in Education of New Staff Members

To achieve the objective of a staff education program—the development of each staff member to her highest potential—learning activities are individually planned. Professional nurses, especially, have widely varying educational backgrounds. This is less true for practical nurses and aides. All professional nurses realize there is a wide difference in the product of the three types of professional nursing education programs: collegiate, three-year diploma, and two-year associate degree. Evaluation of the product is made by nurses in terms of that which they expect of a graduate nurse and that which they consider important. A well-known and highly competent nursing service administrator in a large general hospital has spelled out the differences in capabilities, as she and her associates see them, among new graduates of the three types of professional schools.[1] Her judgment is as true and her ideas are as applicable today as at the time they were promulgated. Excerpts from her paper follow:

The graduate of the associate degree program has "ability to relate easily to patients and their families, to gain their confidence readily, and to meet their emotional needs. . . . She is uncertain about some technique and, although familiar with principles, may be lost in the gadgetry. . . . She is able to use the plan of nursing care started by the team leader and makes valuable additions that are helpful to the evening and night staff."

Because the associate degree graduate has had a limited amount of practice and has cared for only one or two patients at a time it is advised that "emphasis need be placed on techniques and on planning care for more than one patient. Therefore to capitalize on her skills and help her develop to meet the demands on nurses in a busy hospital service, she (the team leader) will start her with small assignments and increase them until the young graduate can carry the heavy load expected in hospitals today."

In describing the graduate of a hospital diploma program, Miss Brackett states that "she is skilful at doing procedures and handling complex equipment. . . . She has demonstrated ability to carry a fairly heavy assignment and get medications and treatments done on time. She demonstrates manual dexterity in making patients physically comfortable. She seems to have less skill in talking to patients, in interpreting what the patient says in relation to his feelings" than do the graduates of associate degree and collegiate programs. The diploma school graduate "needs help in using time to good advantage when there is nothing to do physically for a patient. She is not at ease if her hands are not busy. She feels guilty and thinks she is 'wasting' time."

The team leader should therefore try to give the new diploma school graduate a "fairly small assignment so that she may stay longer with" the apprehensive patient "and thereby give him the reassurance and security he needs." The team leader or head nurse will also try to help this young graduate learn to feel at ease in conversing with the patient when there is nothing physical to be done for him.

The collegiate graduate needs to have an assignment which will "tax

[1] Mary E. Brackett, Hartford Hospital, Connecticut. Nursing Service Utilizes Graduates of Various Nursing Programs, an unpublished speech for New Jersey League for Nursing, Committee on Citizen Participation, May 11, 1961.

her technical ability." Her need for assistance with procedures and comfort measures should be recognized and provided. Her assignment should be gradually increased until she is capable of carrying a full load.

The collegiate school graduate has "some insecurity, but . . . an eagerness to learn and a desire for knowledge." She "uses the ward library more frequently than other nurses. . . . This nurse readily sees implications resulting from a patient's apprehension and has good suggestions for dealing with him. She seeks help with technical equipment and at the . . . team conference she reports many observations." The collegiate school graduate recognizes the need for adaptation of schedules and variation in care for individual patients. She is "quite successful in assessing individual needs and working out plans to meet such needs. . . . This nurse's manual skills are less well developed than were some other nurses'." She has some difficulty in handling a large assignment of patients.

Miss Brackett points out that nurses cannot be stereotyped to the degree these descriptions imply. "No one nurse is typical of all nurses from the same program." She has attempted, however, "to show some of the expected differences." She has also indicated the kind of help likely to be needed by individuals in these three groups and the type of assignment they should be given to develop their potential.

Variations in Experience of New Staff Members

A wide range of experience is present in all groups of nursing personnel. The head nurse must always bear in mind that the graduate nurse who has just come to her division may have been a student yesterday or last week. The older nurse may not have practiced her profession for twenty years. The nurse may have had all her experience in a rural or semi-urban community. The amount, type, and recency of experience have a marked effect on the nurse's knowledge of modern medical and nursing practice, her ability to adjust to a new situation, her competency in caring for an individual patient or in handling a large assignment.

Assessing Capabilities

It seems obvious that, in order to help develop new staff members through guided experiences, the head nurse must know a great deal about the background of each individual. Certain information she can obtain from the department administrator or the nursing office. Before she can plan orientation or an initial assignment for a new member the head nurse should know the person's immediate past nursing experience. Within a day or two, preferably on the day of arrival, the head nurse plans a conference with the newcomer. It is important to learn how much the new nurse knows about the care of patients on the services represented on the division. To gain this knowledge the head nurse outlines for the nurse the diagnosis, medical regimen, and nursing care plan of several patients presently on the division. How familiar is the nurse with this kind of care? How recently has she cared for a patient with this type of medical program? The head nurse will wish to know whether the nurse has been assigned to this unit because she knows and likes the service or whether she has come because she realizes she has certain deficiencies and wants to learn. Perhaps she has been sent here because help was needed. She may have no special liking for this type of nursing and may even dislike it. The head nurse will also want to know whether the new staff member has had experience in team nursing and as evening or night charge nurse.

In her initial conference with the head nurse the new nurse or aide should be free to express herself. The nurse who feels threatened in any way will be hesitant to admit that she needs help, say, in the care of a tracheotomized patient. She may fear to let it be known that she has never had contact with patients following neuro- or thoracic surgery. The head nurse will do well to take the attitude that no new nurse is expected to know the way everything is done in this hospital.

The interview guide. An interview guide devised by the head nurse for use with each category of personnel during the initial conference is a useful tool. A list of questions about the individual's past experience prevents forgetting important points. Statements of the abilities the individual will need in order to function on this division are helpful. If copies of the interview guide can be mimeographed space may be left for answers and comments. Examples of questions and statements which might be included in an interview form for new nurses on a gynecologic division are:

Type of experience:
   Date of graduation from school of nursing
   Type of school
   Experience since graduation
     Where
     Length
     Type (staff nurse, head nurse, other)
     Recency
Amount of experience and feeling of adequacy
   In patient care
     Hysterectomy
     Radium insertion

Exenteration
Other
In nursing care
Dealing with emotional needs of patients and families (those facing sterility, inoperable carcinoma, death)
Giving formal instruction to patients and families
Carrying responsibility for critically ill patients
Caring for dying patients and assisting their families
In technical procedures
Radium removal
Catheterization
Douche
Assisting with pelvic examination
Other
Team member
Team leader
Conducting conferences
Planning assignments
Preparing nursing care plans
Evening duty—charge
Night duty—charge

The way the interview form is used is highly important. It is not a questionnaire to be given to the staff member to complete. The head nurse and new member, preferably together, fill it out during the conference. It is especially necessary that the new staff member feel comfortable, welcome, and at home. The way the form is used can add or detract from this feeling.

Planning Learning Activities

In the initial interview it is well for the head nurse and new staff member together to map out a program for the newcomer. Experiences which both feel are necessary or desirable should be checked on the interview guide. From this list they plan the type of assignments and the supervision which the nurse needs. If the collegiate school graduate needs experience in organizing and giving care to a group of patients she should recognize this fact and, if at all possible, help decide on the rate at which she can increase her load. She may need help in seeing how individualized care can be given when she is assigned to six or seven patients. Under no circumstances should she be caused to lose her ability to meet the human needs of patients as a result of having less time to devote to each person. With proper guidance this will not happen.

The nurse who has problems in talking with patients and discovering their fears, worries, apprehensions, will not learn these skills just by being assigned to only one patient. She needs a great deal of help from a person who has scientifically grounded behavioral skills. If the head nurse does not possess this ability she herself should seek help (see Chapter 20).

GUIDED LEARNING FOR THE REGULAR STAFF

Learning activities are planned for regular staff members as well as for new ones, for they need to grow in service. Some were inadequately trained in their basic programs. Likewise tremendous changes are taking place in health services. New and improved methods of medical and nursing practice are being developed, making it imperative that each staff member continue to learn if she is to remain competent in the face of change. Nurses on a division need also to develop a common philosophy of patient care. It is the head nurse's responsibility to exert leadership which will result in the growth and development of her entire staff. Understanding, tact, and ingenuity on her part are needed if experienced individuals, especially professional nurses, are to see a need for help. Deficiencies should seldom be directly pointed out. A group approach is often more effective. The entire staff may study methods and content for patient instruction, the approach to a "difficult patient," and other aspects of comprehensive nursing. Ideas are exchanged in conference. Following such a study each nurse is assigned the care of patients requiring skills she feels she needs to develop. If the head nurse conveys to the staff nurse that meeting the patients' needs is a mutual responsibility, that they are both working for the same ends, the nurse will be prompted to seek help and guidance.

Many activities related to the care of her patients will be of interest to the nurse. With planning, it is sometimes possible to arrange for the staff member to go to the physical or occupational therapy department, to the operating room, or to x-ray with one of her patients to observe the treatment, surgical procedure, or test he is receiving. Likewise, a visit with the public health nurse to see one of her patients who has been discharged will give the nurse new insight into the importance of teaching and referral. Observation of an autopsy on a patient for whom she has cared can also be of value. Others on the staff will benefit from the nurse's experience in any of these areas if she is given an opportunity to report her observations. She will take pride in having something of value to contribute to others.

Gaining acceptance of the need for guided experience creates no problem when nurses are involved in the care of patients undergoing a new type of surgery or a new therapeutic or diagnostic procedure instituted by the medical staff. The nurses who will be responsible for the care of the patients want the opportunity to become proficient in psychologically preparing patients, in performing the new procedures, in making accurate observations and judgments. Thus, when open-heart surgery was first performed in some hospitals, nurses on the division where the patients were housed were given special instruction. All nurses on the unit, day, evening, and night, plus the department, evening, and night administrators met with the surgeon, who described the surgical procedure. He outlined the preoperative and postoperative measures to be carried out by the nurse, the importance of emotional support, the observations to be made and their significance, possible complications and their symptoms. Following this introduction each nurse on the staff, starting with the head nurse, was assigned to care preoperatively for a patient who was to have open-heart surgery. She then observed the operation and, with a house medical officer in constant attendance, specialed the patient through the postoperative period. She cared for him thereafter until he was discharged. All nurses on the unit followed the progress of the patient daily and participated in planning his care. Only when the entire professional staff of the division had been prepared to nurse patients having open-heart surgery was this experience made available to graduate and senior basic students.

There are innumerable activities which will stimulate the interest of the nurse, increase her knowledge and understanding, and thus help her to grow. To mention a few, the following opportunities are available in many places: attending conferences of the health team especially when one of her patients is being discussed; making rounds with the attending physician or attending medical "grand rounds" in a teaching center; visiting another hospital in the vicinity to observe their methods of patient care; attending professional institutes, conventions, and other meetings; reading a nursing article of special pertinence to their patients and reporting on it to the staff.

APPLICATION OF PRINCIPLES IN PROVIDING GUIDED LEARNING

In planning learning activities the head nurse must keep in mind the principles brought out in Chapter 12 on assignment planning, notably those related to continuity in patient care and the need for sufficient practice to become skilled. She should also understand that, although one learns by doing, economical learning results only if the doing is supervised and evaluated (See Chapters 17 and 18). As has been seen in Chapter 12 the staff nurse acting as team leader needs a great deal of instruction in the team method, help in making assignments, conducting team conferences, and preparing nursing care plans. Guided experiences, then, are essential in developing staff members *to their highest potential.*

Lest there be misinterpretation of the expression "develop to their highest potential" which has been used several times in these pages, it will be well to clarify it. The statement means that the staff member should be helped to grow to her fullest capacity *within the limits set by licensing laws and by the particular hospital,* for persons in her role. In other words the practical nurse should be helped to become the best *practical* nurse which her particular talents permit. Because she is a highly intelligent, capable practical nurse, however, is no reason for her to be given professional nurse responsibilities or even responsibilities which her licensure permits but which the hospital does not. For example, practical nurses are taught to give medications, and laws of some states permit her to do so, but the hospital in which she is employed may for certain reasons not permit it. Nevertheless, regardless of hospital policy, that which the practical nurses and aides are taught, expected, and permitted to do on a patient care division depends very largely on the head nurse's concept of the professional nurse's responsibility. If the head nurse believes one of her practical nurses is sufficiently competent and trustworthy to care for the critically ill or the patient with many personal problems and assigns her to such patients, the head nurse is teaching this practical nurse to assume professional responsibility for which she has been neither prepared nor licensed. The head nurse should give serious thought to the possible consequences of such action. She should realize that in planning a guided learning program it is very important that objectives for the individual's growth be established in terms of the potential for persons in her role.

Another illustration also points up the fact that the head nurse's concept of the professional nurse's responsibility influences the learning activities she plans for her staff. If she considers that the professional nurse's primary function is to give technical care and to work with the gadgetry, and if she believes that giving comforting physical care to meet patient's personal needs is of less importance, nurses and aides alike will consider the ministering function to be "aides' work." The entire staff is influenced by the philosophy and attitudes of the head nurse in this regard. Her plans for guided experience and her assignments will reflect her beliefs. The learning of the staff member is determined in large measure by the assignments the head nurse plans for her. If the staff is to continue to develop the head nurse must have for each member a clear picture of her possibility for growth, the limits on her activities, the staff member's personal goals, and the experiences available. Only then can the head nurse plan worthwhile learning activities.

SUMMARY

Guiding the new staff member's experience involves the assessment of her knowledge and ability in relation to the requirements of the patients on the division; planning with her the experiences which will increase her proficiency; assigning experiences according to principles already enumerated; supervising and evaluating the staff member's performance until she and the head nurse are confident she can function competently. The regular staff must have guided experiences also to keep them abreast of change in medical and nursing practice. Goals for each person in terms of her potential for growth within the limits of her role as set by law and hospital policy, should guide the head nurse in planning learning activities.

QUESTIONS FOR DISCUSSION

1. How feasible is it for the head nurse to determine the background of a new staff nurse and her capability for functioning in the situation in which she has been placed? How feasible is it to plan for her to receive needed experience and to provide for her supervision? Give reasons for your answers.
2. In what areas of practice would the nurses on your division profit from planned learning activities? Would it be possible to make and carry out plans for this learning? Justify your responses.

EXERCISES

1. Imagine yourself a new staff nurse in a service no longer familiar to you. List the special competencies you think you would need in order to function in the service, and have your list checked by a nurse who knows the requirements. Plan a program of guided activities which you feel would prepare you to care for patients safely and competently.
2. If you are a head nurse, confer with one of your staff who seems

interested in learning, to find out areas in which she would like experience. Ideas from this chapter may suggest possibilities. Plan the learning activities if at all possible. Together with the nurse evaluate the results.

REFERENCES

Drulias, Fotine J., and Sitler, Beverly. A reorientation program, Amer. J. Nurs., Vol. 61 (February 1961), p. 71.
Three admitting room head nurses, who had been in the hospital nursing service for an average of 27 years, were given an opportunity to see other areas of the hospital as well as several community agencies. The results of a carefully planned program were gratifying.

Frye, Lillian B. An on-duty inservice experiment for aides, Nurs. Outlook, Vol. 13 (August 1965), pp. 60-61.
A night supervisor held "on-duty review" meetings for nurses' aides. The night nurses and aides participated in the planning and evaluation. As a result nurses spent more time with the patients and felt greater satisfaction in their work.

Gowin, Joan. Staff development in the operating room, Amer. J. Nurs., Vol. 65 (May 1965), pp. 117-119.
Orientation and carefully planned learning activities make it possible to handle a constantly changing staff with relative ease.

Marshall, Minna H. Inservice programs require effective follow-up, Nurs. Outlook, Vol. 12 (August 1964), pp. 42-44.
A successful inservice program is influenced by ward climate, morale, attitudes. These in turn are influenced by follow-up of instruction or orientation and the way in which the follow-up is carried out.

Randall, Carol E., and May, Florence E. Skills the new graduate needs, Nurs. Outlook, Vol. 9 (April 1961), pp. 232-233.
A list of skills nursing service administrators expect of new graduates and a description of what the new graduate expects of the hospital employing her. Challenging for the head nurse.

Wood, M. Marian. From general duty nurse to team leader, Amer. J. Nurs., Vol. 63 (January 1963), pp. 104-105.
An inservice program for team leaders is described together with a description of their responsibilities.

J. Nursing Admin 4. 31 May/June 74

Management — Nur. Mirror 138: 62 Mar. 22 74.

Nurs Outlook 22: 394-7 Jun 74

Nur. Res. 23 307-18 Jul/Aug 74

Nur. 74 4: 51-8 July 74

Nurs Times 70: 57-9 Insert aug 22 74

Journal Nur. Admin 4: 19-25 Sep/Oct 74

AJN 51: 257 April 1957

AJN 51: 665 Nov. 1951

chapter 17

SUPERVISION OF PERSONNEL

Before considering the head nurse's responsibility for supervision of personnel it will be well to have an overview of the entire supervisory process in nursing at the division level. This process has ten facets, some of which have been previously discussed. The overall supervisory process involves:

1) Establishment of long-range objectives for the quality of care desired for patients on the unit.
2) Assessment of needs for improvement in the care given.
3) Determination of immediate objectives.
4) Planning methods for meeting the immediate objectives.
5) Assessment of needs of individual staff members for improvement in light of the objectives for patient care.
6) Establishment of personal objectives by staff members.
7) Planning methods for achieving personal improvement.
8) Carrying out the plan under supervision.
9) Evaluation of results and making new plans.
10) Continuous evaluation of the effects of individual effort on the quality of care given patients on the division.

It will be recognized that points 1 through 4 and 10 were discussed in Chapter 13, Supervision and Evaluation of Patient Care. Suggested also in that chapter were the values to staff development of participation in the supervisory process. These values cannot be overemphasized.

PURPOSES OF SUPERVISION

Desired outcomes of supervision were also stated in Chapter 13, namely: 1) a high quality of care for each patient and 2) the development of each staff member to her highest potential. Since these outcomes are considered desirable they become the purposes or objectives of supervision. For clarity, the two purposes and methods for achieving them are considered individually in this text. However, it should be recognized that administrative and educational supervision cannot be separated *functionally*. The two

369

are correlative and complementary functions. By increasing the ability of the staff, nursing care is made better. When patient care is of a high quality the staff who share in it continue to grow. Improved morale also results from good supervision. However, the latter is not an objective to be sought directly.

PHILOSOPHY OF SUPERVISION

"Inspection and direction have been discredited"[1] as methods of supervision. Instead, the head nurse in her supervisory role works with the staff to establish worthwhile objectives toward which all strive. Supervision, then, can be defined as working together to achieve common goals. Inherent in the process is evaluation of outcomes. Supervision is a kind of teaching. It involves advising, helping, inspiring, leading, liberating.[2] The supervisor (head nurse) is a counsellor rather than a superior officer. She cooperates with the staff and serves its needs. Leadership is substituted for authority.

Who is a supervisor? Many people supervise who are not called supervisors. Head nurses and instructors have supervisory functions. When the term "supervisor" is used in this chapter, it may relate to any one of these individuals. It will refer primarily, however, to the head nurse in her supervisory relationship with the staff members assigned to her service.

PRINCIPLES OF SUPERVISION

A principle is a law or proven truth. Principles underlying modern concepts of supervision, some of which have been discussed previously, may be summarized as follows:

1) Good supervision is focused on improvement of the work rather than on upgrading the worker.

2) Good supervision is based on the needs of individuals which have been cooperatively determined. It employs techniques which provide for self study by staff members, as a starting point in their growth and development. In nursing this means the staff member with the help of the head nurse studies her own ability to give the kind of patient care the staff has

[1] William H. Burton and Leo J. Brueckner. *Supervision, A Social Process,* 3rd. ed., New York, Appleton-Century-Crofts, Inc., 1955, p. 80.
[2] John Alexander Rorer. *Principles of Democratic Supervision,* New York, Bureau of Publications, Teachers College, Columbia University, 1942, p. 218.

established as its goal and determines her need for further development. Only if both share in the assessment will they be able to coordinate their efforts.

3) Good supervision is cooperatively planned. Objectives, methods of supervision, and criteria for judging success in the attainment of goals are jointly established. The plan is based on the needs of the individual staff member and is varied as her needs change. Supervision is continuously adapted to the changing situation on the division.

4) Methods employed in good supervision are democratic in nature. They are adapted to the experience and ability of the staff member and to the existing situation. There is no one technique suitable for all persons or all circumstances. The method should be selected to achieve the desired outcome.

5) Good supervision stimulates the staff to continuous self-improvement. Stimulation results when the individual's interests are aroused so she responds with enthusiasm. Supervision needs to be continuous, not periodic. It assumes that staff members are competent, that they can and want to improve their competency. It encourages and challenges the individual to greater endeavor through adequate approval and commendation and by recognition of work well done. Supervision creates in the staff member a desire for help in the attainment of her objectives. If she has been aided in achieving success, her attitude toward supervision is improved. She returns to the supervisor for further assistance. Good supervision recognizes that even the excellent staff member needs supervision to continue to grow. It provides freedom for experimentation, self direction, and self evaluation,[3] but this does not mean the counsel and assistance of the supervisor is unnecessary.

6) Good supervision respects the individuality of the staff member. It "accepts idiosyncrasies, reluctance to cooperate, and antagonisms as human characteristics just as it accepts reasonableness, cooperation, and energetic activity. The former are challenges; the latter, assets."[4]

7) Good supervision helps create a social, psychological, and physical atmosphere in which the individual is free to function at her own top level. This principle was discussed previously and will not be elaborated here.

Although it is recognized that not all staff members are receptive to change or see the need to improve, that many work only because they need to do so, nevertheless, the principles stated are sound. If improvement is to be made either in patient care or in the individuals who give it, the improvement will likely result from application of these principles of super-

[3] Rorer, *op. cit.*, p. 222.
[4] Burton and Brueckner, *op. cit.*, p. 85.

vision. A recent study [5] showed that "the quality of care given to patients and the general tone of nurse–patient relationships was related to the quality of supervision and teaching that the head nurse provided." Many head nurses are autocratic, lack skill in leadership, have their minds centered on getting the work done rather than on providing high quality care and fostering the growth of the staff. It may be possible to challenge these head nurses to improve the quality of their leadership. If not, they will eventually be replaced by nurses who are being educated in modern concepts of supervision.

METHODS OF SUPERVISION

Methods of supervision are many. Those which are effective when used by one head nurse may be quite unsuccessful for another. Keeping principles in mind, each must continuously experiment to find methods which are effective for her. These she must adapt and change to suit the individual whom she is supervising. A few methods which have proved effective for experienced supervisors will be enumerated here to stimulate the thinking of head nurses who may be searching for ways to assist their staff members. At all times it is necessary to keep in mind that the supervision of experienced persons should not be detailed or directive. The head nurse who is used to working with students may need a special reminder in this regard. Two other points should be remembered when reading this description of methods. *First,* supervision must be in terms of the objectives and criteria for patient care on this division; *second*, the methods described are based on the principles which have been stated.

Cooperative Determination of Staff Member's Needs

When objectives for nursing care have been formulated by the staff and the weaknesses delineated (see Chapter 13) it should be assumed that each member will wish to improve the quality of her own nursing. This will require self evaluation and assessment of her personal needs. If relationships are good between the head nurse and her staff, the staff members

[5] Elizabeth Hagen and Luverne Wolff. *Nursing Leadership Behavior in General Hospitals,* New York, Institute of Research and Service in Nursing Education, Teachers College, Columbia University, 1961, p. 136.

will often welcome the help of the head nurse in making the assessment. The process, if successfully begun in the initial conference, can easily be carried over to the evaluation of further needs at a later time. Regular conferences for assessing each individual's need for growth are necessary. Out of the discussion should come not only recognition of her needs but realization that the head nurse has a good deal to offer which can help the individual in her professional development. The desire to satisfy a recognized need becomes the staff member's personal objective.

While supervisory conferences such as those described above are usually instigated by the head nurse they may also grow out of a request from the staff if its members are in earnest about reaching the specific goals for nursing care which they have formulated. Whether conferences are suggested by the head nurse or by the staff is immaterial as long as some acceptable way is found to bring about individual consultation for reviewing the member's needs. Each person should be helped to *want* assistance from the head nurse in self appraisal and in planning ways to increase her ability. If the head nurse proves capable of stimulating, inspiring, and liberating her staff to think creatively, members will come to her freely for assistance in assessment, planning, and evaluation.

The head nurse must be aware of needs of nurses and aides whether or not the staff member recognizes or is willing to admit them. Time may be required for the individual who has been a member of the staff for a long time to feel free to discuss her shortcomings and request assistance. The head nurse needs to give opportunity for the staff member, without fear of embarrassment or criticism, to say she wishes help. Sometimes the head nurse can offer it and the assistance will be gladly accepted. If both individuals are primarily concerned for the patients' welfare it should be possible to get the staff member to consider and discuss her need for development. The head nurse, of course, must have special abilities which the staff member does not have and which she recognizes as desirable.

Cooperative Planning for Supervision

When a nurse or aide is given a new assignment she may be insecure about parts of the patient's care. Then, there are times when the nursing care of a patient is intricate, requiring delicate or specialized skills in physical handling, in organization and management, in observation and interpretation of symptoms, and in understanding the patient's special needs. A staff nurse may be inexperienced in coping with the problems presented.

Unless the head nurse is sure of the individual's ability and self-confidence in the situation, she needs to discover the extent of the nurse's understanding through judicious questioning. If the nurse has an understanding of scientific principles, is skilled in the use of her hands and in organization of assignments, a conference with the head nurse before the nurse starts to care for the patient may suffice. They discuss the patient's nursing needs, the objectives for his care, important observations to make and record. If there is a plan for the patient's care it is reviewed. If not, the head nurse and staff nurse evolve one. If indicated, the head nurse makes suggestions for approach to the patient and the adaptations in procedure which are needed. It is important that new nurses know how to give the necessary care in *this* hospital to *this* doctor's patient. In each situation new to a staff member, she and the head nurse together decide on the parts of the patient's care with which the individual needs or wishes assistance. This help may be in turning a patient on a Stryker frame, helping with gastric suction, bathing a patient in a pelvic sling, or instructing a patient, preoperatively, to cough and deep breathe. There are many other ways in which the staff member may need help. The amount and type of assistance required depends on the ability and experience of the individual.

There are many instances when the amount of help which the head nurse can give in conference or in assistance with portions of the patient's care is insufficient for the staff member's needs. When the individual is new or young in experience the head nurse might well plan to have a competent nurse with her throughout the entire care of a patient who presents new and difficult problems. A new staff nurse, for example, may need this type of help in caring for a patient who has had an intricate operation or for one who is in a respirator. A practical nurse may need help with a patient in traction. Before beginning the patient's care the important points which are involved and the results to be achieved are discussed. The experienced nurse with whom the staff member is to work participates in this conference. The head nurse's involvement depends upon the teaching ability of the experienced nurse. A plan of action is made, the new nurse indicating the part she would like to play. She frequently wishes the experienced nurse to take the initiative in the patient's care while she learns from working with the nurse who is familiar with the regimen. A follow-up conference answers any questions which may be in the learner's mind. At this time the amount and type of help she needs the next day is determined.

During the days that follow when the staff member is working more independently the head nurse needs to be available and approachable for help and conference. She will wish to visit the patient while the staff member is giving his care in case assistance is needed. Opportunity to confer with the nurse or aide about her problems, successes, discoveries should be made, especially during each of the first several days. The head nurse will read the nurse's notes on the chart and use them as a point of departure in discussing the patient. When the individual's assignment is changed or the patient goes home, the staff member, in conference with the head nurse, should evaluate the care given, her own learning, and the supervision she received.

Supervision at the Bedside

Some head nurses have expressed a need for assistance in ways to supervise at the bedside. We shall here suggest some possibilities.

The head nurse who herself cares for patients may ask a nurse—any nurse, not just a new staff member—to work with her. The two plan activities together and arrange for both to be doing something for the patient at the same time. One may suction while the other strips the top of the bed. One bathes while the other assembles materials for mouth care. Throughout, the head nurse demonstrates any unusual technical care and, by example, ways of relating to the patient, of determining his needs, and of bringing him into the planning for his care. Before the day is over the two discuss the experience, the head nurse attempting to discern the staff nurse's personal reaction to the experience and to the nursing given. Hopefully the head nurse will have demonstrated a successful relationship with the patient which the nurse will wish to discuss and to emulate.

Whether or not the head nurse has time to supervise by working with staff members as described above, she *must* assist members at the bedside, when this is required for the safety and welfare of the patient or for the learning of the individual. For example, a staff nurse may report to the head nurse that she is having a problem in some aspect of nursing care, or the head nurse may discover such a problem as she is making nursing rounds. In either case the head nurse must act. Perhaps the nurse is having difficulty suctioning a tracheostomy tube, or a confused patient who is supposed to be on bed rest is up walking around and refusing to return to bed. A patient may be unnecessarily exposed during his bath or may be having trouble staying on his side while his bed is being changed. How does the head nurse help under these circumstances without appearing to be critical of the nurse? The relationship between nurse and patient must not be jeopardized by any hint of criticism. In no way should the head nurse indicate that the patient's nurse is incompetent in the situation. If the nurse herself does not feel she is being criticized she will by her manner transmit her feeling of self-confidence to the patient.

The head nurse might enter any one of the situations described with a remark such as, "Would you like a little help?" or "Here, let me give you a hand," or "Have you ever tried it this way?" The head nurse who steps in to help should become a partner in the procedure. She helps to hold or turn the patient, covering him as she does so. She may suggest that the nurse put the catheter further down into the trachea or she may take the suction tube from the nurse if it is offered perhaps remarking, "Let's see what I can do," and reassuring the patient that suctioning will soon be completed. She asks the nurse if she would like her to talk with the patient who will not stay in bed to try to determine his reasons. Or the head nurse may suggest to the nurse that the patient be kept quiet and comfortable in a chair until he can be helped to understand why the doctor wants him to stay in bed. Thus we see that sometimes the head nurse assists the nurse at the bedside, thereby demonstrating desirable methods. Sometimes she demonstrates by taking over an activity if the nurse wishes her to do so. Sometimes she suggests procedure to the nurse. Which method the head nurse employs depends on the nature of the situation, whether emergency action is required, the head nurse's knowledge of the kind of help the particular nurse prefers together with the nurse's ability to function adequately with direction, and the method the head nurse is comfortable in using.

It is usually advisable to follow up bedside supervision with an informal conference to pinpoint the problem the nurse was having and to make sure she understands why the measures tried were successful or unsuccessful. This follow-up helps to strengthen learning.

There will be times when the help needed by a staff nurse would be inappropriately given by the head nurse in the course of her rounds. When this is true, she should make note of the behavior observed, preferably putting the anecdotes in writing, and discuss it with the staff member at a later date. (See Chapter 18.) The purpose of this observation and recording is to aid in the staff member's development, not to find fault or criticize.

We have in this chapter mentioned but a few of the ways in which the head nurse supervises her staff. There are countless others, many of which have been mentioned elsewhere in this text. It can be seen that the supervisor (head nurse) is no longer an inspector and rater. Rather, she is a guide, counsellor, or helper to staff members who, with her assistance, have determined their inadequacies in giving the care the staff has set as its objective. The head nurse is a leader who helps them make plans whereby they can receive the experience and assistance necessary to their growth.

She is a teacher who is kindly, understanding, and considerate, and who has faith in their ability and their desire to improve.

A Supervisory Plan

In the preceding paragraphs we have considered ways in which the head nurse plans with her staff the supervision they wish and noted the fact that the head nurse must convince her staff that she has something to offer them through her supervision. We have discussed ways of working with nurses at the bedside. The same measures can be used effectively with practical nurses and aides.

If supervision of personnel is to be more than a chance occurrence which takes place only when staff needs are glaring or when time is readily available, a supervisory program must be established. Only if supervision is considered important enough to plan will time be found to give it consistently.

The outline below which incorporates the ideas enumerated in this chapter and the two preceding ones may suggest to the head nurse a way to plan her own supervisory program.

A PROGRAM OF SUPERVISION

I. Long Term Plan
    A. For new staff members
        1. Initial interview
            a. Brief overview of objectives for care of patients on this division
            b. Primary features of nursing care on this division
            c. Assessment of nurse's knowledge and ability in relation to care needed by patients housed on this division (use guide)
            d. Planning experiences which are needed
            e. Planning type and amount of supervision to be given
        2. Assign experiences and give supervision planned
        3. Follow-up conferences
            a. Purposes—for evaluation and further planning
            b. Frequency—at least weekly until nurse is oriented to all experiences indicated on guide

B. For regular staff
    1. Regular individual conferences for evaluation, defining goals, planning
    2. Daily conferences as needed to be sure staff member understands rationale of therapy for patients she has not cared for previously
    3. Assign experiences needed or requested for individual development, and plan type of supervision
    4. Assign experience and plan type of supervision in new types of treatment or nursing care, such as use of cardiac monitor or respiratory resuscitation, following group instruction
    5. Informal, unplanned supervision at the bedside

II. Short Term Plan
  A. Each week
    1. Review plans for new staff members
      a. Plan supervisory methods in accord with requests
      b. Plan conferences
    2. Review requests for experience made by regular staff members
      a. Plan assignments
      b. Plan supervision (who, how) with the staff member
      c. Orient assistant head nurse to plan
    3. Review plans for special supervised experiences of regular staff (B4 above) and make schedule for the week (ie, which staff nurses are to have experience that week, who will supervise).
    4. Consider other new types of treatments for inclusion in supervised experience, and plan schedule
    5. Orient entire nursing staff to plan for the week
  B. Daily
    1. Review the day's plans in relation to weekly schedule
    2. Adjust assignments if necessary
    3. Review the supervision needed that day
    4. Head nurse plan her own day's program to include necessary conferences and bedside supervision
      a. Delegate part of supervisory responsibility if necessary
      b. Establish priorities for her own time as needed

FINDING TIME FOR SUPERVISION

Supervision of personnel takes time, but the head nurse who believes it to be important will make opportunity for it. She will also find ways to share the supervisory load with her professional staff. When team nursing is used the leader will naturally carry considerable responsibility for supervision. She, however, may have had no experience of this kind and need a good deal of assistance in the application of principles. If there are no teams, a staff nurse should be called on to assist the head nurse, as indicated above. Assumption of this responsibility is a means of staff development for the nurse, and neither she nor the head nurse should fail to capitalize on its values.

The responsibility for developing her staff through supervision should be accepted as a challenge by the head nurse. She may not be able to do all that is here suggested, but with forethought and planning she will find that she can do more than at first she thought possible. She is already doing a great deal of supervision. It may take little more time to do it in a better way. Without a carefully planned and executed supervisory program, staff development will be considerably slowed and may be seriously hindered. As a new role for the head nurse is developed and she is relieved of non-nursing functions, she will have more time to devote to the development of her staff. A planned program of supervision is one way by which she can bring about greater growth. This, as we have seen, will lead to a better quality of nursing.

Evaluation of staff development resulting from supervision and other methods used to stimulate growth will be considered in Chapter 18.

SUMMARY

The two objectives of supervision—improvement of patient care and development of the staff—have been considered individually in this text although they cannot be separated functionally. Neither can be achieved without the other.

The philosophy of personnel supervision has changed in recent years. Inspection and direction as methods have given way to mutual effort on the part of supervisor and supervised to reach a common goal. In the new concept, supervision is a kind of teaching and involves advising, guiding, helping, leading. Principles of good supervision call for cooperative effort by the head nurse and individual staff member to determine the member's needs for growth and to plan supervisory and evaluative methods which will be acceptable and fruitful. Good supervision stimulates self-improve-ment, respects the individuality of the staff member, and helps to create an atmosphere in which individuals are free to grow.

Methods of supervision vary with each head nurse and need to be individualized for each staff member. They should be based on principles of good supervision. If methods are flexible and continuously evaluated, the head nurse will discover those which for her are the most effective. She should, however, never stop experimenting with new methods based on sound thinking.

Good supervision is time-consuming but is of such importance that opportunity must be made for it. Having a plan facilitates its accomplishment. The head nurse should share many supervisory activities with members of her professional staff. It is important for her to recognize that these members require guidance and help in their supervision of others but that the experience for them is a means of growth.

QUESTIONS FOR DISCUSSION

1. Should aides be given opportunity to help decide the kind of supervision they are to receive in doing something which is new to them? Explain reasons for your answer.
2. Would it be practical in your situation to have a planned program for supervision? Could a workable plan be made? Under what circumstances would it be effective?

EXERCISES

1. Attitudes toward the head nurse are reflected in the thoughts of staff members when the head nurse arrives on the scene at a time when everything is going wrong. These thoughts might be, "Thank goodness you are here!" or they might be, "Why did you have to come at this particular moment?" Have you had both kinds of thoughts? If so, describe the differences in the two head nurses which influenced your reaction. How does a staff member react to you under similar circumstances? How does the individual's reaction correlate with your reaction to the situation in which you found her?
2. If you are a head nurse try out an interview guide adapted from the one suggested in Chapter 16, developing with the newcomer a plan for her supervision in some unfamiliar patient care activity. This might be the care of a patient whose needs she wasn't sure how to meet or a procedure with which she was unfamiliar. Take time, after filling out the interview guide, to think of possible ways to supervise the staff member in an area in which she wants help. Then you will be ready to present

her with alternatives. Follow through, giving the planned supervision. It will, of course, be necessary to see that the new person gets the experience and supervision she indicates she needs even though for this exercise you are dealing with only one small area of need. Evaluate results, including the individual's reaction, in relation to pre-established criteria. If possible have someone else find out from the new member her reaction to the supervision and how well she feels she learned.

3. Make a plan for evaluating the supervision given by either the head nurse or by the department administrator. What is the first step in the process?

REFERENCES

Argyris, Chris. Personality and Organization, New York, Harper and Brothers, 1957, Chapters 1 and 2, pp. 1-53.
The characteristics of human personality discussed in these chapters should help the head nurse to understand herself and her staff members.

Bellaby, G. Hospital internal communications: The Hawthorne experiments, Nurs. Times, Vol. 61 (September 3, 1965), pp. 1213-1214.
A review of famous experiments, the first to document the effect of interpersonal relationships on work output.

Blake, Florence. The supervisor's task, Nurs. Outlook, Vol. 4 (November 1956), pp. 641-643.
If students are to learn to be understanding and supportive of patients they need to experience understanding and support from their supervisors. Only purposeful practice in an environment conducive to learning will prepare the nurse to be aware of other's feelings and help her to acquire the capacity to communicate with and help patients and families. Excellent.

Georgopoulos, Basil S., and Mann, Floyd C. The Community General Hospital, New York, The Macmillan Company, 1962, Ch. 9, pp. 613-621.
The effect of supervisory behavior on the satisfaction of personnel, on the coordination of activities, and indirectly on the quality of patient care are dealt with in a very interesting manner.

Hughes, D. M. Management training in nursing, Part I, Nurs. Times, Vol. 61 (August 13, 1965), p. 1120; Part II, Vol. 61 (August 20, 1965), pp. 1149-1150.
A training officer in an industrial plant in England discusses the importance of training for all levels of management. He suggests abilities needed by a manager (Part I) and content of a training program (Part II).

Lambertsen, Eleanor C. Staffing problems emphasize need for better supervision by R.N.'s, Mod. Hosp., Vol. 106 (March 1966), p. 146.
If even minimum standards of patient care are to be realized, graduate nurses must be aware of their responsibility for supervising members of the various categories of nursing personnel.

Mooth, Adelma and Ritvo, Miriam. Developing the Supervisory Skills of the Nurse, New York, The Macmillan Company, 1966.
This small book clearly describes the characteristics of the adult learner and should be useful to the head nurse in the supervision and development of her nursing staff. "Cases" describing supervisory situations are thought provoking.

Perdue, Barbara Lee. To be an effective supervisor, Nurs. Outlook, Vol. 13 (September 1965), pp. 65-66.
The qualities of a good supervisor are summed up in the statement: "The effectiveness of the supervisor is directly correlated with her ability to develop good head nurses."

Rorer, John Alexander. Principles of Democratic Supervision, New York, Bureau of Publications, Teachers College, Columbia University, 1942.
A highly organized, clearly presented report on an investigation of principles of supervision together with the author's conclusions relative to principles. Excellent.

Sells, Annabel C. The first line supervisor and human relations, Canad. Nurse, Vol. 61 (April 1965), pp. 283-284.
The writer has brought together the ideas of many people to make this an interesting article.

Strauss, George, and Sayles, Leonard K. The Human Problems of Management, Englewood Cliffs, New Jersey, Prentice Hall, Inc., 1960.
Chapter 1, The meaning of work, pp. 1-31: One of the keys to effective supervision is understanding what subordinates want from their work—what satisfactions they seek. Chapter 2, Technology and job satisfaction, pp. 32-55: Describes ways in which the workers can gain the satisfaction in their work necessary to productivity. Part 2, Supervision, pp. 103-192: This section of the book is especially valuable in its description of *general* as opposed to detailed supervision of personnel. Part 3, Supervisory skills, pp. 193-237: Has a helpful chapter on interviewing.

chapter 18

EVALUATION OF PERSONNEL PERFORMANCE

PHILOSOPHY AND PURPOSES OF EVALUATION

Achievement can only be evaluated in relation to objectives or goals —the personal goals of the individual and the institution's objectives. These should be in harmony. In other words, in meeting her own goals the staff member should contribute to the attainment of the broader institutional objectives, or at least should in no way interfere with their achievement. Evaluation helps the individual determine her progress and assists her in bringing it about.

Without evaluation it is not known whether goals have been reached or to what extent objectives have been attained. Without evaluation progress is slow, interest lags, there is little motivation for improvement, little challenge. Evaluation is not something that should happen at periodic intervals. It should be a continuous process carried on jointly by the head nurse and the staff member.

Evaluation is more acceptable when appraisal is of the nursing care given rather than of the nurse or aide. A person who is committed to her work and eagerly striving to achieve specifically formulated objectives *wants* her work evaluated. She also *wants to participate* in the appraisal. Self-evaluation is essential to an individual's development and should be encouraged by every means possible. Some persons may be self-sufficient in judging their progress and determining their needs for growth. The vast majority, however, needs or profits from the help of an individual skilled in the areas in which the staff member wishes to improve. For this reason, evaluation of the performance of nursing staff members should be a joint undertaking of the head nurse and the individual member.

Although the head nurse is usually called upon to evaluate personnel for the administrative purposes of promotion, salary increases, and the like, here focus will be on evaluation for the purpose of developing the staff.

OBJECTIVITY IN EVALUATION

Regardless of who does the evaluating—the individual herself or the head nurse—the results will be useful to the extent the appraisal has been

383

made objectively. Evaluation is inaccurate and, therefore, of little worth if it is colored by the feelings of the rater toward either the individual or the situation, for under such circumstances one does not get a true picture of the person's progress. It is a disservice to a staff member to be given cause to believe she is doing much better or much worse than is the case. Inaccurate evaluation is also a disservice to the hospital which may promote an unqualified person to a more responsible position or may withhold advancement from one who could make a larger contribution. If the head nurse realizes the importance of objectivity in evaluating the performance of her staff and the ease with which subjectivity can creep in she will make a practice of testing her evaluative judgments. Many little ways by which the head nurse can strive to make her evaluations objective will be suggested throughout this chapter.

In certain areas it is not possible to be entirely objective. Some outcomes can be *measured*, others cannot—at least not as yet—but they can be *evaluated*. Knowledge of facts can be measured fairly accurately by objective tests which yield quantitative data. For example, the nurse's knowledge of the symptoms of congestive heart failure can be measured by various types of tests. The head nurse, however, is more concerned with judging the way in which the nurse uses her knowledge and how she behaves than in determining the nurse's factual knowledge. Does she report increasing cyanosis? Does she employ nursing measures to relieve dyspnea and support the weight of the arms? Does she reassure the patient by frequent visits to his bedside? By observing the staff member's behavior, the things she does and says, the head nurse is able to *evaluate* her understandings, her skills, and her appreciations. Evaluation is more subjective and less precise than measurement. However, if evaluation is based on records of observed behavior the gap between it and measurement becomes smaller, and greater objectivity is possible. For example, observation of a staff nurse sitting down listening intently and comforting the wife of a patient who is in the operating room would lead the head nurse to believe the nurse is understanding and has skill in human relationships. However, before she could be sure the head nurse would need to observe the nurse in many different situations which required that skill and would have to note the effects of the nurse's attempts to comfort on patients, families and others. Objective measures for evaluating the quality of care is one of nursing's greatest needs.

Personality characteristics, interests, attitudes, ideals are more difficult to evaluate than abilities because subjective judgment is involved. It is not easy for the observer to leave out her own feelings and her personal opinion when making judgments concerning personality traits. Every effort must be made, however, to be objective. The head nurse should attempt to evaluate only the *effect* of the nurse's behavior. Behavior *reflects* her attitudes. For example, in attempting to evaluate a staff member's empathy the head nurse notes what the individual said to the patient, her manner, and the effect of her behavior on the patient.

SOURCES OF INFORMATION FOR MAKING EVALUATIVE JUDGMENTS

In general there are four sources upon which the head nurse needs to draw in evaluating the work of her staff. *First*, she has general information about each person—her education and experience—and knowledge of what can be expected of aides, practical nurses, registered nurses with various types of preparation, and of individuals with different amounts and kinds of experience. *Second*, the head nurse uses her own observations and notes on individual conferences with the staff member which she should have compiled in an anecdotal behavior record. *Third*, the head nurse should have access to the anecdotal notes of assistant head nurses or team leaders with whom the staff member has worked. *Fourth*, the staff member's objectives and recorded notes of experiences should be available to the head nurse.

If records have been adequately kept these sources provide a wealth of information useful to the head nurse in evaluating the quality of work achieved by members of her staff.

THE ANECDOTAL BEHAVIOR RECORD

One of the aids to evaluation most suitable for use with hospital personnel is the anecdotal behavior record. An anecdote is a brief account of some incident. An anecdotal behavior record is a compilation of anecdotes which describe behavior. Significant incidents which portray personality traits and the presence or absence of skill or understanding, or which picture the quality of work produced, are written down at the time of their occurrence. The following anecdote indicates the interest, initiative, and resourcefulness of the practical nurse, Miss James.

Cared for Mr. C_____, elderly Italian, who speaks no English. Patient frightened. Ate little breakfast. Refused bed bath. Miss James requested

Italian porter to talk with patient. Moved patient next to another patient of same nationality. Stated she plans to look up common words in Italian dictionary.

If anecdotes are accurate, well selected, and well written, the anecdotal record gives a clear picture of the degree to which the staff member is meeting objectives. When the number of anecdotes is large, they serve as excellent source material for self evaluation by the staff member and for counselling and guidance by the head nurse.

Choice of Anecdotes

The keeping of anecdotal records can become exceedingly cumbersome and time consuming both in their writing and in summarizing the material for use. Every effort must be made to keep them simple. Of the many incidents which are constantly occurring the head nurse must learn to choose those which have meaning and value. Some incidents are trivial and some are significant. For selection of incidents a guide is needed which describes broad areas of concern in which the behavior of the nurse or aide should be observed and recorded.[1] The areas relate to objectives. In general, incidents which portray the attitudes, understanding, and relationships of the staff member should be selected as well as those indicating technical competence. Following is a list of areas in which observations of professional nurses should be made. Incidents depicting behavior in relation to these points are important to be included in the anecdotal record of a staff nurse:

Initiative and skill in recognizing and meeting patients' needs (physical, emotional, spiritual, social).
Precautionary measures used to safeguard patients and personnel.
Patient-nurse relationships.
Initiative in assuming professional responsibility.
Accuracy and judgment in carrying out medical orders.
A questioning attitude.
Evidence of scientific understanding of nursing principles.
Adaptation of procedures and environment to needs of patients.
Accuracy in observation and professional judgment.
Emergency situations.

[1] The critical incident technique describes a scientific method for delineating areas of concern. See: John C. Flanagan, Doris Gosnell, and Grace Fivars. Evaluating Student Performance, *Amer. J. Nurs.,* Volume 63 (November 1963), pp. 96-99. Reference was made to this technique in Chapter 13.

Skill in making patients comfortable.
Teamwork.
Organizational skill.
Accuracy in recording.
Promptness in reporting.
Neatness of workmanship.
Manner and appearance.

The ability to recognize behavior which is significant develops with practice. The head nurse needs to keep in mind the characteristics and abilities which she expects the individual to possess. Frequent reference to the objectives and criteria is a necessity. Incidents which are important in the staff member's development should be chosen, not those primarily of importance to the head nurse, such as getting the work done.

To avoid the negative effect which anecdotal records sometimes give, it is important that the head nurse write down not only those incidents which are displeasing or undesirable but to make a point of having more favorable than unfavorable incidents written about an individual. No incident should be recorded which produces an emotional reaction in the head nurse for she will be unable to picture it objectively. Certainly the record should not be used to justify the head nurse's actions. The head nurse herself can be evaluated by the anecdotes she writes, for they portray the behavior and attitudes which she considers important.

Opportunities for Observation of Behavior

The head nurse has many opportunities to observe the staff member. Her best field of observation is at the bedside of the patient. She also sees the individual and observes her behavior in the workrooms as she prepares for treatments and cares for equipment. She observes her in the nurses' office as she obtains her assignment and orders, does her charting, and gives reports. Is she methodical in collecting information? Does she put away charts and forms when she is through with them? The head nurse notes the kinds of questions the staff member asks, the thoroughness of her reports, the comments she makes about patients, her co-workers, and her assignments. Her relationships with visitors, doctors, staff members, and other hospital personnel are observed. Does she volunteer to assist other staff members? Does she go to the assistance of a visitor, doctor, or orderly who is looking for someone to whom to speak?

The head nurse includes in her anecdotal records evidence of interest, judgment, and other important characteristics which she observes in the nurse outside her regular time on duty. It is important to record that the nurse came to the floor during off-hours to study patients' records, that she volunteered to come back to special a patient who needed extra care, that the aide brought flowers and magazines to lonely patients. Significant behavior may be observed in the dining room, the corridors of the hospital, on the street. Perhaps the nurse may be overheard talking about patients in the elevator or on the bus.

Content of Anecdotal Records

There is some disagreement as to whether the report of an incident should be wholly objective or whether it should include some interpretation. Interpretation is the observer's opinion of the *reason* for the behavior. Some authorities insist that the anecdote should be a cold statement of fact. They object to interpretation because it explains behavior on the basis of a single incident. Other educators believe that on occasion the observer's interpretation is very helpful because there are times when an anecdote could be interpreted in more than one way. It is fairly well agreed that any interpretation which accompanies an anecdote should be separate from the facts and that the observer should be well aware that she is using interpretation. Records are more valid if it is necessary to interpret only a few of the incidents. The following anecdote is interpreted, the interpretative statement being separate from the incident.

Critical of the fact that Mr. T_____, a patient with congestive heart failure with orders for bed rest, had been getting out of bed and going to the bathroom. Stated concern for his safety and that if he fell she would be held responsible. Had no plans for circumventing the problems this behavior raises other than explaining to the patient that he must remain in bed.
Interpretation: Miss R. seems to think nurses should "make" patients follow orders and that if she does not do so she will be blamed for the consequences.

This notation is objective except for the last paragraph which is interpretative. Without the final statement the anecdote could be interpreted in another way.

Some observers include evaluation in their records; that is, they indicate that the action was good or bad, as for example:

Gave excellent care to Madeline, a 15-year-old girl who had an adrenalectomy yesterday. Gave patient good explanation of postoperative procedures and obtained her cooperation. Wisely spent time just talking with Madeline, who was quite apprehensive.

Without the evaluation the statement would read:

Cared for Madeline, a 15-year-old girl who had an adrenalectomy yesterday. Explained the need to cough, deep breathe, and turn in simple terms and obtained the patient's cooperation. Spent time just talking with Madeline, who was quite apprehensive, about things interesting to teenagers—school friends, vocational plans.

The reader of the second statement is permitted to make her own evaluation in the light of all the facts. She is unbiased by the opinion of another. The head nurse, reading the record at a later date, is not influenced by her own earlier judgment. The staff member upon reading the record can judge for herself the significance of her behavior.

Probably one of the most common faults in writing anecdotal records is the tendency to generalize. Behavior is described as though it happened frequently or was characteristic of the individual. A statement of this type is the following:

Miss Grant makes suggestions to the charge nurse about patient's need for changes in nursing care plans.

In this instance the head nurse made a general statement whereas an anecdote is a single incident. She should have recorded the characteristics of Miss Grant's charting for the day the observation was written. It would be more accurate to state:

Suggested that her patient who had been critically ill with congestive heart failure was beginning to assert herself and that the nursing care plan should be changed so that all will know the amount and type of activity permitted.

The most useful anecdotal record specifically describes an incident. It includes a brief statement of the situation or setting and tells what the individual and other people did and said if these are significant:

Miss Jones was one of two nurses who came on duty this morning, the other three having reported ill. The second nurse was disgruntled and complained that the two of them could never care for all 26 patients. Miss Jones, however, cheerfully suggested a plan for starting the day's work, said it would be fun to see what two people could do. She soon had the other nurse enthusiastically entering into the plan.

Had the situation not been described in this case, the incident would have been meaningless. If no mention had been made of the attitude of the second nurse, Miss Jones' quality of leadership would not have been shown so clearly. There are times, however, when a statement of the situation is unnecessary. A simple description of significant behavior stated objectively is all that is necessary.

Cared for Mrs. A, terminal uremia. Manipulated oxygen equipment with ease and checked frequently so that a new tank of oxygen would be ordered on time.

We get an indication of this nurse's skill and sense of responsibility. It is not necessary to know about other things which were happening on the division.

Nursing activities which are not performed well, if important in the individual's development, are recorded. For example, the unwise handling of a patient's worries or complaints, the failure to record important information or to take needed precautions are significant. Since such mediocre workmanship should be discussed with the individual at the time, it is necessary for the head nurse, in writing the anecdote, to include the staff member's explanation regarding her performance. The explanation may cast an entirely different light on the situation. The nurse may say that she forgot to record the patient's headache, that she didn't think it significant, or that the night nurse had recorded it and she believed it unnecessary to repeat the information. The reasoning of the nurse may be just as important as the incident itself. Of significance also may be the nurse's attitude toward her failure to remember to record the headache, that is, whether her reaction is one of casualness, defense, of shocked surprise, or of deep concern.

Following a poor performance, the head nurse makes a point of observing the nurse in similar situations to determine whether improvement has been made. Such follow-up observations are recorded so that in reading the series of anecdotes progress or lack of it can be recognized.

Method of Recording Anecdotes

The anecdotal record for each individual is kept in chronological order on cards or in a notebook. Each entry is dated and if more than one individual writes anecdotes each entry is signed. It is possible in this way to follow the staff member's progress. Needless to say, anecdotal records are highly confidential and must be kept in a safe place, preferably under lock and key, where they will not be a temptation to inquisitive individuals.

The clinical instructor, department administrator, assistant head nurse, team leader, the evening and night nurse administrators as well as the head nurse should write anecdotes. Each may wish to keep her own separate record or there may be a composite record for each staff member made by all individuals who observe her work while she is on a particular division. It is important that the head nurse keep records of student nurses regardless of how many other people are also keeping them. As the person responsible for nursing care she sees and knows the importance of some actions which have less meaning for those working in other capacities. She sees the results of the behavior of nurses on the total management of the division. She knows better than anyone else the results of a nurse's failure to record narcotics, to keep an accurate record of intake and output, or to remove the dentures of a patient going to the operating room. In each instance the head nurse is held responsible for the failure of one of her staff members.

Anecdotes must be written promptly if they are to be accurate. The head nurse in all probability will not have time or opportunity to write up an incident the moment it occurs. However, she can spot an incident as worthy of recording, make a mental note of the contributing factors, and write down enough to remind her of the details when she sits down to write her records later in the day. Time needs to be planned in each day's program for the writing of anecdotes. Anecdotal records should be kept on all staff members but are imperative on those who are in need of special help. If they are to serve their purpose anecdotal notes must be consistently and conscientiously written on those for whom they have been undertaken.

Anecdotal records take time and they take thought. It is often very difficult for the head nurse to find time to write them. However they are invaluable aids in understanding and helping nurses, and the head nurse cannot afford to omit them. Practice makes it easier to simplify them and to include only the essentials. The more skill the head nurse develops in observing behavior and recognizing its importance the easier the task becomes. With the help and encouragement of her department head the head nurse should persist in keeping anecdotal records to the extent of her ability and time. Once she has formed the habit she will not be willing to relinquish the practice and will manage to find the time for writing them. She will be rewarded by the grateful appreciation of her staff, their continuous growth in ability and desirable attitudes, and the improved quality of nursing care on her unit.

Use of Anecdotal Records in Evaluation

Evaluation is a three-fold operation: 1) determining the objectives and criteria, 2) observing and recording the facts, 3) evaluating the data collected. The first two have already been discussed. Anecdotal notes contain the data which must be evaluated if staff members are to be helped and the head nurse is to know how successful she has been in the development of the personnel. How is the data used to arrive at an evaluation?

In general, evaluation consists of an analysis of all the available information about the individual and making a value judgment as to the quality of performance in terms of established criteria. For example, the staff member's personal written notes about her work and the head nurse's anecdotal record may show several instances in which patients and families for whom the individual had cared had become less fearful and anxious. Unless there were several other instances in which the staff member's patients had not been helped or had become more anxious, it could probably be concluded that she relates well to people and has a gift for reassuring and for inspiring confidence. The important point to remember is not to generalize, that is, not to make a value judgment on too little evidence. If objectives are clearly defined and are greatly desired, behavior which evidences progress toward the goal or that which interferes with the desired development can be easily detected. When this evidence is written down over a period of time by the staff member and the head nurse, then looked at sequentially, evaluation is not so difficult.

It is usually best for the head nurse and the staff member separately to study the anecdotes and for each to make her own evaluation. They can then compare their judgments. The head nurse will probably need to help the aides and practical nurses and perhaps the professional nurses analyze the meaning of their behavior. Following the analysis and drawing of conclusions future plans should be made. Objectives may need to be revised and enlarged. Ways for meeting them should be reviewed. From the anecdotes, new criteria for evaluation can be formulated which will help in continuing appraisal. Both head nurse and staff member will review their efforts to attain the objectives and to be alert to indications of success or failure.

The head nurse may find it very helpful in drawing conclusions from evidence found in anecdotal records to *rank* her professional nurses (or practical nurses or aides) in a given characteristic. To make a judgment concerning the nurse's ability to make a patient comfortable, the head nurse compares the members of her professional staff, placing them in rank order. The one who shows the greatest skill is listed first; the one who shows the least is at the bottom of the list. Others are placed in rank order according to their functioning in this one area—making the patient comfortable. The next step is to analyze what the one in top place does that is different from that of the others and so on down the line. Evidence available in anecdotal records helps prevent subjectivity in the process. Needless to say individuals are compared with those in the same category. An aide is not compared with a nurse, at least not in areas where the nurse is expected to excel. Junior students are not compared with seniors.

Rating staff members on the degree to which they achieve objectives is another aid in evaluation. An objective is the goal or end result one desires to attain but all persons do not achieve the objective to the same degree. Levels of performance are sometimes difficult to determine. In establishing criteria for evaluation it is helpful if these levels are spelled out in descriptive phrases. For example, social acceptability is an objective. One in whom this quality is highly developed could be said to inconvenience herself willingly in order to help others. Another who meets the objective a little less well may plan her work with thoughtfulness for others. Such descriptive phrases may be placed in an ascending or descending scale at intervals along a line to indicate degree of attainment. The middle of the line is considered average and indicates a sort of standard. The individual is rated on the scale. She need not be checked at a regular interval but any-

Social Acceptability	Willingly inconveniences self to help others	Plans work with thoughtfulness for others	Friendly and helpful to others	Does own work paying little attention to others	Inconsiderate of others

where along the line to indicate degree. When setting up descriptive phrases for rating there tends to be greater accuracy in scoring if some are arranged on an ascending scale, others on a descending scale. Although the head nurse may not feel competent to establish levels of performance she may be asked to use a form which gives descriptive phrases, such as the one illustrated above, for evaluating members of her staff. The better forms leave space for the head nurse to give illustrations to substantiate her judgment. For this purpose she should use conclusions drawn from her anecdotes. If in a report on social acceptability a practical nurse was checked "plans work with thoughtfulness for others" the following illustration would explain the head nurse's judgment:

Routinely makes rounds to see that patients are comfortable and that they have their personal needs met before she goes off duty thus reducing the demands on the staff of the next tour of duty. Plans her work to have patient ready for x-ray, physical therapy, and other departments at the time scheduled.

PERSONAL NOTES OF STAFF MEMBER

It is important to reiterate that the staff member should have her own objectives simply stated and clearly in mind. If an objective for a surgical division is to send patients to the operating room in a confident frame of mind, the nurse's personal objective is to have the ability to free the patient's mind of ungrounded fear and give him confidence. In addition to her objectives related to the high quality of patient care which have been established as a goal by the staff, the individual staff member may have other goals of her own. For example, if she has recognized problems in interpersonal relationships she may have as an objective the ability to work harmoniously with staff members. Criteria for judging outcomes (see Chapter 13) should be used by the nurse or aide as a check list for self evaluation. She will wish the head nurse to use the same criteria in appraising her work.

Instances illustrative of behavior will seldom be remembered unless they are put in writing at the time they occur. If the staff member has real goals for herself she will be aware of times when she meets criteria and the occasions when she does not measure up to her own standards. Writing down briefly her successes, frustrations, and failures and her analysis of the situations will help her review her progress. When she knows these descriptive notes will not be used against her in any way it is hoped she will be forthright in picturing her failures and not hesitate to have the head nurse review them with her.

Although it is hoped, as pointed out in Chapter 17, that the members of the staff will recognize their own limitations and ask for help, this does not always happen. The head nurse may realize a problem exists which the staff member does not recognize or does not admit. The head nurse, in these circumstances, needs to identify the problem and take steps to diagnose the situation before she can be of any help to the individual.

DETERMINING A STAFF MEMBER'S NEED
FOR ASSISTANCE

Symptoms Which Indicate That a Problem Exists

Indication that a staff member needs help may be noted in the behavior of patients as well as in the actions of the individual nurse or aide. The following examples of patient behavior are suggested as possible symptoms indicating that something is amiss: The patients assigned to the staff member in question may be exceptionally restless, have their signal lights on frequently, appear unhappy and disgruntled. They may complain about little things, appear critical and disgusted with their treatment. Family members may appear uneasy and lacking in confidence as evidenced by the manner in which questions are asked and the kinds of things they do in the way of care for the patient and his surroundings. Do members of the family, after greeting the patient, immediately come out and ask for fresh water, that his ice bag be filled, that the patient be made comfortable? Do they start straightening up the room, bringing out dead flowers, old newspapers, extra dishes?

Symptoms which the staff member may display are complaints about little things, chronic fatigue, or irritability. She may show poor relationships with other staff members or evidence poor planning and disorganization. Perhaps she is habitually absent from staff meetings. She may come to work late or fail to show up on holidays.

The alert, conscientious head nurse who is striving for comprehensive nursing care on her division is aware of things which interfere with its achievement. She notes that the staff member needs some kind of help. The department administrator is called upon for counsel and assistance in detecting evidence that the staff member is not functioning at her best.

Determining the Cause of the Problem

If the department administrator and head nurse believe a member of the staff is having real problems they should make a preliminary investigation of the situation to determine factors which may be contributing to the problem. This would include such things as division and hospital policies, general morale, and smoothness of the administration of the division. Preliminary study would also include a review of the individual's background and any personal problems which may be accentuated by the existing situation. Has she had previous experience in caring for patients with the conditions represented on this division? Has she been prepared to give comprehensive nursing or only technical care? How many years has she nursed? Has there been a recent interruption in her experience? Was she well oriented to the division?

The head nurse will also wish to look at the present situation to determine possible reasons for any apparent lack of satisfaction. Has her nursing load been especially taxing? Do certain unit practices irriate her? Has she had an excessive amount of night duty? Has there been lack of continuity in her patient assignments? Was she expecting a promotion which she did not receive? Do family problems make heavy demands on her time, energy, and emotions?

This preliminary survey having been made and any necessary remedial measures adopted, the next step is to observe the staff member in all types of situations. Anecdotal notes should be kept on observations of her relationships with patients, visitors, and personnel; on her general behavior, the situations which seem to bother her, and the things which trigger undesirable behavior. The evidence is analyzed and her nursing evaluated. A hypothesis is made relative to the cause of the staff member's failure to function adequately. The next step is to test the hypothesis (see illustration below).

At this point the head nurse has enough evidence to be sure that the staff member needs help. This is the time to confer with the individual to ascertain her feelings about her work, her attitudes, interests, problems as she sees them. The head nurse may be able to help the nurse or aide establish objectives that are very real to her and through anecdotes assist her in self evaluation. Observation and notation of behavior in conferences and following them may give sufficient information to test the hypothesis and determine the cause of the individual's behavior. On the other hand the fact finding may be too complicated for the head nurse. The department administrator or a trained counsellor may be needed not only to determine the cause of the individual's problems but to help her recognize and deal with them. The head nurse, however, has a real responsibility to see that needs are recognized and met insofar as possible using all available resources.

IDENTIFICATION OF A PROBLEM:
AN ILLUSTRATION

It was clearly evident that a staff nurse, Mrs. Post, was not happy in her work and that her attitudes were reflected in her patient care. In a preliminary investigation by the head nurse and the department administrator it was recognized that Mrs. Post had recently returned to nursing after twenty years of married life and child rearing. Financial reverses had made it necessary for her to return to work. Nursing and medical care had changed markedly during the twenty years she had been away. No longer did professional nurses give all the care to patients. Nurses' aides and practical nurses were doing many things which were to her the job of the nurse.

Nursing teams were being used. Her first day on the division, after a brief orientation to the geography of the units and to the patients, she was made team leader. She was told she was responsible for the supervision of the aide and practical nurse on her team and for the care of the patients to whom they were assigned. Because the team members could not give medications she must do so. She had not heard of most of the drugs ordered, and having been taught never to give a medication unless she knew the purpose, action, favorable and unfavorable symptoms which might result from its administration, she spent much time reading the pharmacology reference book on the division.

When the circumstances were considered, the head nurse and department administrator realized that the nurse had been inadequately oriented to modern nursing and to the team concept. Arrangements were made to change her from team leader to team member, to reduce her assignment, and to spend time helping her learn new therapeutic methods and discussing the philosophy of the team and her problems and questions in relation to it.

Following this period of instruction and guidance Mrs. Post was once more made a team leader. Her relationships with team members and others on the staff were closely observed. The quality of her patient care was evaluated in terms of the criteria for good nursing. Anecdotes were kept and after a few weeks it was thought some of the problems previously observed still existed and the anecdotes seemed to indicate that Mrs. Post failed to give leadership to her team members. There was also evidence that she related well to the patients for whom she herself cared but that she had little contact with those assigned to the aide and practical nurse. When she gave the team members their assignment she asked if they knew how to care for the patients. If they gave an affirmative answer she left them alone. They asked their questions of other staff members instead of seeking out the team leader. Team conferences were short and consisted merely of asking whether the members had any problems.

From this evidence it was hypothesized that Mrs. Post was failing to exert leadership because she did not understand and accept her role as team leader.

The head nurse consulted Mrs. Post in an effort to learn her attitude toward team nursing, her feeling of responsibility for patients assigned to the team and her concept of good nursing. In a nonjudgmental way she was asked to evaluate the nursing being given the team's patients and was helped to see wherein she had not measured up to her responsibilities. With the help of the head nurse she set two goals for herself: 1) to get to know the needs of all the patients assigned to the team, and 2) to make sure each patient received the care ordered and was satisfied with it. Methods for achieving the goals were. established. First, Mrs. Post would study the patient's chart, become personally acquainted with him, and make a plan for his care. Secondly, the level of care required (professional nurse, practical nurse, or aide) would be decided with the help of the head nurse, and team members assigned according to their ability to meet the needs of the individual patient. Third, Mrs. Post would determine and give the supervision needed, and finally, each patient's physical, mental, and emotional reaction to his care would be observed.

The head nurse realized that if Mrs. Post succeeded in developing a real nursing team and patient care improved markedly as a result, her hypothesis would have been correct. Mrs. Post *could* be a good leader. She was failing because she had not understood and accepted her responsibilities as a team leader.

EVALUATION REPORTS

Reports on a staff member's competence to hold her position, her readiness and worthiness to be promoted to a higher one, are important to the individual herself and also to the nursing service administration. Since the head nurse is the person most closely associated with staff nurses and aides her evaluation is important. Usually a report on a new staff member is requested at the end of the first month and at periodic intervals thereafter.

Preparation of Reports

Evaluation reports should be prepared jointly by the head nurse and staff member. If the member's self-evaluation has at any time been used against her she will not be free to express herself. She will also resent the writing of anecdotes by the head nurse and others. If on the other hand both head nurse and member have kept records which they have periodically analyzed and the member believes the head nurse's purpose is to help and not blame, she will not fear to be honest in the evaluation of her strengths and inadequacies. In case she is not measuring up she will already be aware of it. If her shortcomings interfere with her satisfactory functioning she should be told by the head nurse and know that this will be included in her report. If she is making progress this too should be indicated. In this way the staff member knows exactly where she stands. (See Chapter 19 for description of evaluation conference.)

The head nurse who has had no experience in helping a nurse or aide with self-evaluation and the preparation of a report may herself need help from the department administrator or from someone skilled in evaluation. A clinical instructor, used to helping students in analysis of their strengths and needs, if available, may be willing to assist the head nurse.

Uses of Written Evaluation Reports

A series of well-written evaluation reports on a staff member, made over a period of time, can be very helpful to the nursing service or department administrator in counselling the individual relative to the type of work for which she is best suited. Such reports should indicate a nurse's potential for leadership and help the administrator decide whether she should be encouraged to obtain further education to prepare for a position of greater responsibility. Decisions regarding promotion, transfer to another service, or special counselling will be based in part on the evidence of competence and growth expressed in evaluation reports.

Permanent, cumulative evaluation records are a valuable source of information for purposes of recommendation which nursing service administrators are frequently called upon to provide to other hospitals and to universities. It can easily be seen that these uses are a benefit to the individual staff member herself.

Criteria for Good Evaluation Reports

A report which is suitable for any of the uses indicated gives the head nurse's reasons for the mark on a scale, the answer to a question, or the statement of judgment. Why does the head nurse think that a nurse has outstanding ability to organize her work? What behavior has she shown to give the head nurse this impression? As mentioned earlier *a good report gives illustrations to substantiate the head nurse's judgment.* For example, the head nurse selects from the individual's anecdotal record evidence in relation to her organizing ability. On the evaluation form she lists a few examples:

Handles full assignments with apparent ease. Makes a practice of methodically gathering equipment as she goes down the hall. Uses spare minutes to perform necessary tasks such as distributing fresh drinking water. Dovetails work, but when patients are left their care is complete.

Failure to attain desired standards can often be illustrated by suggestions for ways to improve:

Further improvement in ability to plan the day's work is needed. Remembering to care for the most uncomfortable patients first, to assemble equipment before beginning care, and to arrange the unit for convenience in working will aid in providing time for unexpected interruptions.

Illustrations of this type not only help the individual but they describe to the director of nursing specific characteristics of the staff member. For students the anecdotal records of the nurse are sometimes clipped to the evaluation form when it is sent to the office.

It is essential that the report be reliable, that is, that it show consistency of the same head nurse at different times. If the report is reliable the head nurse who used the same anecdotal records or other evidence would make the same judgments next week that she has made this week when writing the report. A reliable report is objective. It is based on specific observations, uncolored by the emotions and personal prejudices of the head nurse, rather than on mere impressions. It is very difficult for the head nurse to attain the desired objectivity if she maintains social relations with the staff member. It is important for her to know the nurse or aide but not so intimately as to allow favoritism to color her judgment. Likewise if she is to attain objectivity the head nurse should not try to write reports when she is unusually fatigued or distraught or when she has recently been emotionally affected for good or ill by the individual. A good practice is to lay the report aside for a day or so after writing it and then to see if it conveys the meaning intended. A report which shows bias of the head nurse is usually discounted in entirety by the reader.

In evaluating the work of individuals the head nurse needs to be very sure that she is judging the qualities she is purporting to judge. In other words *the report should be valid.* It may be evident that an aide, Betty, possesses greater skill than another aide, Anna. This is important. However it is also important to recognize that Anna made more progress in the development of skill although in the end she did not possess as much as Betty. Betty showed more natural skill whereas Anna displayed an unusual amount of persistence in the attainment which she made. In evaluating these two aides their achievement should be judged. So also should their natural abilities, their effort, and their progress, but the characteristics should not be confused with one another.

The tendency for one or two outstanding characteristics to color the judgment in relation to other characteristics is termed the "halo" effect. The fact that Anna put forth greater effort than Betty should not influence her score on achievement. That another aide, Yolande, is a rapid worker is no indication that she is thorough. Because she is well liked by patients the head nurse cannot necessarily assume that she uses good technique. Good or poor work in one or two respects does not guarantee good or poor work in other respects. The "halo" effect is one of the greatest known limitations to accuracy in reports. The head nurse finds it possible to avoid the "halo" effect if she evaluates a group of individuals in the same category on one characteristic at a time.

Another criterion for a good evaluation report is accuracy. It should give a correct picture. No rating will be accurate in which the individual is compared with persons of unequal experience. A practical nurse should not be compared with a professional nurse or with an aide but rather with other practical nurses. The head nurse, as we have said many times before, must know what she expects of individuals at different levels of preparation. A practical nurse may be doing high quality work consistent with her preparation whereas if she were giving the same performance as a professional nurse it might be considered mediocre. An individual head nurse sometimes tends to rate consistently higher than others, which clearly implies that the standards for those traits are lower in her mind than they are in the minds of other head nurses.

A head nurse should never score a staff member on a characteristic when she has no basis for judgment. Although it is true that individuals tend to fall in the average range, there is a tendency on the part of head nurses who do not wish to admit lack of knowledge to rate an individual average. Sometimes also the head nurse marks a person average because she is too lenient or does not have the courage to mark her low. This, too, makes for inaccuracy and such ratings have little value.

A composite opinion of several individuals is more likely to be accurate than the judgment of one person. The head nurse, department administrator, team leader, the assistant head nurse, and the person herself should collaborate in evaluating the work of aides and staff nurses. The report should indicate all persons who participated in making the appraisal.

Well-written reports *show progress* made by the individual. Reports should not be influenced unduly by the happenings of the first week, nor should they be based wholly on the observations of the last week before the report was written. The fact that progress was made and that it was slow or rapid characterizes the person better than a mere report of final achievement. It is significant that a new staff nurse adjusted slowly, requiring two weeks to develop sufficient confidence, skill, or knowledge to carry as much responsibility as was expected of one of her experience. Important also is the fact that when she "found herself" she proved to be dependable and able not only to carry well a large assignment but to change her plans, surmount interruptions, and take on additional work resulting from new orders.

The *manner in which a report is expressed* may affect the receptivity of the individual to its criticism. Since there are favorable observations to make concerning every person it is psychologically sound to begin with commendatory comments and to end on a hopeful note. In general a report which is couched in positive terms is more acceptable than one which contains negative statements. Instead of writing "she often did not realize the relationship between the patient's nursing care and his condition," the statement could read, "she often needed more understanding of the relationship between the patient's nursing care and his condition."

Evaluative statements should be based on the degree to which the staff member succeeded in relation to her own ability. Although the head nurse in making judgments of an individual's work must compare it with that of others, she should avoid comparative statements in the written report. It should not matter to the individual that she didn't measure up to the achievement of another provided she put forth effort and has made as much progress as she is capable of making. Each individual should be concerned with the quality of her own work in relation to her ability.

A report can serve to stimulate the staff member to greater effort in overcoming her deficiencies, but if it is to do so it must be written with that thought in mind. A report designed to challenge the nurse or aide will indicate measures which she may take to improve herself instead of specifying things which someone needs to do for her. For example, a young nurse may need to give greater attention to observing and recording symptoms. Obviously she should receive help in learning to do so. Her report, however, had best read:

Miss London will do well to study and to apply her knowledge of symptoms to a greater degree in the care of her patients and in recording her observations.

rather than:

Miss London needs help in applying her knowledge of symptoms and in recording her observations.

Meaningless expressions such as "her neatness of working is above average," even though amplified with illustrations, are to be avoided. What does "above average" mean? Should it matter that she is a little better than someone else if she is or is not as neat as she might be? Statements that "her surgical technique is not perfect" or "she needs more manual dexterity" are obvious when they refer to young students and should be replaced by statements that are more specifically descriptive such as:

Surgical technique is not yet a habit but requires conscious effort which she occasionally forgets to make, especially when under tension.

Another may read:

Her finer manual skills (handling clamps, controlling irrigating flow) are slow in development and will require persistent effort before they can be performed with ease.

The use of hyperbole weakens rather than strengthens statements. Excessive use of the expressions *always, never, very, most, usually, exceptionally* are usually exaggerations which may label the entire report inaccurate.

The best report forms have space for a *general statement or summary.* Too often after reading the various characteristics of the staff member one is left with no impression of her as an individual. Each trait has been analyzed but the picture of the person possessing them is somewhat nebulous. A final statement summarizing her strengths, her needs, and her progress serves to synthesize into a composite whole the elements which make up the person. The summary should also indicate any unusual conditions which existed on the division during the period covered by the report, since the situation influences the quality of performance which can be expected. A statement explaining any variance in evaluation between the head nurse and the staff member should be included in the report which should also indicate that it was jointly prepared.

Confidential Reports

A word might be said in closing this chapter about the place for confidential reports. There are times when a staff member shows personal qualities which in the eyes of the head nurse make her unsuited to nursing or to the position she holds. It may be an apparent lack of personal integrity,

, or physical stamina or insufficient theoretical knowledge ᴜᴜ intelligently. She may possess a personality which antagonizes ᴘₐₜients and co-workers alike. Any one of these problems may be too big for the head nurse to handle. She might easily do the individual infinite harm in trying to do so. In a confidential report the head nurse can give evidence for her judgment and state her observations. The administrator of the department or of the nursing service after a careful analysis of the staff member's entire record will either deal with the situation herself or advise the head nurse in the best method of helping the individual.

SUMMARY

Evaluation, an integral part of supervision, is a continuous process. It serves as a guide to tell the head nurse and the staff member whether objectives are being met. Most individuals want evaluation if they have meaningful goals. They want to participate in the evaluation of their work but they also want help from individuals whose judgment they respect and whom they know have a personal interest in them. Evaluation is not only necessary to growth; it is a means through which growth occurs.

Self evaluation with guidance is essential for rapid growth. Materials which aid in the process are notes written by the staff member relative to her own ideas of her progress supplemented by anecdotal records kept by the head nurse and others. These notes are evidence of behavior. To be useful in evaluation, incidents to be recorded must be carefully selected, the notes specific and objectively written. The individual's record and the anecdotal notes of the head nurse together serve as an excellent basis for self evaluation. Records of this type need not be kept for all staff members though they are essential for new ones, for those who are having problems, and for students.

Recording behavior is only one step in the evaluative process. It is essential to know objectives and to keep them in mind when observing and recording behavior. A second vital step is the analysis of the evidence to determine its meaning for the individual's growth. The third step is the evaluation. Ranking and rating are aides in evaluation. Judgment expressed in these should be substantiated by illustrations gained from anecdotal records.

An evaluation report is preferably jointly prepared by the head nurse and the individual being evaluated. There is, however, a place for a confidential report when the head nurse is uncertain of her ability to evaluate accurately. Every effort should be made to write meaningful reports which will be helpful to nursing service administration and benefit the individual herself. To serve its purposes a report must be valid, reliable, objectively written. It should be illustrated and give a clear picture of the individual as differentiated from others. Although many nurses will see the need for help through evaluation some will not seek it. If the head nurse is aware of a need, she must, with the department administrator, analyze the situation and the individual's background in order to diagnose the cause of the person's behavior or poor workmanship. The obvious causes are removed or corrected if possible. A hypothesis relative to the problem is formulated and is methodically tested in conferences with the individual and by observations, analysis, and evaluation. The needed assistance is given all along the line. When the problem is too big for the head nurse to handle it is referred to the department administrator who in turn may need to call on a trained counsellor.

QUESTIONS FOR DISCUSSION

1. How did you feel about evaluation reports as a student? as a staff nurse? What made you feel as you did?
2. Is the use of anecdotal records practical in today's busy hospital divisions? If you think not, what would you substitute that would achieve the purposes of both stimulating growth and measuring it?
3. Should anecdotal records be discussed with the staff member? If so, who should participate in the discussion? Give reasons for both answers.
4. Have you ever helped to write your own evaluation report? If so, how did you feel about it? If not, would you like to? Do you think a staff nurse should write her own evaluation and the head nurse add a brief note or just sign the report?

EXERCISES

1. Think of an experience in your life which meant a great deal to you and which required considerable taxing preparation on your part. How was evaluation handled during the learning process? Did you consciously evaluate your own performance and progress during the preparatory period? Did you have to meet someone else's standards as well as your own? Who was the more severe task master—you or the person help-

ing you? How was evaluation given? Did you appreciate it at the time? later? What would results have been without this help? What conclusions can you draw from this experience which could help you as a head nurse? From the review of this experience, summarize the elements you found to have been essential to successful evaluation.

2. Consider a staff member on your division who presents problems. Specifically state the chief problem in terms of *effects* on other people. (For example, not that she comes late to work but that she holds up report for four other people or that the head nurse must spend time going over with her the part of the report she missed, or the like.) Itemize briefly all the information you have about the staff member which may account for her behavior. Does the behavior seem in any way justified? If so, can the situation be modified? Validate your hunches with the staff member and get her suggestions for a solution. If you can see no justification, note conditions which precede or seem related to the individual's undesirable behavior. Modify the conditions if possible and test the effect of the change. If the problem still exists, make a point of showing special interest in the staff member and, in a *noncritical way,* suggest that you and she talk about the way she feels about her work. See if this leads to self-evaluation and improvement over a period of time. Organize a report on your study and present it to a group of your peers for discussion.

3. a. Select a staff member who will be willing to work with you. Together prepare a list of simply stated objectives which she wishes to achieve. The guide in this chapter may help in formulating her goals. Ask the staff member to keep brief notes of her activities which indicate whether or not she is progressing toward the objectives. You keep anecdotal records. Both should review objectives daily to make sure that all are being considered. After two or three weeks, each one should independently analyze both sets of notes and draw conclusions using the notes as evidence. Compare your findings. Was this a useful means of evaluating the staff member's performance? Did you manage to avoid personalities and to evaluate outcomes objectively? How did the staff member feel about the experience?

b. Using the criteria for well-written anecdotes stated in this chapter, evaluate each of your anecdotal notes. Were they objective? Were any of them evaluative? How many gave interpretation? Did they have enough information to make possible a judgment? Were any too detailed? Select your best stated anecdotes to present to the class. Select those which need improvement, change them and present both editions to the class for evaluation.

c. How many anecdotes did you have pertaining to each objective? enough to draw any valid conclusion or to suggest a judgment? What are the implications of this finding for use of anecdotes in evaluation?

REFERENCES

Angus, Monica D. Evaluation: a constructive or a destructive force?, Canad. Nurse, Vol. 62 (July 1966), pp. 26-28.
Evaluation of nursing personnel as sometimes practiced can lead to stagnation and lack of growth. However, if nursing establishes the criteria for graduate nurse performance and takes responsibility for seeing that only qualified persons perform evaluations, it will help protect nurses from the oppressiveness that could result from periodic evaluations in a bureaucratic organization.

Argyris, Chris. Personality and Organization, New York, Harper and Brothers, 1957, p. 24.
Since an individual's personality is more than a sum of his traits, merit ratings that attempt to score an individual's personality by adding up the parts can't get an over-all score.

Clissold, Grace K. and Metz, Edith A. Evaluation—a tangible process, Nurs. Outlook, Vol. 14 (March 1966), pp. 41-45.
Through description and illustration, this article clearly expresses the need to observe what a learner is actually doing if evaluation is to be meaningful and useful.

Ellsworth, Robert B., Butler, Grace, Ernst, Jane, and Gurel, Lee. The APEV Scale: a study of aide performance as perceived by nurses, aides, and patients, Nurs. Res., Vol. 11 (Winter 1962), pp. 15-20.
A very interesting study in which an Aide Performance Evaluation Scale was designed. There was high agreement between scores on the form completed by head nurses, evaluation by the aide's peer group, and patient evaluation of certain qualities. The form is specific enough to be useful in counselling.
Another study utilized this form and developed a different set of groupings of qualities based on factor analysis. See: Mulaik, Stanley A. and Dobson, William R. A factor analytic investigation of the Aide Performance Evaluation Scale, Nurs. Res., Vol. 13 (Spring 1964), pp. 167-169.

Flanagan, John C., Gosnell, Doris, and Fivars, Grace. Evaluating student performance, Amer. J. Nurs., Vol. 63 (November 1963), pp. 96-99.
The critical incident technique described here is also valuable for evaluating staff nurses' performance. The staff nurse as well as the student can be helped to identify areas of weakness and with the head nurse develop a plan for improvement.

Gettys, Elaine, and Stephan, Frances M. Nursing quiz on the wards, Amer. J. Nurs., Vol. 64 (December 1964), p. 103.
Paper and pencil tests are used for experienced staff nurses on the wards when problems arise. The majority of the nurses like the quizzes and find that they help identify their strengths and weaknesses.

Gorham, William A. Methods for measuring staff nursing performance, Nurs. Res., Vol. 12 (Winter 1963), pp. 4-11.

Head nurses will find the conclusions of the report on this study of special value. The emphasis is on the need for a different philosophy toward evaluation by both head nurses and staff nurses—an attitude that "improved patient care is the primary goal of the profession, and that one of the best ways to attain that goal is through a constant reevaluation of current practice and nursing effectiveness."

Heslin, Phyllis. Evaluating clinical performance, Nurs. Outlook, Vol. 11 (May 1963), pp. 344-345.
A splendid discussion illustrating the principles of evaluation.

Kellogg, M. S. Appraising the performance of management personnel. Reprinted in Koontz, Harold and O'Donnell, Cyril. Readings in Management, New York, McGraw-Hill Book Company, Inc., 1959, pp. 166-175.
In the industrial concern's evaluation process which is described, each individual to be rated prepares for his position a "responsibility summary" which is used by his immediate superior to evaluate the worker's performance. Good ideas for nursing are to be found in this document.

Palmer, Mary Ellen. Our students write their own behavioral anecdotes, Nurs. Outlook, Vol. 11 (March 1963), pp. 185-187.
Student nurses in one school write descriptions and evaluations of their work and become increasingly skilled in doing so. The many values are presented by the writer. If graduate nurses could be helped to write such reports on themselves they too would benefit.

Schultz, Frances K. Evaluation: Signpost or judgment?, Nurs. Outlook, Vol. 12 (September 1964), pp. 57-58.
The system used in evaluation of student performance and growth could be adapted for use by the head nurse and her staff. Observation and practice of patient care by instructors in the clinical setting, anecdotal records, and self-evaluation by students are some of the methods and tools used.

Smith, Kathryn M. Discrepancies in the role-specific values of head nurses and nursing directors, Nurs. Res., Vol. 14 (Summer 1965), pp. 196-202.
It was found in this study that discrepancies in nursing role values exist between head nurses and nursing faculty. "To a significant extent these groups used different criteria to evaluate the performance of the nurse." This creates a difficult situation for student nurses.

Strauss, George, and Sayles, Leonard K. The Human Problems of Management, Englewood Cliffs, New Jersey, Prentice-Hall, Inc., 1960, Ch. 23, pp. 527-548.
Sample evaluation forms are shown and methods of evaluation are illustrated and discussed. Very useful for the head nurse.

Tate, Barbara L. Evaluation of clinical performance of the staff nurse, Nurs. Res., Vol. 11 (Winter 1962), pp. 7-9.
Since head nurses are in the best position to evaluate the staff nurse and since head nurses are the persons called upon to write evaluation reports, a group of 450 head nurses from all over the United States participated in workshops in which they selected traits important to be evaluated and decided on behavior statements to illustrate each trait.

———— Evaluating the nurse's clinical performance, Nurs. Outlook, Vol. 10 (January 1962), pp. 35-37.
Although evaluation of clinical practice remains a difficult problem, collection of behavioral descriptions of practice promises to be a useful device. One must know *what* she wishes to evaluate and *why*.

Tribou, Marita. The incident process in teaching, Nurs. Outlook, Vol. 13 (January 1965), pp. 36-39.
An interesting illustration of this method of teaching which can be used effectively with nursing staff as well as with students.

chapter 19

THE RESPONSIBILITY OF THE HEAD NURSE IN CLINICAL INSTRUCTION

Educational programs for many different groups are carried on in the clinical divisions of hospitals. The new staff nurse and the nurse's aide, the student nurse and the medical student, to mention a few, all may have organized programs of clinical instruction for which the facilities of the patient care division are used. Whether or not she realizes it, the head nurse influences the education of these individuals to a marked degree. She is often the determining factor when a division is selected for student [1] experience.

At or near the patient's bedside much semi-formal teaching goes on in addition to the more organized instruction given in conferences, clinics, rounds, and demonstrations. *The extent to which the head nurse shares in the formal* teaching on the division depends upon the demands which other activities make on her time, her interest in teaching, and her instructional ability. If she likes to teach and believes the head nurse can and should make a contribution to clinical instruction she will develop her ability and find the time to do it. Regardless of the degree to which they participate, all head nurses need to know teaching methods and the essentials for effective clinical instruction. This is important, *first,* because each head nurse does a certain amount of teaching even if she is in an administrative role. *Second,* since in all first-rate hospitals someone—for example, a clinical instructor for student nurses, director of inservice education for staff nurses and aides —teaches on the division, the head nurse is in a position to help or hinder the educative process. If she understands what is going on she will undoubtedly be more in sympathy with the program. *Third,* if the head nurse is familiar with instructional methods it is likely she will do more teaching.

ESSENTIALS FOR GOOD CLINICAL INSTRUCTION

To determine the essentials for good clinical instruction it will be helpful to consider the criteria the instructor of student nurses, new staff

---

[1] In this chapter *student* refers to anyone who is having a planned program of instruction. The nurse in charge of any such program is referred to as the *teacher* or *instructor.*

nurses, or nurses' aides uses in choosing the division to which to take her students for clinical practice. The instructor must, of course, select units on the basis of the clinical conditions and nursing problems presented by the patients in relation to the student's educational needs. However, when she has a choice between units offering comparable experience she considers the following points.

First and vitally important, she selects a unit where the patients receive good care. This means the head nurse knows and believes in comprehensive nursing, is capable of giving it, and sets high standards for her staff. *Second,* the instructor considers whether the head nurse is understanding of the needs of students and other inexperienced individuals, and sympathetic to the educational program which aims to develop these individuals to a high level. *Third,* she selects a division on which the head nurse will cooperate in every way possible to provide opportunity for the instructor to teach and the student to learn. *Fourth,* the instructor tries to find a division with a head nurse who is interested in attending and sharing in the discussion in nursing care conferences, nursing rounds, and other sessions where patients are discussed.

Another essential for good clinical instruction is, of course, a competent teacher. Her selection is the responsibility of the administrator of the nursing service (for personnel) and of the school (for students). Each of these criteria will be discussed in detail in terms of the part the head nurse can play in meeting them.

Patients Receive Comprehensive Nursing Care

This criterion has been extensively developed and little more needs to be said. Students learn good nursing by participating in a nursing service which provides a high level of care to all its patients.

The Head Nurse Understands the Needs of Students

The head nurse needs to realize that to achieve desired results an educational program must be organized. In the hospital situation, the instructor of any group needs to be free to carry out her plans. This means she may place her students on the division at the time when needed experience is available and take them off the division for experiences elsewhere when this is desirable. The head nurse should of course expect that prearrangements will be made by the instructor relative to the time students will be present on the division. If patients are to receive good care, the head nurse has to be able to plan it and delegate responsibility for it. This is especially true in relation to student nurses. There are enough irregularities in staffing without the nurse instructor adding to the confusion by pulling students out of the situation for experience elsewhere at a time the head nurse is counting on their service. Learning activities for students must be carefully planned by the instructor but if the experience is to be of maximum value the student must actually make a contribution to nursing service. In gaining her education for service, the student must serve. It follows logically that the head nurse who is immediately responsible for the nursing of patients must know in advance the part the participants in that service will play. She must know when a student will be on her division, for how long, and what responsibility she will assume. It is important that the student identify with the staff and feel herself an important part of it even though she is on the division a limited number of hours.

The head nurse who understands the educational needs of students permits them to care for patients who will provide needed learning opportunities. Selection of patients for whom students are to care is a joint responsibility of instructor and head nurse. The instructor knows the capabilities and experience needs of the students. The head nurse is familiar with the patients and their requirements and is therefore in a position to aid the instructor in making assignments to students. Both the head nurse and teacher should be aware of and sympathetic with the objectives of the other. The head nurse should approve the assignment from the point of view of the patient, the instructor from the point of view of the student.

The understanding head nurse accepts the fact that students are learners. The senior student nurse is not a finished product although she may have developed a great many skills. If she is ready to practice as a staff nurse with minimal supervision she should be graduated and have opportunity to work for remuneration. Since she is still a student she needs a planned program of instruction and carefully selected activities to meet specific objectives. Every learner is developing new skill and new understandings. That this is a slow process the head nurse must realize. Students need opportunity to practice according to the principles and procedures they have been taught. The learning of motor and organizational skill, skill in talking, listening, and evaluating, thinking through problems and seeing relationships, all take time and concentration. The head nurse who understands and accepts this fact will realize that if the student is to develop desirable attitudes and gain true understanding she must have an assignment small enough to permit her to practice thoughtfully, to try out new ideas and evaluate them.

The head nurse should recognize that not only do individuals differ in native ability but they also vary in their motivation. Hence, no two students will develop the desired skills at the same rate or to the same degree. Patience and understanding are necessary if slow learners are to feel accepted. Learning will be still further retarded if the individual feels the head nurse lacks faith in her ability to achieve. Learners are often nervous in new situations and need help in gaining self-confidence.

It is also important that the head nurse recognize and accept the fact that individuals who are learning will make errors in judgment. To avoid serious consequences, responsibility is gradually increased and the student is not expected to make decisions until she has background sufficient to prevent dangerous mistakes.

The Head Nurse and Instructors Cooperate with One Another

The head nurse who understands and accepts the educational needs of students will do all in her power to make the educational program effective. Her cooperation is important to its success. Important also is the attitude of the nurse instructor toward nursing service. All too frequently in nursing education teachers and students work independently and in isolation, with the head nurse having no part in the educational program. Seldom do student nurses know the head nurse since their association with her is so limited. Often she neither expects nor receives reports directly from students who have been caring for patients. Instead students report off to their instructor. One might well ask what this manner of functioning teaches students about responsibility for and to nursing service, what attitudes are thereby engendered in young nurses, and whether these attitudes might be the cause of some of the problems common among new graduates. If nursing education is to prepare men and women to give nursing care in a service organization, student nurses need the contact with head nurses which is described in this chapter. Much responsibility rests with the head nurse to make a place for herself in the educational programs of both student and graduate nurses.

Cooperation between head nurse and instructor is essential. They must see one another's problems and each show consideration for the other. Students and clinical instructor are expected to adhere to the hospital and nursing policies of the institution which they are using as a practice field. The clinical instructor depends upon the head nurse to tell her of changes in these policies as well as in nursing procedures because such changes will affect student instruction.

Student nurses, especially, but other groups of new workers to some extent, have relatively short practice periods while much time is spent in classes and conferences. The cooperation of the head nurse is needed in getting students off to these sessions on time. The instructor usually makes patient assignments for students taking into account the individual's ability and the time available for practice. However, it is not always possible to estimate correctly and the assignment may prove to be too large for the learner to complete in the allotted time. The student may not have been able to plan around interruptions, she may have been slower than anticipated, or the assignment may have been too large or complicated. These occasions may be frequent because the student's ability in new activities cannot be accurately gauged. At such times the head nurse must be willing to have someone else complete the assignment and free the student to attend her class on time. On the other hand the student should feel her contribution to nursing service is important and that it does make a difference to the staff that she is there and that she completes her assigned work. Her contribution will not seem important if she can casually walk out leaving her work unfinished and the head nurse says "Oh don't worry, the aide will finish up." The head nurse needs understanding and skill to make the student who does not complete her assigned work feel comfortable about leaving when circumstances are beyond her control, yet not causing her to feel that the assignment was so easy or trivial that it mattered little whether or not she completed it.

If the instructor consistently misjudges the amount of responsibility her students can assume in a given period of time the head nurse should interpret to her the burden this places upon the staff. It is usually more difficult for staff members to add to their assignment in the middle of the morning than to plan for an extra patient at the beginning of the day. The head nurse's attitude toward uncompleted work by students will affect the attitudes of the staff toward students and the educational program. If she is generous and understanding they are likely to feel the same way.

Evaluation of the student's clinical work should be made by the head nurse as well as by the instructor. The head nurse's criteria for good nursing for each patient should be known to the instructor who interprets them to the student. The instructor evaluates the student's performance, the head nurse the care of each patient. Both evaluations are in terms of the criteria. In preparing for her evaluation conferences with the student the instructor will wish to make use of the head nurse's observations. If the head nurse has kept good anecdotal records they will be invaluable to the student and teacher (see Chapter 18).

Another way in which the head nurse cooperates with the clinical instructor is in keeping her informed about patients. It is helpful, too, if she passes on information concerning new drugs and therapeutic measures which are being used on the division.

The cooperative head nurse helps the instructor find a place to teach if necessary. She then makes sure that the staff knows that a conference is going on in that place. The most desirable place in which to hold conferences is a room adjoining the unit so that as little time as possible is required to reach it. It needs to be near enough for the group to go to see patients and return during the period of the class. Proximity is desirable when patients or equipment from the division need to be brought into the classroom. The place which is used for teaching should be quiet and free from interruption. A room which is used by doctors and nurses in the course of their unit activities is not a suitable place in which to hold a class or conference. The solarium is sometimes cleared for the purpose. This, however, deprives patients of its use, and is therefore educationally unsound since the purpose of the education is to teach good nursing.

The place selected must not be so close to the patients that they or their visitors will overhear the discussion. If no other space is available, occasionally the end of a corridor can be screened off for the conference. Whatever location is used, chairs are an essential. Preferably they are arranged around a conference table but if that is not possible chairs with arms for writing are satisfactory. Although note taking is not always necessary, such procedure needs to be made convenient should the student wish to take notes. There is an air of informality when the teacher and the students are seated so that each is able to see the other. Good lighting and ventilation are important and the room should be warm enough for comfort but not overheated. A blackboard is a desirable addition to the classroom. If a room with all these requirements is not available it is necessary to use the best place possible. Freedom from interruption is most important.

The Head Nurse Participates in Conferences

The head nurse has direct access to information about patients which others do not possess. She knows the plans for medical care and is familiar with diagnostic findings. This information the head nurse passes on to the nurse or team members responsible for the patient's care. However, her personal interpretation is invaluable when patients are discussed in conference or nursing rounds. The good head nurse knows her patients and their families well and takes the opportunity in conferences to share her knowledge with students and teacher. She has a great deal to contribute to planning nursing care which is often the objective of a student conference. Likewise, by participating in conferences the head nurse lets the students know of her vital concern for nursing care and her interest in their learning to give it. It is most unfortunate for students to get the impression that conferences in which care of patients is considered are wholly for the students' benefit rather than primarily to meet the patients' nursing needs. The presence of the head nurse helps to focus attention in this direction.

The Head Nurse As an Effective Teacher

It has been noted that the head nurse has much of value to contribute to students' knowledge and understanding of patients. Before attending a conference she needs to have read the last progress note and latest laboratory report on the chart and to have thought through the understandings and attitudes she wishes to convey to the students. In other words she goes to a conference prepared. Much that she has to say may be brought out by the students, in which case she may merely emphasize the most important points and answer questions which may be put to her. The head nurse will be more convincing in her contributions if by her manner she conveys her interest in the patient and her eagerness that his needs be met. If she thinks the things she has to say are important she should transmit this to the students by speaking with conviction. Her standards of care will be evident not only in what she says but in the way she says it. Her enthusiasm and earnestness will be infectious. The more frequently the head nurse participates in conferences the more she will realize the needs of students and the more interested she will become in their education. The clinical instructor, who will conduct most of the conferences, can usually help the inexperienced head nurse evaluate the part she has played. The head nurse can learn a great deal about effective methods of teaching from observing an experienced instructor.

Many times the head nurse is not invited to participate in nursing conferences, perhaps because it has been assumed she is too busy or is not interested. If the head nurse has not been asked it is not out of place for her to tell the instructor she would be interested in attending. The teacher will, in most instances, welcome her warmly.

METHODS OF CLINICAL INSTRUCTION

Today clinical teaching is a regular part of the instructional program for students in schools of nursing. It is customary for the instructor to hold two or more clinical conferences a week for the students assigned to each division. In some institutions conferences and other methods of clinical instruction are used in the staff development program. The more common methods of clinical instruction will be briefly described to familiarize the head nurse with their purposes and uses. Many of these methods the head nurse will wish to use in helping her staff to develop. Familiarity with methods will at least help her to appreciate the teaching which takes place on her division.

Conferences

Group conferences. By definition a conference is the act of consulting together. It always involves a two-way flow of conversation. An individual conference involves two persons while a group conferenct includes more than two individuals. The group should be small enough to permit each member to participate. If properly conducted, team conferences, nursing care conferences, initial, and evaluation conferences are two-way discussions, that is, they are true conferences. However, the term *conference* is loosely used to mean any coming together of two or more individuals in an informal meeting for the purpose of giving or exchanging ideas. ideas. Often the flow of conversation is mostly one-way rather than two-way. Thus nurses speak of orientation conferences and conferences preceding demonstrations. These are not confereces in the true sense of the word because they consist primarily of giving information rather than discussing ideas.

Conferences with the staff can be profitably used for many purposes. Some, as previously discussed, are held to set objectives and criteria for nursing care on the division, to plan methods for improving care, to solve problems which interfere with good nursing care, to evaluate results of efforts. Nursing team conferences were described earlier as was the joint conference for medical, social service, nursing, and other health personnel.

The latter group is often referred to as the health team. Each of the conferences mentioned above is directly or indirectly related to patient care and has for its purpose the planning or improving of that care for an individual patient or for the patient group. All but the team conferences are led by the head nurse and should involve the entire staff including, if possible, students currently assigned to the division. To reach all members—the night and evening staff and those who are off for the day as well as the day staff—the conference must be held more than once.

Conducting the staff conference. The purpose of the conference, that is, the reason it is being held and that which it is expected will be accomplished, should be clear to all. Since ten or fifteen minutes may be all the time that can be spared the subject for consideration must be limited in scope. The head nurse as leader should open the conference by briefly stating its purpose even though the staff should already know the problem or subject to be discussed. She starts the discussion by asking a carefully thought-out question or making a statement designed to bring out ideas, suggestions, or problems of the various staff members. For example, the head nurse may open a conference thus: "We are all aware that intake and output records on our floor are inaccurate, yet we know how important these records are both in diagnosis and in the treatment prescribed. There must be some reason why we fail to do what we know to be vital to our patients' welfare. Let us look at the reasons why you personally find it difficult to record intake and output."

If the staff is motivated by the head nurse's concern that solutions to problems be found and by her appeal for their help, they will be eager to present their ideas. The head nurse should accept each person's suggestion as worthy of consideration, make a note of it on a blackboard or small pad. Each member should be encouraged to express her thoughts. The head nurse then summarizes the suggestions. A group decision is usually in order. This may be to give further thought to the matter and consider it again after consulting other individuals such as the department administrator and the head nurse on another division, or the decision may be to try out one of the suggestions made. The head nurse ends the conference by stating the next step or steps and delegating any responsibilities that may be entailed.

Decisions about unit procedures frequently must wait until the second group of staff members (evening and night nurses and others) have met and expressed their ideas. Under no circumstances should these individuals be left out of staff discussions and decision making.

Needless to say evaluation conferences should be held periodically following the institution of any change in division policy or procedure. There may be need for further change. Under any circumstance, the group's judgment relative to results of their decisions is of great importance if other problem-solving conferences are to be entered into seriously.

Nursing care conferences. Nursing care conferences are extensively used in basic nursing education. Usually a single patient is discussed although comparisons may be made in symptoms, therapy, and nursing care of two or more patients. The nursing care conference may have one of two purposes. One is to portray the nursing problems typically associated with a particular disease or disorder, or with such factors as age, social or ethnic background, and to picture the related nursing care by associating the problems and the care with a specific individual. The second purpose is to learn problem-solving methods through attempts to identify patients' problems and needs, their origin or causes, possible methods of alleviation, and the nurse's role in the entire process. In achieving the second purpose the student must learn about the condition or disorder from which the patient is suffering. Emphasis, however, is on utilization of the experience and the thinking of group members in finding solutions to problems and in preparing a plan for the patient's care. For this reason the head nurse is a very important participant.

The statement of purposes indicates to some extent the method of conducting the conference. The first, *to portray,* implies that someone is telling others. If this is all that happens then the term *conference* is a misnomer even if two or three students in the group are reporting on various aspects of the patient's care. If, following such a presentation, the student or the instructor or head nurse leads discussion in which all in the group are freely participating by asking questions or making suggestions, the conference method is being used. This is not to say that reports of nursing care studies are lacking in value. They make a distinct contribution to learning if they are well presented and the group is interested and attentive. The instructor tests understanding through thoughtful questioning which calls for application of knowledge in a new situation.

The second purpose, to learn problem-solving methods, implies concerted activity in a seeking process. The patient to be discussed is selected because he has needs which his nurse wishes help in identifying and meeting. All pertinent data relative to his medical and personal history, his condition, progress, therapy, and nursing care are presented by the nurse who has been caring for him. She then states the difficulties she is having in identifying and meeting his needs and asks for help from the group. Under the skilled leadership of the instructor the problem is stated, a hypothesis is formulated, and a plan made for testing the hypothesis.

For example:

Mr. Agar was an extremely courteous gentleman until his third postoperative day when he became irritable and told the student nurse with whom he had apparently established a very good relationship to "get out and stay out" when she went in to perform his irrigation.

In discussing his action in a nursing care conference later that morning the students wondered why his behavior had suddenly changed. They were doubtful that their classmate should continue to care for him if he had "turned against her." In the course of the discussion it was brought out that the patient had learned the preceding afternoon that his colostomy was to be permanent. The instructor helped the students think through the probable reason for Mr. Agar's behavior. They thought he might be worried about going out in public, retaining his job, living a normal life. He might have these concerns, they thought, because he would feel so cially unacceptable due to odors, irregular elimination, and so forth.

The students decided, therefore, to try to find out why Mr. Agar's behavior had suddenly changed and whether their hypothesis that it could be attributed to a feeling of social unacceptability was correct. Their specific purposes were 1) to determine, if possible, just how he felt, 2) to help him see that his disability need not be a handicap, and 3) to observe his behavior during and following this attempt. If he accepted his colostomy and resumed his former courteous, outgoing manner they could deduce that his irritability had been due to his concern about his future. The following plan[1] was made:

The same student will continue to care for Mr. Agar. She shall be very accepting of his behavior. No annnoyance or hurt feelings will be shown because of his behavior toward her. To determine how he feels about his colostomy she will listen for clues from him and his wife. These she will pick up by asking appropriate questions or reflecting statements which seem significant. His attitude toward visitors will be noted. By her interest in his comfort and the creation of a relaxed atmosphere, Mr. Agar will be encouraged to express his feelings. The student's observations will be reported to her instructor and classmates in conference in which it will be decided whether the evidence supports their supposition that Mr. Agar is concerned about his social acceptability.

During the time the student is attempting to learn Mr. Agar's feelings she will also try, through her own actions, to help him accept his colostomy and understand that it need not be a handicap to him. She will change Mr. Agar's dressings promptly and will take care to give no sign that the procedure is distasteful to her. She will observe his actions while dressings are being changed. He will not be asked to look at his stoma or assist with the irrigation. The possibility of regulation through diet will be explained. When it seems appropriate the student will tell Mr. Agar about

---

[1] This plan could be followed through by students only if they had opportunity for continuity in caring for the patient. The plan could have been made in a nursing team conference to be carried out by the staff. However, continuity would be important in this instance also.

another patient with a colostomy who has lived a normal life for many years and ask Mr. Agar if he would care to talk with him.

If Mr. Agar begins to speak about social acceptance, ask questions concerning his dressings; if he becomes willing to observe and then assist with his irrigations, it can be assumed he is beginning to accept his colostomy. If he begins to visit freely with other patients, to encourage calls from his friends, and to resume his previous courteous behavior, it can be concluded that his discourteous manner had resulted from fear of being socially unacceptable due to his colostomy.

It can be seen how important it would be for the head nurse to participate in these conferences. Not only would she have a contribution to make regarding her own observations, but she should share in plans being made for the patient's care and be able to interpret them to the rest of the staff, both day and night. Consistency in treatment and behavior on the part of all personnel would be very important in a case of this kind.

The preceding paragraphs have dealt with nursing care conferences mainly for student nurses. The primary purpose of these conferences is educational although students' attention should be focused on providing the best possible care for the patient being studied. Nursing care conferences may also be conducted by the head nurse for the entire staff or by the team leader for her team members. Purposes of conferences for the staff relate primarily to the patient, his needs, his care, while the educational value to this group is a secondary consideration. Because the staff members usually know the patient under discussion and the nurses in the group have some understanding of his pathophysiologic condition, less time than is needed by students may be spent discussing medical history, physical findings, and the prescribed medical care. In the staff conference attention can frequently be focused entirely on the nursing history, the nursing care plan, and the nursing problems presented by the patient.

Bedside clinic. A bedside clinic is a modification of the nursing care conference. In this method the group visits the patient or the patient is brought to the conference room for part of the session. This method is used when some members of the group are unfamiliar with the patient or when there are special observations which need to be made to give the discussion more meaning. The point in the conference when the patient is to be visited is predetermined. The class knows the purpose of the visit and what they are to observe. Frequently the patient is engaged in conversation. This too should be purposeful. He should feel at ease. Nothing should be said or done to embarrass him. The patient must know the group is coming and what is expected of him. He will be more comfortable if his person and his unit are neat and in good order. No more than four or five individuals should visit a patient in his room. This is about all that can get around a bed. If the group is larger it should be divided or the patient brought to the conference room.

Individual conferences. Conferences are held with individual staff members and students for planning and for evaluation. The purpose and content of these have been discussed elsewhere (see Chapter 18). The success of the evaluation conference depends largely upon the preparation made by the head nurse and the individual concerned, the head nurse's knowledge of the staff member, and her skill in handling the discussion. To prepare for the conference the head nurse reviews the notes on all preceding conferences, studies and evaluates the staff member's anecdotal record. She plans what she expects to achieve in the conference and the points which she wishes to make. She thinks through a tentative plan for an introduction to the conference which will put the individual at ease. It may, of course, be necessary to change the plan.

A time and place for the meeting convenient for both the head nurse and the staff member are arranged. Neither of them is able to attain the desired relaxation if she feels pressure from impending work. Fatigue is a deterrent to objectivity making it unwise, often, to hold conferences at the end of a busy day. The place where the conference is to be held should be quiet and free from interruption. Comfortable chairs add to the atmosphere of ease. There should be a good light but no glare. The head nurse will have a clear view of the expression on the staff member's face if the member is seated facing a window or light. It is unlikely that a room with all the desirable attributes is available on the division. If there is no conference room nearby the best possible place will have to be chosen for the conference. The most important requisite is that the room be free from interruption. Evaluation conferences should be held in the atmosphere of the hospital and not in the living quarters of either the head nurse or the staff member where it is difficult to remain impersonal.

Prior to the conference, preferably the preceding day, the head nurse gives the staff member her anecdotal record to read and arranges a place on the unit where she can study it without being disturbed. She asks the individual to evaluate her work and her personal development in terms of the objectives which she established for herself. The nurse or aide uses all the anecdotes which have been written and her own notes in making her judgment and comes to the conference prepared to discuss her progress.

In conducting the conference, it is important that both the head nurse and the staff member be relaxed. Mutual confidence should exist. The head nurse must be able to keep the discussion on an objective level and at the same time convey to the individual her personal interest. The staff member is encouraged to talk first and to evaluate her own work. Often the head nurse's suggestions grow out of questions and problems raised by the member of the staff who many times can suggest a solution to her own problems or shortcomings. The head nurse needs to be a good listener but she should be responsive and encouraging in her manner. She needs to guide the discussion to keep it on the subject and should not permit it to drag along for an extended period. If it is necessary for the head nurse to criticize, her criticism should be directed at the nursing done and not at the nurse or aide.

During the conference further objectives are established and a plan for their achievement devised, a plan largely formulated by the individual herself and one which she is willing to accept. At the close of the conference it is well for her to summarize the plan and the goals which have been established.

When the conference is over the head nurse writes down in a notebook or on cards the highlights of the conference. Her notes should include the date, evidences of the attitude of the staff member, her chief problems, and the goals established. This information is reviewed before the next conference and serves as a measuring rod of progress. The head nurse helps to increase her ability to conduct conferences by reviewing and evaluating her methods in terms of the reactions of staff members and their progress in reaching goals.

Conferences to help the staff member plan care for her patients must also be thought through by the head nurse. If the nurse feels she is helped by conferences of this type she will be eager for them. Many of the principles for a successful evaluation conference are also applicable to planning conferences.

Special Reports

Daily reports are given by the head nurse or team leader on patients who are admitted during the past 24 hours and include diagnosis, brief medical history if known, nursing history and diagnosis, and medical orders. The plan for the nursing care of the patient is briefly discussed thus helping the nurses to anticipate nursing care which is needed. A method used by some head nurses to keep their personnel up-to-date is the brief special report on a timely subject. A staff member may be asked to look up and report on the uses and effects of a new drug currently prescribed for a patient. Routines for x-ray series, basal metabolism tests, and other diagnostic measures may be reviewed in relation to specific patients having such tests that day. New hospital or division routines should be carefully explained *before* they are instituted if they involve participation by nursing personnel. Likewise, it is well to describe changes in nursing procedures. If possible equipment should be shown and some aspects of the procedure demonstrated. Review of procedures which are unfamiliar or which are not being performed well may also be presented by a member of the staff.

Most staff members will need some help in preparing reports until they have given two or three. The head nurse should emphasize brevity, selecting essential points and organizing them, speaking distinctly and with conviction.

Rounds

Nursing rounds. The purpose of nursing rounds is to acquaint the staff with all patients on the division in order that better understanding and more purposeful care may be achieved for each patient. Rounds are especially useful in situations where assignments are made to provide continuity of care, for by continuous assignment to the same patients the staff members tend not to know the other patients on the division. Nursing rounds are a means by which all personnel may know something about all patients. Rounds have sometimes been used with student nurses who, because of limited assignments, have almost no opportunity to know other patients. Rounds are very useful for the staff on larger divisions where there are no nursing teams or where it is difficult for members to know patients with whom they are not involved. In the present system of hospital organization a staff member might be called on to do something for any patient on the division. If the nurse or aide knows even a little about an individual, there will be less chance for error or misjudgment in response to questions or requests. Many nurses are not comfortable if they are uninformed about any patient with whose care they might become concerned.

Rounds should be held often enough for the staff to become acquainted with new patients. Weekly nursing rounds are highly desirable. For them to be of maximum value, each staff member must have been on the division long enough to know most of the patients by name. Professional nurses should be in a group by themselves. If time prevents making rounds on all the patients, the new ones may be visited and also those in whose condition or therapy there has been a marked change.

There are many variations in the way nursing rounds are conducted. In true rounds the head nurse with a small group of staff members goes to the patient's room. Outside his door but out of his hearing his diagnosis, condition, progress, medical regimen, and nursing care are briefly presented. His history is included only as background. The patient's nurse should present this material if possible. She should then take the group to the patient's bedside and introduce him. Special observations to be made will have been pointed out in the preliminary presentation. The head nurse should be prepared to present each patient whose nurse is not present. Since time is at a premium the content to be included must be carefully selected, well organized, clearly and interestingly presented. Only three or four minutes can be spent on each patient. If more than this brief picture is needed arrangements need to be made to discuss the patient at another time, perhaps following the night and afternoon reports.

If staff members know all patients by name and sight, "rounds" can be held in a conference room. The procedure is the same except that the patients are not visited.

When nursing rounds are well presented staff nurses find them exceedingly interesting and valuable. They learn many things they have forgotten or have never known about laboratory findings, pathology, the details of therapy, the importance of nursing to each patient. If time does not permit making rounds with all members of the staff, effort should be made to provide this instruction for the professional nurses. Perhaps the head nurse can take this group and the team leaders make rounds with the members from one another's teams.

Other types of rounds. There are other types of rounds of value to professional personnel including the head nurse. In a medical center teaching rounds for interns and medical students are conducted daily. This is an excellent opportunity for the nurse to gain insight into the thinking of the medical group relative to the patient's care and prognosis. These rounds are usually long but on occasions when the work load is light the head nurse who is looking for ways to keep her staff interested and alert will free the members, in turn, to attend them.

In a teaching hospital an attending or resident physician is often glad for the opportunity to take professional nurses on rounds and discuss the diagnosis and therapy of the patients. In this way, points in nursing care considered important by the medical staff are emphasized. Nurses enjoy the opportunity to ask questions and to learn. Arrangement for medical rounds for nurses are planned by the head nurse or department administrator.

Other individuals from whom nurses can learn a great deal are the medical social worker, the physical therapist, the nutritionist, and the psychiatrist if they are full-time members of the hospital staff. Rounds conducted by these individuals, when they know all or most of the patients, are very helpful in understanding patients' behavior, in teaching them, and in observing their symptoms. While members of other professions participate in these rounds, focus is on nursing, and either the head nurse or the department administrator provides the leadership. Although there is a limit to the time nurses can spend in this way the head nurse and nursing service administrator must recognize the motivating factors involved when interest is taken in staff members' development. The time spent may be repaid many fold through greater interest, improved morale, and better understanding.

The Demonstration

The purpose of a demonstration is to show method. The head nurse may wish to show the nurses on her division a newly accepted method for performing a procedure, the adaptations to be made in a procedure for a particular patient, a procedure which is new or unfamiliar to the group or to a new staff member. She may feel that it is necessary to review a procedure which is being performed ineffectually. Before a demonstration is undertaken the head nurse must review the accepted method of the hospital for its performance. It is very confusing for staff and particularly for students, in going from floor to floor, to find the same procedures performed in different ways. Certain variations are necessary, to be sure, to meet specific needs of certain patients, but insofar as possible methods should be the same throughout the institution. They should be based on sound scientific principles.

A more economical use is made of the head nurse's time when she demonstrates to groups of nurses rather than to individuals. The size of the group depends upon the type of demonstration and the place in which it is to be held. It is essential that all those present be able to see. For some procedures this requires that the nurses gather around the bed of a patient. Four to six people are all who can be accommodated under these circumstances and even that number may crowd the room and be disturbing to the patient. If the procedure is one which is embarrassing for the patient it should be demonstrated individually. Catheterization and colostomy irrigations and dressing are of this nature. Regardless of the individual patient's modesty or lack of it, nurses will not learn desirable attitudes and appreciations unless consideration is shown for the sensibilities of all patients.

A demonstration may be a separate presentation or it may be included as a part of some other teaching project such as a nursing care conference or bedside clinic. A demonstration may show the functioning of a piece of equipment such as the respirator, an oxygen tent, Wangensteen

suction, or it may show some part of patient care as suctioning, turning a patient in a body cast, irrigating the suture line following cleft palate repair, the application of restraints to a child. Demonstrations on patients should be preceded and followed by a group conference, whereas in the demonstration of a piece of equipment the entire discussion may accompany the demonstration. Except when demonstrating to individuals who need to learn the location of equipment and the way it is assembled, time is saved by having all equipment gathered and ready before the demonstration begins. It may be of value to demonstrate the entire procedure although if certain parts of it are familiar they may be omitted, especially for graduate nurses or senior students. The aftercare of equipment may be demonstrated, merely discussed, or its consideration may be omitted entirely depending upon the needs of the group. Important aspects of charting regarding treatments are usually of sufficient significance to be included in the discussion.
Preparation for the demonstration. First the head nurse decides on the content which is necessary to achieve her purpose, organizes it, and determines the length of time which will be required. She selects the most suitable time for the demonstration from the point of view of the patient, the individuals who are to attend, and the unit activity. Patient care demonstrations should be given at the time when the care is needed or when the treatment is due.

A suitable place on or near the unit is planned for the conference which is to precede the demonstration. Chairs are arranged and visual aids assembled. If the demonstration is to be a long one, it may be preferable to bring the patient to the place where the nurses are gathered rather than following the usual procedure of taking the group to the patient's room. In this way the nurses may be seated for part of the demonstration or for all of it.

The patient's permission is, of course, obtained before his care is made the subject of a group demonstration. Most patients enjoy the unusual attention and are glad to be of help in the education of staff members if they are approached in a proper manner. The doctor is consulted if there is any possibility of his scheduling a test or treatment at the time of the demonstration. The nurse who is assigned to the care of the patient must know the time and plan for the demonstration in order to have the patient properly prepared. The porter and the maid need to know that they should have the room cleaned and ready.

The patient and the head nurse should both know what to expect in the demonstration. For this reason, the head nurse makes it a point to perform the procedure prior to the demonstration. If she has not performed the treatment recently her skills are likely to be imperfect no matter how familiar she is with the technique. A demonstration should be a work of art, perfect in every detail. Practice also helps the head nurse to decide on the best method to use for the particular patient and the most convenient arrangement for equipment.

Equipment is assembled long enough in advance to know that it is obtainable and is functioning properly. It is necessary that it be in perfect working order, clean and attractively arranged. Accessory equipment such as that found in the patient's stand is examined for cleanliness and condition. All equipment is checked again at the last minute before the demonstration to make sure that none of it has disappeared. It is highly embarrassing as well as disrupting to the smoothness of the demonstration to find a part of the equipment missing.

In a demonstration the patient is playing host to a group of guests and wishes to look his best. He should be proud of his personal appearance and that of his unit. The head nurse, therefore, sees that he is clean and well groomed, his bed freshly made, the room swept and dusted, and all excess equipment removed. Other patients in the room are also clean, comfortable, and neat. The patient is told when to expect the group. It is necessary to see him a few minutes before the demonstration to be sure his personal needs are met and that all is in order. His bed and unit are arranged ready for use and he is placed in the desired position.

Conduct of the demonstration. It is important to begin on time. If the group is small all should be seated, preferably in a circle for the preliminary conference. It is especially important that the head nurse be in view of each one. If she uses notes they should be brief, topical ones written on inconspicuous cards. This lends to informality. A teacher who is bound to her notes is not very inspiring. If she is unable to remember subject matter without constant reference to notes the material seems to the staff unimportant for them to learn.

In contrast to a nursing care conference, only enough information about the patient is given, preliminary to a demonstration, for the nurses to gain a concept of his personality and to understand the purpose of the treatment. She gives an overview of the procedure including its purpose, the results expected, and a broad picture of that which the treatment entails. A detailed account of the steps in a procedure serves only to confuse the listeners. Details are best learned by seeing them, not by hearing them enumerated.

It is often helpful to display during the introductory conference the equipment which is to be used in the demonstration. The nurses thus have an opportunity to examine it, ask questions, and gain an understanding of its use before going to the bedside.

The conference usally takes from 5 to 15 minutes. Before proceeding to the patient's room instructions are given concerning subjects which should not be discussed in the presence of the patient. Staff members are told the part they are to play and particular points to observe. They are instructed to return to the conference room at the end of the demonstration.

It may be a rather strained moment for the patient when the head nurse comes in the room with a group of nurses or aides no matter how well he knows each one individually and even though he is prepared for their coming. He doesn't know quite what to expect and may be a little tense or embarrassed. The skillful head nurse immediately puts him at ease by some friendly, casual remark which breaks the tension for all. It is hoped that members of the group will enter into the brief preliminary conversation. From the beginning to the end of the demonstration the patient is the center of attention, one of the group, not an outsider who is being talked about as though he were an inanimate object. This is true even though the patient is unconscious. The head nurse talks to him, tells him what is going to be done. "We are going to turn you over now, Mr. Green. Will you help us?" One never knows how much an unconscious patient hears. He often responds in some way, and whether or not he does staff members learn that all individuals are treated with consideration and thoughtfulness. Desirable attitudes are more important in the long run in the development of the nurse than is the understanding of techniques which are learned from the demonstration.

During the course of the demonstration when the patient is at ease, he may be asked to tell about himself, the history of his illness, the sensations he receives from the treatment, its effect from his point of view. He must not be embarrassed by the questions which are asked or by unnecessary exposure. If the patient is embarrassed the nurses react in similar manner and the experience holds little satisfaction for anyone.

Every effort is made to make the demonstration a perfect performance. It should look smooth and easy and the treatment should be carried out in the way in which the head nurse expects the nurses to perform it. When a procedure is poorly demonstrated, the head nurse can expect a poor return demonstration by those who observed it.

While performing the treatment, the head nurse may describe or comment upon the steps for the benefit of the group, provided that which is said will in no way cause the patient to worry or become disturbed. Discussion of the procedure may not be necessary if the nurses have been told previously what they should observe. Always in demonstrating, positive action should be stressed, that is, the desirable way in which to perform the act. The demonstrator needs to be sure that no important points are missed by the observers. In order that attention may be directed toward the performance of the procedure, extraneous conversation is avoided during the actual demonstration. By what she says and by her actions the skillful demonstrator directs attention to the most important parts of the procedure. All persons in the room must be in a position to see the entire demonstration.

No matter how carefully the head nurse has planned the demonstration, unpredictable things may occur. This is true especially with children. Unexpected occurrences must be met by the head nurse as they arise. The way in which she does so may be the most important teaching done that day! The understanding with which she meets the patient's unusual requests, her use of unexpected teaching opportunities, the way in which she handles an accident with equipment show the head nurse's resourcefulness and set an example which may be remembered long after the demonstration is forgotten.

It may not be a practical expenditure of time for the group to stand around and observe while the room is returned to its normal condition. The observers, however, must be satisfied that the patient is comfortable when left and that he is told that his nurse will be in soon to complete his care. Equipment, if not removed, is left in order with trays covered. The patient's belongings and signal are placed within his reach. When the patient is left he is graciously thanked for his participation.

Following the demonstration the group returns to the conference room. If no provision is made for a follow-up conference, the full effectiveness of the teaching is often lost. It is important that all points are perfectly clear. There should be an opportunity for questions by the members of the group and the head nurse may wish to ask a few questions to test understanding. This is usually the time to discuss the care of equipment and the charting. A desirable way to close the discussion is for the head nurse or one of the nurses in the group to summarize the most important points in order that all may leave with a clear concept of the entire procedure.

Unplanned demonstrations. When possible, observation of uncommon treatments is planned in advance and made the subject of a demonstration. If the treatment is of an emergency nature or is unexpected, this may not be possible. In this circumstance, students and staff nurses who are unfamiliar with the technique, should have the treatment briefly explained. They are then, if possible, sent one or two at a time to observe the treatment in progress. Needless to say, the patient's feelings are given every consideration. Particularly, if the procedure is painful or frightening, the confusion of people coming and going may be very distressing. It is more important that a nurse be taught consideration for the patient than that she observe an unusual technique. An opportunity should be made at an early date for the group to discuss the treatment and ask questions concerning it.

SUMMARY

The patient division is the center of clinical instruction for many groups especially in teaching hospitals. The head nurse contributes in a variety of ways to the educational program for student nurses and nursing service personnel. In fact, she may be the determining factor in the selection of a unit to be used as a practice field for student nurses.

The head nurse who has students (basic, graduate nurse, or aides) assigned to her division contributes to their education if the quality of care the patients on her division receive is good. It is also important to education that the head nurse understand the needs of students, that she and the instructor be cooperative in their relationship with one another. Her participation in the instructor's conferences for students is invaluable.

The head nurse can profitably use conferences for many purposes. The true conference is a two-way conversation. Frequently in a conference the group is trying to find the solution to a problem. As leader the head nurse should make sure the purposes are clear to all, that everyone feels free to participate, that discussion is to the point, that results or decisions are summarized. In preparation for the conference she needs to plan how to begin the conference and to formulate leading questions which will start discussion. Since conferences on nursing and nursing service problems concern the entire staff they should be repeated so that all personnel can be reached.

The nursing care conference for student nurses is conducted by the clinical instructor. A single patient is usually presented by one or more students for the purpose of gaining a concept of the nursing involved in a particular disease or condition. Nursing care conferences may also be held in an attempt to identify nursing problems in the care of a patient and to suggest possible solutions. In both types of conference the head nurse has a contribution to make. In the latter, especially, her participation is highly important. Not only should she share in suggesting solutions to problems but she needs to have full knowledge of any plans made for patients and the reasons for them. Although nursing care conferences for students are held primarily for educational purposes, the learners should understand that the real objective of the conference is to contribute to better care for the patient. When nursing care conferences are held for staff members the entire emphasis is on finding ways to nurse the patient better. The head nurse, however, realizes that through such conferences the staff learns and grows professionally.

Individual conferences are held primarily to help staff members establish personal objectives and ways for meeting them and to evaluate outcomes. The ability of the head nurse to put the nurse at ease will determine in large part the success of these conferences.

Other methods of instruction the head nurse can use profitably with her staff include special reports on subjects related to patients presently on the division and nursing rounds to keep the entire staff informed about all patients. The staff can also benefit from attending medical rounds and rounds for nurses conducted by members of the other health professions. Another method, the demonstration of a procedure or piece of equipment, teaches attitudes as well as techniques. The head nurse's objectives must be clear and her preparation detailed if a demonstration is to be successful.

QUESTIONS FOR DISCUSSION

1. Would a clinical instructor be shirking her responsibility if she asked the head nurse to conduct a nursing care conference for student nurses? Would you give the same response if the department administrator asked the head nurse to conduct a nursing care conference for the staff? Give reasons for your answers.
2. If you were planning to give a demonstration of patient care for staff members, what positive concomitant learnings would you wish to achieve? What negative concomitant learnings would you try to avoid?
3. Can you remember a demonstration involving a patient at which you were a participant observer? If yes, how much did you learn from the demonstration? What impressed you about it, so that you now remember it?

EXERCISES

1. Try to find an opportunity to *observe* (not participate) a teaching conference where there are a leader and at least two "students". Make a list of criteria for a good conference using the text as a guide, and after listening to the conference evaluate it in terms of the criteria. What were the objectives of the conference? Were the students aware of them?

How do you know? Do you feel the objectives were attained? What makes you think so?

Realize that in the first instance you are setting criteria for the *conduct* of the conference. In the second, you are considering the objectives of the conference, that is, what the instructor hoped to achieve by it. How are the two purposes related?

2. Make a list of the ways you believe the head nurse on your division could contribute to the education of the student nurse if she had time and opportunity. Be specific in relation to your own situation. In how many of these ways *is* the head nurse contributing? Under what circumstances would it be possible for her to contribute in the other ways?

3. List subjects which would be appropriate for a special report and which would have value for the staff on your division. If you are a staff nurse, prepare one such report and request the opportunity to give it for the staff. Have the head nurse help you evaluate your presentation. (Objectives and criteria are, of course, necessary.) If you are a head nurse, ask one of your staff to prepare a report which both you and she think will be helpful and interesting to the staff. Give her a time limit and, if she needs it, help in organization. Evaluate the presentation independently, then compare your judgments.

4. Thinking of the types of problems which patients on your division face because of the nature of their illness or disability, make a list of possible ways a member of another health profession—dietitian, physical therapist, social worker, public health nurse, doctor, or other—could help the nursing staff better understand the problems, needs and/or prescribed therapy for the patients. The list might be quite general or it could relate specifically to a few individual patients. Review the list with the nursing staff to see if they have additions and would be interesting in having a member of the particular specialty come to talk with them. If so, confer with this person, present your request, and arrange for rounds. Evaluate the results.

REFERENCES

Brackett, Mary E. Hospital nursing service—a practice field for nursing students, Nurs. Outlook, Vol. 8 (October 1960), pp. 556-559.
    The purposes of nursing service and nursing education are not the same. Their philosophies must be in agreement, however, if the two are to have har-

monious working relationships in the same institution. Clearly depicts the relationship between the head nurse and instructor in clinical instruction. Excellent reading.

Fosberg, Gordon C. Teaching management skills in a team nursing setting, Nurs. Outlook, Vol. 15 (April 1967), pp. 67-68.
A plan for teaching leadership skills to senior students.

Hanebuth, Lorna. Nursing rounds—a teaching method, Amer. J. Nurs., Vol. 64 (July 1964), pp. 116-117.
Nursing rounds with a difference! Students set objectives, selected and presented patients, with the result that patients' problems were identified and plans made to deal with them. A method that would also be effective with staff.

Loder, Eileen F. "Group" inservice with the evening shift, Nurs. Outlook, Vol. 13 (July 1965), pp. 31-33.
Regular unstructured group meetings between the evening supervisor and nursing assistants has not only improved patient care but has markedly increased staff satisfaction.

Mercadante, Lucille T., and Ross, Vivian. Nursing grand rounds, Nurs. Outlook, Vol. 12 (October 1964), pp. 33-36.
A full description of the way in which nursing grand rounds for the nursing staff are used to improve patient care and stimulate the staff. Although members of other disciplines participate, rounds are focused on nursing and the leadership comes from nursing.

Monteiro, Lois A. Tape recorded conversations: a method to increase patient teaching, Nurs. Res., Vol. 14 (Fall 1965), pp. 335-340.
The method described helped students to increase the content of their teaching. (Does this have implications for inservice education of staff?)

Muller, Theresa G. The head nurse as a teacher, Nurs. Outlook, Vol. 11 (January 1963), pp. 46-48.
The head nurse has a place all her own in the education of the student.

Pohl, Margaret L. Teaching activities of the nursing practitioner, Nurs. Res., Vol. 14 (Winter 1965), pp. 4-11.
Opinions of 1,500 nurses engaged in clinical practice showed a lack of preparation to teach. Implications are that basic nursing education should prepare students for informal teaching of patients and co-workers; that students in baccalaureate programs should be prepared for structured teaching.

Rohweder, Anne W., and Hart, Betty L. How attitudes are taught and caught, Amer. J. Nurs., Vol. 60 (June 1960), pp. 806-809.
Illustrations of ways to teach students, in the clinical situation, an understanding of patients' behavior and ways to give support. Excellent.

Schumann, Delores M. An improved method of making clinical assignments, Nurs. Outlook, Vol. 15 (April 1967), pp. 52-55.
Many values resulted from assignment of students to patients anywhere in the hospital rather than to a unit in accord with a rotation schedule. Problems which resulted are also presented.

Schwartz, Doris R. Research in patient care, Nurs. Outlook, Vol. 10 (February 1962), pp. 108-110.
Basic collegiate students should have instruction in the components of research. In one school the outstanding student may elect to participate in ongoing research in nursing care or may carry out a small isolated study of limited scope.

chapter 20

THE HEAD NURSE'S SELF DEVELOPMENT

It should be apparent from the discussion in the preceding chapters that the head nurse position is not one for an individual ungrounded in the principles of organization, supervision, and teaching. One who is to assume such important responsibilities needs adequate preparation for the position and must have several years of experience before the greatest possible contribution can be made.

The young nurse who wishes to become a head nurse should give serious consideration to her preparation. It is unfortunate when a new graduate is forced by circumstances to assume the duties of head nurse with little or no previous experience as a graduate nurse. In most schools of nursing today emphasis is rightly placed on the acquisition of scientific and clinical knowledge, development of understanding and judgment, skill in human relations, growth in desirable attitudes, and the appreciation of health and disease as factors influencing not only the mind and body of the individual but affecting also the society of which he is a part. During her period in the school, the student's practice in nursing is limited. Communication and manipulative skills are only partially developed. Judgment does not have time to mature. Upon completion of her program there is much yet for the nurse to learn from continuous experience in caring for patients.

One to two years of general staff nursing not only helps the prospective head nurse acquire the skill, confidence, and maturity which she sorely needs but also helps her to understand the problems and point of view of the staff nurse. Although there are advantages in having her first work experience in the familiar surroundings of the hospital in which she was educated, it is highly desirable for the nurse to have some experience in another hospital. This not only gives her an opportunity to compare standards of care and to learn new nursing methods but it familiarizes her with different medical practices. If her student experience has been in a large metropolitan hospital or a teaching institution, experience in a smaller community hospital would help her to see the difference in nursing service problems. If, on the other hand, she has had her basic education in a small hospital where clinical experience is limited, it would be highly advisable for her to have staff nurse experience in a large hospital where there is more variety in the conditions which bring patients to the hospital, where all types of surgery are performed, and where medical research is being undertaken. The quality of medical and nursing care given in the institution should be investigated as should the opportunity for professional growth. Ways to determine these characteristics will be considered later in this chapter.

Experience in public health nursing or in an outpatient clinic is essential if the head nurse is to understand and appreciate the broader concepts of health, realize the effects of illness on family life and of family life on health. It is almost impossible for a nurse to meet the nursing needs of patients whose home environment and cultural background are completely different from her own unless she has had guided experience in working with such families.

The prospective head nurse will profit from a six to twelve months' experience as an assistant head nurse before assuming the responsibilities of head nurse. The head nurse in whose professional preparation staff nurse and assistant head nurse experience were omitted will not likely be willing to go back at a later date to secure these experiences. The day may come when she will recognize that having missed the ground work is a continual handicap to her. The head nurse as an administrator of nursing care, supervisor, and teacher needs to be thoroughly grounded in basic nursing skills and to have the understanding which comes only from having done well those things which she is expected to teach to others.

Many nurses, however, have become head nurses without having had the desired preliminary experience. Others have had good staff nurse experience but no preparation for the responsibilities entailed in the head nurse position. Still others, with varying degrees of success, have been head nurses for many years. All have room for growth even if only to keep up with change. Hospitals in increasing numbers are recognizing the need to employ prepared head nurses if available or to educate them for their positions through programs of orientation and staff development. In some institutions, however, the head nurse receives almost no help with her own development from nursing service administration. Under any circumstances, a large share of the responsibility lies within herself.

Where possible, hospitals, especially teaching hospitals, are employing as head nurses, men and women who have preparation which includes a liberal education strong in the biologic, physical, and social sciences. As indicated in Chapter 6, if the head nurse is to change her role to one similar to that described, her education must be broad and deep enough for her to be accepted as a partner of the physician.

ASSESSING THE QUALITY OF THE
HEAD NURSE'S WORK

Before considering the ways in which the head nurse can bring about her own professional and personal development it will be well to look at methods for assessing the quality of the work she is now doing. This may help her understand her needs. In general the head nurse herself, the department administrator, the nursing director, the nursing staff, the doctors, the community say that the head nurse is *good* when:
1. Patients are well nursed, families shown consideration.
2. There is a concerned, yet relaxed atmosphere or climate on the division.
3. Care given by nurses is well organized and administered.
The purpose of this volume has been to present the ways in which these attributes can be achieved. By way of summary a few questions will be asked and briefly answered.

In What Ways Is the Head Nurse Responsible for the Quality of Patient Care?

Although the head nurse in her present role does not employ her staff nor determine its number and composition, within the limits of that with which she has to work, she implements the standards of nursing care established by the institution. For instance, the leadership she exerts influences the attitudes and motivation of her staff which in turn affect both the quantity and quality of their work. The use she makes of personnel through appropriate delegation of responsibility, her supervision of patient care and personnel, the orientation and teaching program for the staff—whether thorough or sketchy—determine to a large extent the quality of care which patients receive.

How May the Atmosphere on a Division Be Described?

The atmosphere may be *tense and uneasy*. Individuals are afraid of upsetting others, especially the head nurse. They also fear making mistakes, hesitate to interrupt the head nurse because she is so busy and preoccupied. The opposite situation sometimes exists and the atmosphere is described as *casual*. No one seems to be very much concerned that things get done on time, that patients' personal needs are met. Individuals whether patients, families, medical staff, or personnel from other departments never feel quite sure that requests will be remembered or honored. The *coldly efficient* atmosphere gives the impression that getting things done by a certain time (for example, care of all patients completed before doctors' rounds) is the paramount goal. All else is pushed aside to meet this goal. Patients are hurried through their baths. There is no time for them to talk or ask questions. The nurse's mind is on the next task to be performed rather than on the patient for whom she is caring. Each staff member is expected to work to the limit of her endurance.

Sometimes there is an air of *indifference*. Why bother to do anything well, to do more than the mere essentials? No one in authority really cares what happens so why should I? Another kind of atmosphere is one which is *undignified*. Relationships tend to be too personal. Talk is about outside affairs. Behavior is more suited to a social gathering than to the serious business of caring for sick individuals and helping their worried families.

Last, there is the *concerned yet relaxed* atmosphere in which interest is patient-centered; each member of the staff is purposeful in her activities. Individuals feel free to ask for help when necessary. There is no fear of punishment for a misstep. When this climate, which is obviously the one to be desired, exists the most important work gets done, the staff has a feeling of accomplishment, there is less fatigue because nervous tension is minimal.

These descriptions may have been somewhat exaggerated. However, they exist to varying degrees and are not mutually exclusive. The head nurse should try to observe the atmosphere on her division objectively and to think through its effect on various groups, especially the patient and his family. How do the attitudes of the staff which are displayed in the existing atmosphere affect the confidence and comfort of the family of a critically ill or suffering patient?

By What Means Can the Work of the Head Nurse Be Evaluated?

Criteria for evaluating nursing care have been enumerated in Chapter 13. The quality of care given patients is the ultimate test of the head nurse's effectiveness. But by what means can this quality and the factors which affect it be evaluated? The department and nursing service administrators and the head nurse herself need ways to determine whether criteria for good nursing are being met. Sophisticated measures are badly needed. Without them, certain indications give clues to those who wish to judge the effectiveness of the head nurse.

Some evidence that criteria for good nursing are being met exists if the best staff nurses indicate a desire to work on the division, patients and families write commendatory letters—spontaneously, not in response to a questionnaire. More indicative of the head nurse's competency is the report she makes to the nursing administrator relative to patients and their care. Does she show interest and concern for their rehabilitation and for their happiness as well as for their immediate physical needs? When the nurse administrator makes rounds on the unit are the staff members most frequently found with patients rather than visiting in the office or in the kitchen over a cup of coffee? Is the general atmosphere purposeful? Are patients socializing with one another and with staff? Are they helping with unit activities, waiting on themselves and on bedridden patients? Do they appear happy or are they bored? Is the physical environment free from confusion and clutter?

There are still other ways by which the department administrator or director of nursing judges the work of the head nurse. Do many accidents or errors in medication occur on the unit? Are these reported promptly and fully? Do the administrators feel that they always have the pulse of the division, know what is happening, feel confident that the head nurse will recognize when she needs help, that she will solve her own problems to the extent she is able to do so and will be specific in expressing her needs for assistance? How many calls for sedative orders which could have been anticipated come to the evening or night administrator from this division? Are there complaints from the operating room or other departments that patients are inadequately prepared? Is the time planned for the best utilization of the staff? Does it provide for continuity in patient care and for adequate rest and relaxation for staff members? Is there always a responsible person in charge? Is she well oriented to her responsibilities? When the division is inadequately covered is the department administrator or the nursing office fully aware of the situation?

Are division policies clear, written down, known to the nurse in charge? Is the head nurse consistent in her behavior, not criticizing an act one day or for one person and ignoring it the next time or in another person? Does the head nurse delegate responsibility clearly and permit individuals the authority to function adequately? Does she utilize the special abilities of staff members and help each one to grow through carefully planned activities? Are staff members well oriented to their responsibilities? Are they encouraged to evaluate their own work and do they know the head nurse's judgment of their performance? Are evaluation reports discriminating? Do the head nurse's recommendations regarding readiness of staff members for added responsibility indicate sound judgment? Does the head nurse evaluate the quality of nursing care, organization, supervision, and interpersonal relationships on the unit and her part in making them what they are? Does she ask for help in evaluation of her work?

Affirmative answers to these questions indicate the head nurse has many of the qualities desired, that she is functioning at a high level. She is no doubt a person who would profit from opportunities for further professional and personal development, which will be described later in this chapter. She should be continuously striving to set new and higher goals for herself. When objectives are reached there are always new ones to be attained.

THE ROLE OF THE DEPARTMENT ADMINISTRATOR IN THE HEAD NURSE'S DEVELOPMENT

The head nurse may not know her potential for growth. Hopefully she will have opportunity for professional development in the situation in which she finds herself. She can be helped to acquire new knowledge and skill in interpersonal relationships, to provide better experiences for her staff, evaluate patient care, and institute methods to improve it. A well-adjusted, clinically well-informed department administrator who understands her own role is a real source of help to the experienced as well as to the inexperienced head nurse. There needs to be a close working relationship and frequent personal contact, nonauthoritative in nature, between the two. Mutual trust and understanding are essential for maximum productivity and development. The head nurse needs to be supported in her judgments and to receive sympathetic help in analyzing those in which she may have been ill-advised. She needs someone at all times to whom she can turn with her questions and problems. The head nurse needs leadership from administrators who are interested in her personal and professional development.

It is unfortunate that all head nurses do not receive such leadership and support. They often have to find opportunities for growth without the help of those to whom they are responsible. The head nurse herself must realize there is much to learn both generally and professionally which will enrich her life and make her a better head nurse.

OPPORTUNITIES FOR PROFESSIONAL DEVELOPMENT

Within the Hospital

Many ways to achieve professional development are available to the head nurse in the course of her day's work. If she has an inquiring mind she can learn a great deal by questioning members of the medical staff relative to their patients. The more up-to-date the physician, of course, the more the nurse is likely to gain. Understanding of pathology, significance of laboratory findings, rationale of therapy, action and uses of new drugs, and much more can be learned from studying the patient's record, observing him, and conferring with the doctor. In a hospital where medical students are taught, patients are discussed at "grand rounds." The head nurse who can plan her time to attend these conferences and supplement them with reading will find herself much more alert to patients' symptoms. She can also learn from participation in medical, nursing, and other types of research if she is interested in so doing. From both rounds and research the head nurse will have information to share with the staff and in the sharing will learn methods of communication.

The head nurse who would keep herself informed should read regularly nursing journals, particularly the official ones, as well as other literature which comes to her as a member of her professional organizations. She will also become familiar with medical literature in her specialty and will look up recent publications concerning the disorders from which her patients are suffering. When this is done in conjunction with reading patients' charts the material has more meaning and the planning of patient care is enhanced.

The head nurse is in an excellent position to study nursing care, to find answers to problems. If she is eager to improve this care, she will continually search for ways to do it. She will obtain the help she needs and will experiment and evaluate, utilizing the services of her staff throughout. The head nurse should not expect that her week can be limited to forty hours. No person in a position of responsibility (businessman, teacher, clergyman, doctor, nurse), whether self-employed or salaried, considers his work to be ended with the completion of his regular hours. While many individuals take work home, all should at least expect to give thought to evaluation of the day and to plans for the morrow. Time for reflection away from the pressures, tension, and interruptions of the working atmosphere is important for those who are responsible only for their own work, but thinking and planning are essential for those in leadership roles. The head nurse falls into this category. She cannot expect to attain her potential or advance in her profession unless she works toward the improvement of nursing on her division and this objective can be achieved only if the head nurse is willing to spend some of her own time in reading, thinking, and planning.

Professional Organizations

Membership in professional organizations is an obligation of all nurses. Dues of members help support activities which are important to the profession as a whole. However, paying dues will not help the head nurse to develop her potential. Attending meetings at local, state, and national levels is stimulating and inspirational and brings the head nurse in contact with others in similar positions. An opportunity for sharing problems and experiences should be sought at these meetings. Participation in activities at the local level is especially important for the head nurse. It is here she has the privilege of serving on a committee, planning an institute, studying bylaws, or becoming involved in recruitment or other activities in which she is interested. Organizations are always looking for workers. The head nurse who becomes a member of her District Nurses Association or Local League for Nursing and attends meetings regularly will usually find she is asked to become an active participant. This will bring her into contact with nurses from other agencies and members of allied professions. Broader insights, new interests and points of view will result.

Community Organizations

The head nurse will find still wider interests if she joins and participates in the activities of one or more of the allied health organizations or other community groups. Local Heart Associations, Health Councils, and the Red Cross number nurses in their membership. Participation in any one of these serves to increase the nurse's perspective and widen her professional horizons. She greatly enriches her life when she contributes to the larger community beyond the hospital by taking an active part in its affairs. Hospital nurses especially, unless they live in the community, tend to limit their interest and activities to those of their immediate professional responsibilities and to associate almost entirely with a small group of their nurse colleagues. They little realize how much there is to gain from contact with other groups of people and from participation in community affairs beyond their everyday professional interests. Then, too, nurses can assist in bringing about better health through their association with civic and welfare organizations. They can help their fellow citizens to become health conscious and interpret for them the health needs of the community. Through local organizations nurses are able to stimulate public interest in nursing and to gain support for nursing education. When she accepts a position in a community the nurse should plan to become an active member of that community. This is impossible if all or most of her leisure time is spent out of the city or town.

Educational Meetings

Many institutes and conferences are organized by professional groups for nurses at various levels. The head nurse is often given the day to attend such a meeting if she expresses an interest in it. She must, however, be alert to available opportunities. Probably of more value is the workshop or short course which requires study and active participation. Most of these are conducted by a university or one of the professional nursing organizations on subjects in which there is need and interest.

College Courses

Nurses who live in or near a college or university which has a school of nursing frequently have opportunity to enroll in short nursing courses or workshops which will give them specific help in their work. Courses in methods of teaching, supervision, evaluation, clinical nursing, rehabilitation, team nursing, and improvement of patient care assist the head nurse to gain wider understanding of her responsibilities. Especially important is the opportunity which they provide to share in the thinking of others with like responsibilities and to learn the principles upon which success as a head nurse is based. Also of value to the head nurse are adult education courses given by a university or college in such areas as interviewing, the group process, audiovisual education, educational psychology, and community organization.

The head nurse who has university facilities at hand, the ability to carry college work, and who can obtain the necessary funds should work toward her bachelor's degree in nursing. Programs leading to this degree vary in length but include two or more years in liberal arts and advanced work in nursing practice and leadership. Much of the work for the degree can be done on a part-time basis while the head nurse is carrying her full-time job. Through college study she learns to think better, converse more easily, appreciate good literature. She gains a better understanding of human behavior through the study of psychology, sociology, and cultural anthropology. As a result of this broadening experience the head nurse is better able to understand and counsel patients and staff members. In turn she influences the attitudes of her co-workers toward other people and is able to help them analyze patients' problems, to plan nursing care, to teach and supervise.

Even though the head nurse does not feel she is in a position to complete work for her degree she can profit from taking carefully selected courses in an accredited college or university. It is advisable to get help in their selection from the nurse faculty in a university which has a department of nursing for graduate nurses. Liberal arts courses taken according to a curriculum pattern can usually be transferred should the head nurse later decide she wishes to earn the degree. In this way she will be in less danger of losing credits than if she selected courses at random.

OPPORTUNITIES FOR PERSONAL DEVELOPMENT

Advanced study and participation in community activities develop the head nurse personally as well as professionally. The individual with limited interests has no idea of the new worlds which are opened up through contacts with others through reading, study, and personal association.

Every individual, the head nurse not excepted, needs association with persons outside her profession. Affiliation with a church, philanthropic, educational, or fraternal group is an easy way to make friends. Through personal contact others will learn of the head nurse's interest in art, music, child welfare, bridge, sports, and the like and will help her to assume an active part in such projects. A healthy mental state can be attained through achievement, recognition, and the self-esteem acquired in participating in music, dramatics, handicrafts, and other hobbies. Most communities large enough to have a hospital are near centers where there is opportunity for the head nurse to participate in the League of Women Voters, attend concerts, plays, lectures, and join groups interested in learning to bowl, play tennis, dance or swim. Many communities have adult education classes where crafts, furniture refinishing, painting, gardening, and other skills may be learned. Through outside activities the nurse meets people with common tastes and interests.

Study of the history of the community and visits to interesting places in and near the town make the nurse more intelligent in her contacts with the residents of the locality and help her to understand the people whom she meets in and out of the hospital.

It has been well said that every individual needs emotional security and that if nurses are to give this security to patients they must possess it themselves. A happy marriage and family life provide security to the fullest extent. The unmarried nurse must seek it elsewhere. The head nurse will gain new perspective and will enjoy her work more if the job is not her sole interest in life. Outside interests help her to be sympathetic with members of her staff who likewise have other demands upon their time and attention. The head nurse owes it to herself, those who work with her, and her patients to develop broad interests outside nursing.

FACTORS WHICH INFLUENCE THE HEAD NURSE'S DEVELOPMENT

One who is seeking or considering a head nurse position should realize that her professional and personal development will depend on the job she takes, that is, the richness of clinical facilities, the quality of patient care, the nature of her work, the leadership she receives from the nursing administration, and the amount of freedom she has to use her initiative. It will also depend on the opportunities available in the community for a satisfying personal life and the extent to which the head nurse makes use of them.

Points to Consider in Choosing a Head Nurse Position

It would be naive to think that there is the same opportunity for growth in all head nurse positions. In some situations there is no one capable of giving leadership to the head nurse. In others a prepared head nurse poses a threat to those who supervise her if they have not had adequate preparation. She may not only fail to receive help but stumbling blocks may be put in her road. It is therefore important that one seeking a head nurse position look carefully to determine whether it has the possibilities for bringing her the satisfactions she desires.

Responsibilities of the job. What responsibilities does the head nurse position entail? Are they chiefly administrative wherein the head nurse would spend most of her time coordinating activities with those of other departments, managing the flow of traffic on the division, handling orders and requisitions, checking on details? Or would she have competent full-time secretaries or a unit manager to handle a large proportion of the administration leaving her free to concentrate on the organization and supervision of patient care and the development of her staff? If her chief interest is in nursing practice and administration of nursing care, will she have opportunity for fulfillment? No situation is ideal. However the attitude of the nursing service administrator and her concept of the role of the head nurse will determine whether she works toward the freeing of nurses for nursing, whether she is content with the present state of affairs, or feels that attempts to change would be futile.

If the prospective head nurse is looking for a desk job or one which entails primarily unit administration she will find many positions embodying these activities. Whether the position at which she is looking deals primarily with unit administration or whether it is principally concerned with nursing, the applicant for a head nurse position should try to learn how much chance she will have for using her initiative and creative ability. Will she have the freedom to recommend changes in procedures and hospital practices which affect her work, to institute or participate in a staff development program? If the individuals to whom she will be directly responsible are not interested in change and improvement but are satisfied with things as they are the head nurse might not have opportunity for continuing growth. No head nurse should expect to institute changes before she is fully grounded in the established methods of an institution, has studied the need for improvement, and has won the confidence of her co-workers, all of which require many months. Neither should she be expected to continue indefinitely to follow blind tradition without questioning it and without the privilege of offering suggestions for changes, some of which, at least, she should be permitted to undertake.

Standards of the institution. Before accepting a head nurse position information should be obtained on the quality of nursing care given in the institution, the standards of medical practice, and the caliber of the school of nursing if one exists in the hospital. This information is not always easy to obtain. Standards of the lay public or practicing physicians may not be those of nurses. However, the general reputation of the hospital regarding the quality of nursing may be useful, especially if the calibre is considered poor. A hospital connected with a recognized medical school or one approved by the American Hospital Association meets the requirements for sound medical practice. A school of nursing which is approved by the state board of nurse examiners meets minimum requirements for nurse licensure. If it meets the standards of the National League for Nursing the candidate for a head nurse position is likely to find both the nursing education and nursing service of satisfactory quality. The wise nurse consults faculty members of her own school regarding the reputation of the institution in which she is considering a position. She is also much more sure of the wisdom of her choice if she makes a personal application, talks with the administrator of the nursing service to learn her attitudes toward nursing and nursing service. It is likewise advisable to confer with the department administrator and if possible to spend several hours in the unit to which she expects to be assigned in order that she may observe for herself the spirit that exists among the personnel, the quality of care which is given, the physical facilities which are available.

Living conditions. Comfortable living conditions can make a great deal of difference in one's rest, relaxation, and enjoyment of life and for that reason should be given consideration when accepting a position. The availability of suitable living arrangements in the community should be investigated. The nurse should also know the distance to be traveled to work and to education and recreation centers, and the facilities for transportation. If the nurse is unmarried what are the opportunities for a social life and recreation? Are all nurses with whom she would be working married with families?

Personnel policies. The prospective head nurse should be fully aware of the remuneration she will receive, the hospital policy regarding salary increases, vacation, sick leave, health benefits, working hours, opportunities for college study and cultural pursuits. It is important for her to decide, before accepting the position, whether she can be content with the personnel policies of the institution. If not, she should look elsewhere for a position, for having accepted an appointment she has agreed to the policies of the hospital and thus has no justification for complaint. Insofar as working conditions for all head nurses need to be improved, however, she should work through her professional organization to raise standards.

Obligations Assumed in Accepting a Position

Having taken care in the selection of a position the nurse should consider her obligation to the hospital in which she is accepting a position. Professional and personal growth result from recognition and acceptance of responsibility. No head nurse is mature in behavior unless she realizes that she has definite obligations to the individuals by whom she is employed and the institution in which she is working. It is important for her to realize that no new appointee to a position of leadership makes a very marked contribution to the institution until she has learned well its policies and practices, has mastered her job, has surveyed the situation to learn its needs, and has studied ways of meeting them. Even then she is just beginning to see her way clearly in developing a constructive program. The first year in a new position the head nurse may learn more than she contributes. The hospital does not benefit materially from her services in the first few months. She keeps the division functioning (if that is her responsibility) and the patients cared for. Beyond that she contributes little until she has become efficient in her role. When this time comes she is ready to carry out a program of improvement in nursing practice and in the services rendered to their families and the community.

Length of service. A frequent turnover in head nurses, then, is uneconomical from the standpoint of the hospital. No head nurse can feel justified in leaving her position any time under two years and even then she has just begun to scratch the surface of the possibilities for service. Little do many head nurses realize that a third and a fourth year or more in the same position would repay them both in the experience derived and in the satisfaction of seeing results. Each time her position is changed the orientation process must begin again and the creative experience is postponed. Too many nurses in this country consider the head nurse's position a stepping stone to something else, but what other position in the whole institution is more important? Hospitals and the nursing profession are in large part responsible for the attitudes demonstrated by head nurses. Until adequate preparation for the position of head nurse is demanded, until salaries are commensurate with the responsibilities of the position and with the experience of the nurse, until the position of head nurse carries as much prestige as that of department administrator and instructor, until the head nurse is given sufficient assistance in the form of clerical help and assistants who can relieve her of some of the administrative detail, she will move on to fields of endeavor which she considers more attractive. The nurse who plans to give up her position after a year in order to be married, or for any other reason, is obligated to inform her employer of this fact when she places her application or is offered a head nurse position. If the hospital still wishes to employ her because, all things considered, she appears to be the best choice, it does so with full awareness of all that is involved.

Adherence to accepted methods. The head nurse in accepting a new position does well to think carefully of the effects her coming may have on those with whom she is to be directly associated and to adopt a course of action which is likely to produce desirable reactions upon and win the confidence and cooperation of her co-workers. The head nurse, if she is wise, immediately sets out to learn the methods in current use in the hospital and unit. She studies the nursing procedure book and makes a point of observing the performance of treatments. When she is new no one expects her to know the procedures and routines of a strange institution. If she seeks every possible experience when she comes to the new division she will quickly learn the methods which are used and develop self confidence. Her effort to learn their methods and judicious use of criticism are appreciated by the staff. She need not be hesitant to admit that she is learning and to ask questions freely. After she has been in the position a reasonable time doctors and nurses alike will expect her to be fully informed. There is a tendency on the part of many individuals to evade responsibility for that with which they are unfamiliar. The head nurse does not supervise effectively if she is unsure of her ground. It is only after she has learned the existing situation thoroughly that she can intelligently make suggestions for change. When that time comes she should realize her role as a change agent and be continuously thinking about ways to improve nursing care and nursing care administration. The head nurse more than anyone else is in a favorable position to recognize need for change. She should consider it a responsibility to make recommendations when she believes a new routine or procedure to be advantageous.

Loyalty. When a position has been accepted the nurse is obligated to transfer her loyalty to the institution in which she is serving and to the people for whom and with whom she is working. There are likely to be many things about the new hospital which she does not like, perhaps because they are different and she does not understand them. This will be true in any position which she will ever hold. However, she must believe in the integrity of the institution and its staff, in its aims and objectives. If she cannot honestly do so, she should in all fairness to her conscience dissociate herself from the institution. As long as she is connected with the organization, however, she is obligated to harmonize her efforts with those with whom she is collaborating, and even after she has left the institution she should not criticize the motives and actions of the personnel. The fact that she should be loyal does not imply that she should be a complacent follower but it does mean that she has no right to harm the institution and the people by whom she is employed with malicious or thoughtless criticism. If the criticism is well founded she should act as an interested partner in a joint undertaking and take her suggestions to those who have the ability to do something to remedy the conditions. Although this principle holds true in every employer-employee relationship it is perhaps most important in hospital personnel relationships because undermining the confidence of the public in hospitals can do infinite harm.

If the new head nurse should actually find that patients are poorly treated, that medical or nursing care is unsafe, it is her moral obligation to protest the situation by going through proper nursing channels. If her action brings no results, a report needs to be made to the hospital administrator or if necessary to the board of directors. Decision to take such a drastic step is difficult and should not be hastily or lightly made. Neither should the head nurse shirk a clear-cut responsibility to patients. Statements of protest need to be carefully documented and objectively presented. Reasonable suggestions for improvement are always in order.

SUMMARY

Ideally the head nurse has had staff nurse experience and some academic preparation. However, many nurses have stepped into head nurse positions with no preparation for the job. They were chosen because they were the best persons available. Usually this has meant they had potential for further development. Whether prepared or not, all head nurses have room for further growth. Thinking through the means by which the nursing service administrators and she herself can evaluate the quality of her work is a helpful experience. In this way the head nurse can determine her need for assistance in providing comprehensive care, in creating a concerned yet relaxed atmosphere, and in organization and administration of nursing care. Even though the head nurse may have the help of a department administrator in her professional development, in large part results depend upon her own motivation.

Opportunity for professional development is greater in some institutions than in others. The nurse with an inquiring mind can learn by questioning the doctors about their patients, by reading nursing and medical journals, by participating in research. In a teaching hospital, patients' charts, laboratory reports, "grand rounds," and many other means help the head nurse keep up-to-date in medical developments. Nursing care is greatly enhanced when the head nurse is clinically well informed.

Participation in nursing organizations at the local level, attending state and national meetings give the nurse a new outlook on her profession, bring her in contact with nurses who have common problems and interests. Participation in the activities of other community groups broadens the head nurse's interests. Educational institutes and workshops conducted by professional organizations and universities are within reach of almost every nurse. Many nurses are near enough to a college or university to enroll in courses. These should be taken under the advisement of the faculty of a university department of nursing to avoid the possibility of accumulating credits which follow no curriculum pattern. Professional courses which give specific help in patient care management, supervision, and evaluation are available, as are liberal arts subjects such as psychology and sociology which broaden the nurse's horizons.

Opportunity for personal and professional growth and satisfaction should be given serious consideration whenever a nurse seeks or accepts a position. Personal growth results from many of the activities mentioned but also from development of hobbies, participation in sports, and taking advantage of cultural opportunities. Every nurse needs friends and interests outside her profession to give her perspective.

QUESTIONS FOR DISCUSSION

1. Assuming that membership in professional nursing organizations is an obligation of all nurses, should membership be a requirement of the employing agency? Give reasons for your answer. If you do not believe in such requirements how can nurses be made to recognize and accept the obligation? Be specific.
2. What are the values to the head nurse of membership in professional organizations. Be specific.
3. What unsafe and unethical practices of which a head nurse might be aware could exist in an accredited hospital? If any one of these practices occurred on your division, what should the head nurse do about it? Enumerate the steps she should take.

EXERCISES

1. List the ways suggested in this chapter for evaluating the work of the head nurse. By these means evaluate yourself if you are a head nurse, or evaluate your head nurse. Make a plus and a minus column. Look over the tabulations. Where are the head nurse's strengths? Wherein is improvement needed? Is this a useful exercise for a head nurse?
2. For an hour in the middle of an afternoon or around 9:00 or 9:30 PM

observe the staff on a division with which you are not very familiar. Using the descriptive terms set forth on pages 436, 437, how would you characterize the atmosphere of the division? Substantiate your judgment with illustrations. How did the nurses' behavior appear to affect the patients' behavior and attitudes? Illustrate. Following this observation and evaluation repeat the exercise on your own division. How do the two compare?

3. Investigate opportunities in the community which would be useful to you in preparing for a head nurse position or, if you are a head nurse, in helping you to broaden your preparation. Which items on the list of available opportunities would be possible for you to undertake? Would you be interested in doing so? This exercise would be a worthwhile project for a class or group of nurses.

4. Make an informal survey to find out from your colleagues what professional literature they read, whether they subscribe to nursing journals and which ones, whether they read the periodicals regularly. Are those who read any more interested in nursing practice than those who do not? Are they better nurses? Do they appear more interested in nursing? What was your basis for judgment? What is your conclusion about the importance of reading for nurses?

5. For one or two days be highly aware of evidences of lack of loyalty whether intentional or thoughtless on the part of any staff member on your division. Write brief notes of your observations including the person making the statement, to whom she was not loyal, the content of the statement, in whose presence the statement was made. From this evidence does it appear that lack of loyalty is a problem among your staff? with one or two staff members? As a head nurse, what if anything do you feel you should do about lack of loyalty?

REFERENCES

American Nurses' Association's first position on education for nursing, Amer. J. Nurs., Vol. 65 (December 1965), pp. 106-111.
The A.N.A. takes the position that beginning preparation for professional nursing should be the baccalaureate degree.

Angus, Monica D. The adult education center can serve nursing, Nurs. Outlook, Vol. 13 (June 1965), pp. 66-68.
A thoughtful presentation of the need for continuing education by nurses and a plea that programs be centered in adult education centers rather than in hospitals.

Brown, Esther Lucile. Preparation for nursing, Amer. J. Nurs., Vol. 65 (September 1965), pp. 70-73.
This excellent article points to the direction nursing education must take if it is to meet its responsibilities in the years ahead.

Cooper, Signe S., and Hornback, May. Profile of the continuing learner in nursing, Nurs. Outlook, Vol. 14 (December 1966), pp. 28-29.
Head nurses made up the largest single group attending institutes and workshops conducted by the Extension Division of a state university. A study of nurse participants in these sessions revealed interesting facts.

Coulter, Pearl Parvin. Continuing education for nurses in the unit, Nurs. Outlook, Vol. 10 (February 1962), pp. 113-117.
Continuing education for the nurse is essential because of the explosion of knowledge. The nursing school graduate is not a finished product but must continue to learn. Such learning should not be haphazard but may be less than a sustained degree program. The W.I.C.H.E. program of the Western region is described.

Darley, Ward. The professions and professional people, Nurs. Forum, Vol. 1 (Winter 1961-62), pp. 83-89.
The meaning of the designation "profession" and the responsibilities which professional persons bear.

Davis, Fred, Olesen, Virginia L., and Whittaker, Elvi Waik. Problems and issues in collegiate nursing education. In The Nursing Profession, Davis, F., ed. New York, John Wiley and Sons, Inc., 1966, pp. 138-175.
This essay on the characteristics of collegiate education and the challenge it faces, although of special interest to nurse educators, has implications for the nursing profession as a whole.

Fancovic, Georgianna B. For the doldrums: a workshop, Amer. J. Nurs., Vol. 62 (January 1962), pp. 100-102.
A cleverly written account of the experiences involved in a committee's planning and conducting of a workshop for their supervisor and head nurse peers. Better patient care and improved staff communications resulted.

Hamburg, Alvin Z. Evaluate before employment, Nurs. Outlook, Vol. 13 (March 1965), pp. 45-47.
In seeking a job a nurse should have thought through her goals, interests, aptitudes. It is not fair to herself or her employer for a nurse to accept a position in which she will not be able to utilize her abilities and find satisfaction. The characteristics of the institution and other factors which should be investigated are presented.

Meyer, Genevieve Rogge. Tenderness and Technique, Los Angeles Institute of Industrial Relations, University of California, 1960.
Report of research by a psychologist on the changes occurring in the nursing profession. Four types of nurses were isolated and their interests and concepts studied. Type I is the "ministering angel" type and Type IV the "technical-administrative type." The others fall between. A fascinating study with much of value for nursing education and for nursing service in its choice cf personnel, including head nurses.

Pickett, Barbara L. Is supervision for you?, R.N., Vol. 29 (February 1966), pp. 77-78, 100.
Being a charge nurse or supervisor widens a nurse's perspective, enlarges her scope of usefulness, gives insight into planning. It also makes it possible for the nurse to do "more to help shape nursing's future."

Sister Madeleine Clemence. Existentialism: a philosophy of commitment, Amer. J. Nurs., Vol. 66 (March 1966), pp. 500-505.

An inspiring presentation of the meaning of commitment, demands that personal involvement places on nurses, resulting joys. Each time this article is read it brings new insights.

Strauss, George, and Sayles, Leonard R. The Human Problems of Management, Englewood Cliffs, New Jersey, Prentice-Hall, Inc., 1960.
Ch. 12 (pp. 263-283). The head nurse who is new in her job will do well to read this chapter which admonishes that change should not be made too soon—not until she has won respect for her technical and leadership skills.
Ch. 22 (pp. 509-526) discusses the need for long-range planning for staff development and ways of achieving it.
Ch. 24 (pp. 549-578) is an excellent discussion of the goals and various methods of training for management in business enterprises. A director of inservice education for nursing personel will find many helpful ideas here.

Tosiello, Frank. University-oriented inservice education, Nurs. Outlook, Vol. 12 (April 1964), pp. 40-42.
A thought-provoking presentation of the values in university based inservice education programs for nurses. This type program is essential if professionalism is to be increased.

chapter 21

THE HEAD NURSE—HER OPPORTUNITIES AND RESPONSIBILITIES

Widespread changes in the head nurse role are in view. Others have not yet been conceived. However, the head nurse can be sure they will be continuous and rapid. The purpose of this chapter is to look at the challenging opportunities the future holds for the head nurse together with the responsibilities they place upon her. There is little question that present trends in hospital practice, started by institutions which are in the forefront in providing good service to patients, will spread to other hospitals. In a few years, therefore, the head nurse, in most instances, will find herself in a different role. Her primary responsibility will be to see that patients receive care which is complete and satisfying in every respect. This will entail the development of her staff so that together they may define, analyze, and plan to meet the patient's needs. The head nurse will spend the major portion of her time in giving, administering, and evaluating patient care and in supervising the personnel who help to give it.

Great emphasis will be placed on providing real continuity of care for patients while in the hospital and extending this continuity outside the hospital through the use of well-integrated health services. The head nurse will be responsible for maintaining a highly effective system of communication so this continuity may be achieved. She and her staff will be familiar with the resources of the community and the ways in which they function to serve patients and families.

It should be clear from the foregoing chapters that the head nurse is a key figure in modern health service. If she is to fulfill her obligations she must be willing not only to accept change but to contribute to it. She must move with the times and not cling to outmoded practices of the past. The head nurse must be willing to accept a new role and not be threatened by the necessity to give up cherished responsibilities in which she feels secure.

For many years in many hospitals changes in the head nurse role will involve primarily a shifting of certain non-nursing responsibilities to lay persons and a change in emphasis for the head nurse from unit administration to administration of nursing care. However, a quite different role, such as the one envisioned in this text, will be developed as fast as nursing service administrators recognize the need for sweeping change in organization of the hospital nursing service, and insist on broader preparation for the head nurse.

What does this trend mean for the head nurse of today who is unprepared or inexperienced? It appears that she has three choices: *First,* she can cooperate with changes as they occur seeking opportunity through workshops, special courses, reading, study and practice to improve her nursing and her interpersonal, teaching, and organizing skills. Many will not know how to fill their time when managerial, coordinating, and clerical activities are transferred to a unit manager or director. They have never learned to be at ease in talking with patients and families who have problems. They do not have a scientific understanding of human behavior and therefore are unable to diagnose patient's needs, let alone help the staff to do so. Many head nurses have little understanding of the principles of supervision or the laws of learning. Some have very limited clinical knowledge and little or no concept of organization or administration. Those head nurses who fit this description could take corrective steps *now.* An opportunity under skilled supervision to care for a few patients who have real problems which the nurse could define and with which she could help the patients to deal would be very desirable. Most nurses have not had this type of experience.

The *second* option for the present head nurse is to continue her education on a formal basis earning both her baccalaureate and masters degrees in nursing, the latter to include clinical specialization. This nurse should then be prepared for a head nurse position in a hospital which is making sweeping role changes. *Third,* the head nurse may decide to forfeit her position when a better prepared nurse is available. If she has family responsibilities she may have little choice, in which case she might become a team leader and thereby continue to hold an important post.

Now is the time to plan for the future. There are many opportunities for further development within reach of the head nurse. She may need to leave her home and job for a few weeks to attend a workshop or a university summer session but this is part of her obligation as a professional worker and, especially, as a leader. Educational experiences will be of little value, however, unless the head nurse, on her return, studies her situation and applies her learning in a constructive way.

A systematic analysis of her own needs (see Chapter 20) and a long-range plan for supplementing her basic education is the only way a head nurse can remain competent in a fast changing hospital situation. Such study broadens her outlook and helps her anticipate and accept change as it comes. Unless she is prepared to participate in changing methods of hospital practice she is sure to be passed by. The opportunities in the new head nurse role are great, the satisfactions enormous. To the *good* head nurse the challenge is worth all the effort required.

INDEXES

author index

subject index

Anecdote(s), areas of observation for, on professional nurses, 386-387; as source material for self-evaluation, 386; choice of, 386-387; definition of, 385; illustrations of, 385-386; method of recording, 390-391; putting, in writing, 376; relate to objectives, 386; should portray attitudes, understanding, and relationships, 386; who should write, 391; *see also* Anecdotal behavior record

Assessment, general areas in which, is needed, 312-319; information and knowledge needed for accurate, of situation, 310-311; interview guide used in, 362-363; involves purposeful observation of patients, 312; of capabilities of new staff members, 361-363, 367; of effects of care, 317-318; of needs of patient's family, 315; of patient's condition and needs, 312-315; of patient's environment, 315-316; of patients should be a planned orderly process, 311; of patients takes place during nursing rounds, 311; of personal needs by staff, 372-374; of quality of head nurse's work, 436; of social climate and physical environment of personnel, 319; of the situation, 310-319

Assignment(s), ability is developed through carefully planned, 359; at times may be wise to make a change in, 319; consideration of personal qualities in making, 288; factors involved in making, 288-293; functional method of, 293, 305; geographic location, a consideration in planning, 290; made on basis of patient's nursing needs, 290-291, 305; methods of, for new personnel, 351-353; of personnel to divisions, 170-175; patient method of, 292, 305; planning of, when there are insufficient professional nurses, 291-292; some, take into account physical needs only, 281-282; team nursing as a method of, 294-303

Attitudes, example head nurse sets influences, 338; head nurse attempts to learn, of staff toward patients, 318-319; head nurse's, determine relationships on division, 338, 366-367; what head nurse does and says are indicative of her, 338

Authority, implicit in responsibility is, 134-135

Bedside clinic, 420

Board of directors of hospital, establishes hospital policy, 23; expects medical staff to establish disciplinary procedures for members, 23-24; hospital administrator is appointed by and responsible to, 12; is advised by medical staff, 23; medical staff is responsible directly to, 24-25; members of medical staff must be approved and appointed by, 23; represents the owners, 12; sets standards of medical care, 23; standards of service established by, 12

Cardiac arrest, function of nurse in relation to family of patient in, 47, team, 47

Care-by-parent unit, 53

Centralization, of responsibility, a means of relieving head nurse, 5; problems resulting from, of services, 79-81, 87

Charting, use of, in reporting to head nurse, 157; *see also* Nurses' notes, Nurses' observations

Children, care-by-patient unit for, 53; intensive care section for, 51; needs of, at various age levels, 50; organization of services by age and condition of, 50-51; rooming in by parents of young, 52, 54; services for, and their families, 50-53, 55; *see also* Infants

Clerical work, an activity of the division, 76

Clerk(s), basis for number of, required, 101; computer expected to reduce number of, needed, 101; if, to answer telephone, fewer interruptions for head nurse, 140; is assistant to head nurse, 76; often assists with coordination, 79-80; responsibilities of, 76; *see also* Secretary

Clinical conference, *see* Nursing care conference

Clinical instruction, essentials for good, 409-416; methods of, 416-430; points considered in selecting clinical units for, 410; responsibility of head nurse in, Ch. 19 (409)

Clinical instructor, assigns patients to students with help of head nurse, 283, 413; conducts nursing care conference, 430; head nurse and, cooperate, 412-414; should provide head nurse with information about student, 285

Clinical nurse specialist, responsibilities, relationships, and values of, 48, 55; use of, as alternative to new head nurse role, 120

Clinics, family health care, 35-36; services rendered by, 34

Communication, definition of, 140; developments in, 62; devices, 62; effective system of, 140-141; head nurse will be responsible for effective system of, 444; needs of patient with a problem in, 225; problems of, result from pyramidal organization, 14; types of, in hospital, 140-141, *see also* Messenger service

Community agency, public health agency, 43; referral to, 43, 230-233

Computer(s), can be expected to reduce number of clerks needed, 100; demands on head nurse resulting from, 80; for data processing have contributed to change in hospital services, 61; help of, in time planning, 170; use of, in staffing, 171, 173, 175, 191

Conference(s), as part of demonstration, 427, 429; clinical, space for, 414; conducting staff, 417, 430; content of nursing staff, 364; daily nursing staff, purposes of, 106, 321, 416, 417, 430, 431; definition of, 416, 430; follow-up, for new staff member, 374-375, 376; group, 416-420; head nurse participates in clinical, for student nurses, 414-415; individual and group, as method of supervision, 320-321; individual, purposes and conduct of, 421-422, 431; initial, with new staff member, 362-373; nursing care, 417-420; nursing, during early afternoon, 180; on interviewing for head nurses, 88; regular medical, in which other professional groups participate, 113; supervisory, by whom instigated, 373; unit director and head nurse plan, with new house staff members, 113; *see also* Nursing care conference

Consultation services, offered by medical center, 35

Continuity of care, 292-293; a principle of assignment planning, 365; definition of, 45; desirability of, a factor in assignment planning, 292-293; emphasis will be placed on, 444; head nurse maintains, throughout patient's stay in hospital, 223; maintenance of in progressive patient care, 43, 45; pro-

motes learning, 253; satisfactions of nurse in providing, 45-46; team leader maintains, 294

Coordination, administration and, of patient care services, 103; an integrating function requiring judgment and decision making, 78; basic system of, 12; depends in part on voluntary efforts, 144; factors which facilitate, and cooperation, 136-145; of professional care by head nurse, 96; of staffing by several head nurses, 173-175, 192; of unit and hospital administration with patient care activities, 78, 80, 89; of work and movements of representatives of other departments, 104; problem of, extended by increased traffic, 79; result of head nurse's time being largely taken up with, 80; who should be responsible for, of unit functions, 94

Counselling for parents, of children for whom open heart surgery is recommended, 36-37, 55

Counselor(s), department administrator as, for head nurse, 85; for head nurse and unit director are essential, 117, 118, 121

Criteria, attainment of objective is measured against, 322; developing, for good nursing, 322-325; evidences that, for good nursing are being met, 438-439; for evaluation of nursing procedure, 342; for judging quality of nursing care administration, 145-146; for selection of clinical units for student practice, 410; formulation of, for objectives makes them usable for supervision and evaluation, 84; head nurse and staff should review regularly, 325; head nurse with staff develop, specific for division, 84; list of, 322-323; must be practical and obtainable, 84; use of, in evaluation of nursing care, 326, 328; used by nurses aides in self-evaluation, 394; *see also* Critical incident, Guidelines

Critical incident(s), 323-325; illustrations of, 323-324; sources of 324-325; technique, a means for developing criteria, 323

Data, collection of, a first step in nursing diagnosis, 247; cultural, helps nurse understand behavior, 249, 254; sources of, 247-248, 254

Head nurse responsibility(ies) (cont.)
former, for dietary and housekeeping services and teaching, 3; in clinical instruction, Ch. 19 (409), 412-415, 430; in conceptualized role, 95-96, 100; in planning patient care, 270-273; in providing care patient and family have a right to expect, 204; in relation to dietary service, 76; in relation to her staff, 108-109; in relation to the patient, 105-108; in relation to the physician, 109-115; in relation to unit director, 105; in staffing, 172-174; in team nursing, 300-303, 305; in voluntary, short term, general hospitals, 12; is both professional and administrative, 146; is never to but one doctor, 81; necessitate her being available for consultation, 96; necessitate her being free, 96; need for salary commensurate with, 447; present, 5, 21-22, 26, 80; primary, of the future will be patient care, 444; questions relative to further changes, 6; to decide when patient's welfare might be jeopardized, 86; to help staff become more discerning and understanding, 204; to know teaching methods, 409; to new patient, 202-203; vary, depending upon type of service and ownership of institution, 11; varying degrees of, for non-nursing activities, 76; see also Head nurse, Head nurse role, Relationships of head nurse

Head nurse role, changing, Ch. 1 (3); choices of head nurse in relation to new, 445-446; dual, problems resulting from, 79, 81-87, 89; former satisfactions in, 3; gaining acceptance of new, 116; head nurse must be willing to accept new, 444; historical development of, 3; implementation of new, 115-121, 122; managerial-coordinating, enjoyed by many head nurses, 80; may or may not be changed with appointment of unit manager, 94; need for further change in, 5, 6; new, Ch. 6 (94), 95, 121, 202; new concept of relationship of, to unit director, 97, Figs. 6, 7 (98-99); new, varies among institutions, 95; one concept of a new, 95-100, 121; past changes in, 4; present role, 4-5; problems of dual responsibility suggest new, is needed, 83; procuring head nurses for new, 117-121, 122; qualifications for new, 117, 121;

solutions to problems of dual, 83-87; types of change in anticipated, 444-445; undergoing close scrutiny, 3; widespread changes for, are in view, 454; see also Head nurse, Head nurse responsibility, Relationships of head nurse

Health, insurance provided by government, 32; is right of every human being according to W.H.O., 32

Health services, for those unable to pay and families of moderate means, 32; medical center, a base for, 32; not all hospitals are equable in, they offer, 32

Home care, 42-43, least developed stage of progressive patient care, 42

Hospital(s), administrative organization of, 12-20; changes in design of, have changed hospital service, 61; changes in services of, since World War II, 61; classification of, according to service and ownership, short and long-term care, 10, 26; functions of, 10, 25; organization of, 12, 26, Ch. 4 (61); purposes of, 10; results of expansion and reorganization of, 61; types of, 10, 11, 12

Housekeeper, unit, 102

Housekeeping, a responsibility of separate department, 76; today not a function of head nurse, 3

Infants, new wash technique for, and personnel, 51; special care unit for, 51; see also Newborn special care unit

Informal organization, 16-20, 27; large percentage of work gets done through, 16; small groups which form an, 19

Initial interview, see Nursing history

Inpatient services, 37-53

Inservice education, aim of, 335, 337, 343; approach to, program, 335-336; common procedure in, 335; emphasis in, should be on improving nursing, 337; for practical nurses and aides, 336; for preparation of team leaders, 296; purposes and outcomes of, Ch. 14 (335); responsibility for, 335, 337, 343; see also Staff development, Staff education

Instruction, family often needs, in care of patient at home, 229-230; needed by patient who is going home, 227-230; see also Clinical instruction, Teaching

Orientation (cont.)
tance of, 349, 356; joint, program for
all staff new to hospital, 350; length
of, program, 351; of staff member
familiar with hospital, 354-355; of
staff member new to hospital, 350-354;
purposes of, 349, 356; responsibility
for, of nursing staff, 351; to department of nursing, content of, 351; to division, 351-354; to evening and night
duty, 355-356; to hospital, subjects of
interest, 350; to special experiences,
355-356; unit, 352
Outpatient services, 34-37

Parents' classes, 37
Patient(s), author's concept of, 203; effect on, of reorganization of hospital
services, 61; factors which influence
number of, for whom head nurse can
provide quality care, 107; meaning to,
of admission to hospital, 205-206;
nurse would find it helpful to define
her concept of, 203; rights of, 204, 214,
224, 226, 234; transportation of, 63;
way in which, is conceived by staff determines care he receives, 203; see also
Needs of the patient
Patient care, continuing development of
staff has marked effect on quality of,
343; planning a program for improvement of, 325-327; quality of, patient
and family have a right to expect, Ch.
9 (203); sharing responsibility for, 67-
71; see also Nursing care
Patient care division, activities carried
out on, 75-76; functioning of reorganized, 100-115; hospital and public meet
on, 74; large part of hospital dollar is
spent in, 75; staff of, 100-103
Patient care management, report at time
of transfer of, 157; see also Nursing
care administration
Patient services, administration and coordination of, 103; available today, 32-
33; for children and their families, 50-
53; head nurse's time taken up with
management of, 80; organization of
hospital for, Ch. 3 (32); see also Patient services, types of
Patient services, types of, clinic, 34; clinical nurse specialist, 48; consultation,
35; counselling for parents, 36-37;
emergency, 33; family health care

clinic, 35-36; inpatient, 37-53; life
saving, 47; outpatient, 34-37; parents'
classes, 36; progressive patient care,
37-46; social and diversional opportunities, 49-50
Personnel, see Nursing service personnel
Pharmacist, gains satisfaction from system, 70; more participation by, relieves nurse, 71; new systems place
responsibility on, for preparation of
individual doses, 69-70
Philosophy of team nursing, 293-294; entire staff is influenced by head nurse's,
366-367; hospitals committed to, 295;
understanding and acceptance of, is essential for team leader, 296
Physician, see Doctor
Plan for nursing care, changes are made
in, as necessary, 106; initial interview
helps in formulating, 105; see also
Nursing care plan
Plan, supervisory, see Supervisory plan
Planning, advance, necessary to achieve
long-range goals, 144; long-range, by
head nurse for supplementing her basic
education, 445-446; method of a program for improvement of patient care,
325-327; suggestions for advance, by
head nurse, 144
Planning the care of the patient, Ch. 11
(262); areas of nursing responsibility
in, 264-267; by whom, is done, 262;
head nurse's responsibility in, 270-273;
is continuous throughout hospitalization, 262; is on basis of patient's personal requirements, 262; patient plays
a part in, 262; should be fitted into
long-range plan, 263; see also Nursing
care plan
Planning time, see Time planning
Plant maintenance, changes related to, 66,
71
Policies, development of objectives necessitates review of, 84; of hospital set by
governing board, 12, 23; personnel,
446; responsibility of head nurse in relation to hospital, 84, 85, 144
Policy book, for use in orientation, 355
Portraits, patient, 269, 271, 273, 274, 299
Practical nurse(s), 285-287; inservice education for, 336; pharmacists believe
dangerous for, to administer drugs, 70;
responsibilities for which, are prepared
and ways in which hospitals are using
them, 285-287, 305; role of, has

RT89
B29
1968

NO LONGER THE PROPERTY
OF THE

3 1222 00045 7021

UNIVERSITY OF R. I. LIBRARY